In A Page Signs

Second Edition

In A Page Signs and Symptoms

Second Edition

SCOTT KAHAN, M.D., M.P.H.
Editor-in-Chief
Series Editor
Department of Preventive Medicine and Public Health
Johns Hopkins Bloomberg School of Public Health
Research Fellow, The Johns Hopkins Hospital
Johns Hopkins University School of Medicine
Baltimore, Maryland

REDONDA MILLER, M.D., M.B.A.
Editor-in-Chief
Associate Professor of Medicine
Assistant Dean for Student Affairs
Johns Hopkins University School of Medicine
Vice Chair for Clinical Affairs
Department of Medicine
The Johns Hopkins Hospital
Baltimore, MD

ELLEN G. SMITH, M.D., FAAFP
Director of Education
Harrisburg Family Practice Residency Program
PinnacleHealth Hospitals
Harrisburg, Pennsylvania

Wolters Kluwer | Lippincott Williams & Wilkins
Health
Philadelphia · Baltimore · New York · London
Buenos Aires · Hong Kong · Sydney · Tokyo

Senior Managing Editor: Stacey Sebring
Marketing Manager: Jennifer Kuklinski
Managing Editor, Production: Eve Malakoff-Klein
Designer: Risa Clow
Compositor: Nesbitt Graphics, Inc.
Printer: Data Reproductions Corporation

Second Edition

9 8 7 6 5 4 3 2

Library of Congress Cataloging-in-Publication Data

In a page. Signs and symptoms / Scott Kahan, editor-in-chief ; Redonda Miller, editor-in-chief ; Ellen G. Smith [editor]. — 2nd ed.
     p. ; cm.
     Includes index.
     ISBN-13: 978-0-7817-7043-9
     ISBN-10: 0-7817-7043-2
     1. Diagnosis, Differential—Handbooks, manuals, etc. 2. Symptoms—Handbooks, manuals, etc. I. Kahan, Scott. II. Miller, Redonda G. III. Smith, Ellen G. IV. Title: Signs and symptoms.
     [DNLM: 1. Diagnosis, Differential—Handbooks. 2. Signs and Symptoms—Handbooks. WB 39 I355 2009]
     RC71.5.I5 2009
     616.07′5—dc22   2008001359

DISCLAIMER

This book is intended solely as a review book for educational purposes. It is *not* written as a guide for the intricate clinical management of medical patients. The publisher, editors, and authors cannot accept any legal responsibility for the content contained within this book nor any omitted information.

Care has been taken to confirm the accuracy of the information present and to describe generally accepted practices. However, the authors, editors, and publisher are not responsible for errors or omissions or for any consequences from application of the information in this book and make no warranty, expressed or implied, with respect to the currency, completeness, or accuracy of the contents of the publication. Application of this information in a particular situation remains the professional responsibility of the practitioner; the clinical treatments described and recommended may not be considered absolute and universal recommendations.

The authors, editors, and publisher have exerted every effort to ensure that drug selection and dosage set forth in this text are in accordance with the current recommendations and practice at the time of publication. However, in view of ongoing research, changes in government regulations, and the constant flow of information relating to drug therapy and drug reactions, the reader is urged to check the package insert for each drug for any change in indications and dosage and for added warnings and precautions. This is particularly important when the recommended agent is a new or infrequently employed drug.

Some drugs and medical devices presented in this publication have Food and Drug Administration (FDA) clearance for limited use in restricted research settings. It is the responsibility of the health care provider to ascertain the FDA status of each drug or device planned for use in their clinical practice.

To purchase additional copies of this book, call our customer service department at (800) 638-3030 or fax orders to (301) 223-2320. International customers should call (301) 223-2300.

Visit Lippincott Williams & Wilkins on the Internet: http://www.lww.com. Lippincott Williams & Wilkins customer service representatives are available from 8:30 am to 6:00 pm, EST.

Preface

The idea for this series comes from the difficulty I experienced during medical school and residency in weeding through the massive amount of medical information that confronted me. The problem wasn't that the material was too complex; rather, it was the challenge of separating "the forest from the trees." Indeed, I still often feel overwhelmed by all there is to know.

I wanted a resource that would streamline the abundance of medical knowledge into a manageable nucleus—or, as a resident once described it to me, "a book that tells me exactly what I need to know so my attending won't think I'm an idiot!"

That became the goal of this series: to present medical diseases in a high-yield, understandable fashion that makes it easier for readers to concentrate on the "big picture," without being distracted by the mountain of surrounding detail.

Reviews from medical students, residents, fellows, and other health professionals have been excellent. I hope readers will find the *In A Page* series to be a valuable tool for rounds, for board review, and for independent study. As always, I welcome your questions, comments, and suggestions.

Scott Kahan, M.D.
scott.kahan@gmail.com

Contributors

Michael Awad, MD, PhD
Department of Surgery
Johns Hopkins Hospital
Johns Hopkins University School of Medicine
Baltimore, Maryland

Jon Brillman, MD
Chairman of Neurology
Allegheny General Hospital
Pittsburgh, Pennsylvania
Professor of Neurology
Drexel University College of Medicine
Philadelphia, Pennsylvania

Matthews Chacko, MD
Assistant Professor of Medicine
Johns Hopkins University School of
  Medicine Faculty
Interventional Cardiology and
  Cardiac Care Unit
Johns Hopkins Hospital
Baltimore, Maryland

Harold V. Cohen, DDS
Professor of Oral Medicine
University of Medicine and Dentistry of
  New Jersey
Newark, New Jersey

Lawrence J. Cheskin, MD
Associate Professor
International Health
Division of Human Nutrition
Johns Hopkins Bloomberg School
  of Public Health
Attending Physician
Johns Hopkins Bayview Medical Center
Director
Johns Hopkins University Weight
  Management Program
Baltimore, Maryland

James P. Dunn, MD
Associate Professor of Ophthalmology
The Wilmer Eye Institute
Johns Hopkins University School of Medicine
Baltimore, Maryland

April S. Fitzgerald, MD
Instructor
Department of Medicine
Johns Hopkins University School of
  Medicine
Baltimore, Maryland

Richard Frisch, MD
Department of Orthopedic Surgery
University of California-San Francisco
  School of Medicine
San Francisco, California

Scott Kahan, MD, MPH
Department of Preventive Medicine and
  Public Health
Johns Hopkins Bloomberg School of
  Public Health
Research Fellow, The Johns Hopkins
  Hospital
Johns Hopkins University School
  of Medicine
Baltimore, Maryland

Matthew Kim, MD
Assistant Professor of Medicine
Division of Endocrinology and
  Metabolism
Johns Hopkins University School of
  Medicine
Baltimore, Maryland

Paula J. Kue, MD
Instructor
General Internal Medicine
Johns Hopkins University School of
  Medicine
Baltimore, Maryland

Rafael Llinas, MD
Associate Professor of Neurology
Johns Hopkins University School of
  Medicine
Director of Clinical Services
Johns Hopkins University—Bayview
  Neurology
Co-Director, Neurology Residency Program
Johns Hopkins Medical Center
Baltimore, Maryland

Susan Matra Rabizadeh, MD, MBA
Clinical Instructor
Department of Dermatology
Johns Hopkins University School of
  Medicine
Baltimore, Maryland

Redonda Miller, MD, MBA
Associate Professor of Medicine
Assistant Dean for Student Affairs
Johns Hopkins University School of
  Medicine
Vice Chair for Clinical Affairs
Department of Medicine
The Johns Hopkins Hospital
Baltimore, MD

Pankaj Mohan, MD
Clinical and Nuclear Cardiology
Jefferson Regional Medical Center
Pittsburgh, Pennsylvania
Assistant Professor of Medicine
Drexel University College of Medicine
Philadelphia, Pennsylvania

Albert J. Polito, MD
Chief, Division of Pulmonary Medicine
Mercy Medical Center
Assistant Professor of Medicine
Johns Hopkins University School of
  Medicine
Baltimore, Maryland

Rajnish Prasad, MD
Director, Cardiac Care Unit
University of Maryland Medical Center
Assistant Professor of Medicine
University of Maryland School of Medicine
Baltimore, Maryland

John J. Raves, MD
Assistant Professor of Surgery
Drexel University College of Medicine
Philadelphia, Pennsylvania
Senior Attending Staff
Division of General Surgery
Allegheny General Hospital
Pittsburgh, Pennsylvania

Anastasia Rowland-Seymour, MD
Assistant Attending
Division of General Medicine
Johns Hopkins University School of
  Medicine
Baltimore, Maryland

Philip Seo, MD, MHS
Assistant Professor of Medicine
Johns Hopkins University School of
  Medicine
Co-Director
Johns Hopkins Vasculitis Center
Johns Hopkins Hospital
Baltimore, Maryland

C. John Sperati, MD
Assistant Professor of Medicine
Division of Nephrology
Department of Medicine
Johns Hopkins University School of
  Medicine
Baltimore, Maryland

Catherine Takacs Witkop, MD, MPH
General Preventive Medicine
Johns Hopkins Bloomberg School of
  Public Health
Baltimore, Maryland
Assistant Professor
Obstetrics/Gynecology
Uniformed Services University of the
  Health Sciences
Bethesda, Maryland

Jean S. Wang, MD
Assistant Professor of Medicine
Division of Gastroenterology
Department of Medicine
Johns Hopkins University School of
  Medicine Faculty
Department of Medicine
Division of Gastroenterology
Johns Hopkins Hospital
Baltimore, Maryland

Acknowledgments

The greatest strength of this book is its diverse group of authors. We sincerely thank all our contributors, who have worked so hard to make this book a valuable resource for clinicians.

We are also grateful to the staff of Lippincott Williams & Wilkins, especially Nancy Duffy, Liz Stalnaker, Jennifer Kuklinski, and Eve Malakoff-Klein.

A special thanks to Myron Weisfeldt for his guidance and for helping to get this book off the ground.

Finally, we thank our family, friends, and mentors for their support.

Contents

Abbreviations

A-a	Alveolar–arterial oxygen gradient
AAA	Abdominal aortic aneurysm
ABG	Arterial blood gas
ABI	Ankle-brachial index
Abs	Antibodies
ACE	Angiotensin-converting enzyme
ACL	Anterior cruciate ligament
ACTH	Adrenocorticotropic hormone
ADH	Antidiuretic hormone
ADP	Adenosine diphosphate
AIDS	Acquired immunodeficiency syndrome
ALT	Alanine aminotransferase
ANA	Antinuclear antibody
ANCA	Antineutrophil cytoplasmic antibodies
ASO	Antistreptolysin O antibodies
AST	Aspartate aminotransferase
ATFL	Anterior talofibular ligament
AV	Arteriovenous, atrioventricular
AZT	Zidovudine
BiPAP	Bilevel positive airway pressure
BMI	Body mass index
BNP	Brain or B-type natriuretic peptide
BOOP	Bronchiolitis obliterans organizing pneumonia
BP	Blood pressure
bpm	Beats per minute
BRCA	Breast cancer gene
BUN	Blood urea nitrogen
CAH	Congenital adrenal hyperplasia
CBC	Complete blood count
CDC	Centers for Disease Control and Prevention
CFL	Calcaneofibular ligament
CHF	Congestive heart failure
CIDP	Chronic inflammatory demyelinating polyneuropathy
CNS	Central nervous system
COPD	Chronic obstructive pulmonary disease
CPAP	Continuous positive airway pressure
CPEO	Chronic progressive external ophthalmoplegia
CPK	Creatine phosphokinase
CPR	Cardiopulmonary resuscitation
CRP	C-reactive protein
CSF	Cerebrospinal fluid

CT	Computed tomography
CVA	Cerebrovascular accident
D5W	5% dextrose solution in water
DES	Diethylstilbestrol
DHEA-S	Dehydroepiandrosterone sulfate
DI	Diabetes insipidus
DIC	Disseminated intravascular coagulation
DKA	Diabetic ketoacidosis
DNA	Deoxyribonucleic acid
dsDNA	Double-stranded deoxyribonucleic acid
DSM-IV	Diagnostic Statistical Manual IV
EBV	Epstein-Barr virus
ECG	Electrocardiography
EEG	Electroencephalography
EGD	Esophagogastroduodenoscopy
ELISA	Enzyme-linked immunosorbent assay
EMG	Electromyography
ENG	Electronystagmography
ENT	Otolaryngology (ear, nose, and throat)
ERCP	Endoscopic retrograde cholangiopancreatography
ERG	Electroretinography
ESR	Erythrocyte sedimentation rate
FiO_2	Fraction of inspired oxygen
FSH	Follicle-stimulating hormone
FTA-ABS	Fluorescent treponemal antibody absorbed test
GABA	γ-Aminobutyric acid
GAD	Generalized anxiety disorder
GBM	Glomerular basement membranes
GERD	Gastroesophageal reflux disease
GFR	Glomerular filtration rate
GGTP	γ-Glutamyl transpeptidase
GI	Gastrointestinal
GIFT	Gamete intrafallopian transfer
GnRH	Gonadotropin-releasing hormone
HAIR-AN	Hirsutism androgen insulin resistance, acanthosis nigricans
Hb_{A1c}	Hemoglobin A1c (glycosylated hemoglobin)
hCG	Human chorionic gonadotropin
HIV	Human immunodeficiency virus
HSV	Herpes simplex virus
5-HT	5-Hydroxytyramine
HTLV	Human T-cell leukemia/lymphoma virus
IBD	Inflammatory bowel disease
IBS	Irritable bowel syndrome
ICSI	Intracytoplasmic sperm injection
ICU	Intensive care unit
IgA	Immunoglobulin A
IgE	Immunoglobulin E
IGF	Insulin-like growth factor
IgG	Immunoglobulin G
IgM	Immunoglobulin M

IM	Intramuscular
IP	Interphalangeal
IUD	Intrauterine device
IV	Intravenous
IVF	In vitro fertilization
IVIG	Intravenous immunoglobulin
KOH	Potassium hydroxide
LCL	Lateral collateral ligament
LDH	Lactate dehydrogenase
LFT	Liver function test
LH	Luteinizing hormone
LSD	D-Lysergic acid diethylamide
MAO	Monoamine oxidase
MCL	Medial collateral ligament
MCP	Metacarpophalangeal
MCTD	Mixed connective tissue disease
MDMA	Methylenedioxymethamphetamine
MEN	Multiple endocrine neoplasia
MGUS	Monoclonal gammopathy of uncertain significance
MI	Myocardial infarction
MPTP	1-Methyl-4-phenyl-1,2,3,6-tetrahydropyridine
MRA	Magnetic resonance angiography
MRCP	Magnetic resonance cholangiopancreatography
MRI	Magnetic resonance imaging
NARES	Nonallergic rhinitis with eosinophilia
NASH	Nonalcoholic steatohepatitis
NBT	Nitroblue tetrazolium
NMDA	N-Methyl-D-aspartic acid
NSAID	Nonsteroidal anti-inflammatory drug
OCD	Obsessive-compulsive disorder
ORIF	Open reduction with internal fixation
OTC	Over-the-counter
P_2	Pulmonic second sound
PAS	Periodic acid-Schiff
PCL	Posterior cruciate ligament
P_{CO_2}	Partial pressure of carbon dioxide
PCOS	Polycystic ovarian syndrome
PE	Pulmonary embolus
PEEP	Positive end-expiratory pressure
PET	Positron-emission tomography
PMI	Point of maximal impulse
PMN	Polymorphonuclear cell
P_{O_2}	Partial pressure of oxygen
PPD	Purified protein derivative (TB test)
PSA	Prostate-specific antigen
PT	Prothrombin time
PTFL	Posterior talofibular ligament
PTH	Parathyroid hormone
PTSD	Posttraumatic stress disorder
PTT	Partial thromboplastin time

PUD	Peptic ulcer disease
PUVA	Psoralen with ultraviolet A
RBC	Red blood cell
REM	Rapid eye movement
RF	Rheumatoid factor
RMSF	Rocky Mountain spotted fever
RPR	Rapid plasma reagin
S_1	First heart sound
S_3	Third heart sound
S_4	Fourth heart sound
SIADH	Syndrome of inappropriate antidiuretic hormone
SC	Subcutaneous
SLE	Systemic lupus erythematosus
SPECT	Single-photon emission computed tomography
SPEP	Serum protein electrophoresis
SSRI	Selective serotonin reuptake inhibitor
STD	Sexually transmitted disease
SVT	Supraventricular tachycardia
T_4	Thyroxine
TIA	Transient ischemic attack
TIPS	Transjugular intrahepatic portosystemic shunt
TMJ	Temporomandibular joint
TNF	Tumor necrosis factor
t-PA	Tissue plasminogen activator
TPN	Total parenteral nutrition
TSH	Thyroid-stimulating hormone
TTKG	Transtubular potassium gradient (in kidney)
TTP	Thrombotic thrombocytopenic purpura
TTP-HUS	Thrombotic thrombocytopenic purpura–hemolytic uremic syndrome
UPEP	Urine protein electrophoresis
US	Ultrasound
UTI	Urinary tract infection
UV	Ultraviolet
UVB	Ultraviolet B
V/Q	Ventilation perfusion ratio
VDRL	Venereal Disease Research Laboratory
WBC	White blood cell
WPW	Wolff-Parkinson-White syndrome

In A Page Signs and Symptoms

Second Edition

Abdominal Bruit

INTRODUCTION

An abdominal bruit is a systolic sound heard over the abdomen that may correspond to blood moving at high velocity across a severe narrowing or stenosis in a blood vessel. It is heard best with the diaphragm of the stethoscope, usually over the abdominal aorta or in the flanks over the renal arteries. It can be a sign of atherosclerosis, vasculitis, or fibromuscular hyperplasia. It may also be heard over a large, highly vascular tumor or as a result of partial occlusion of a vessel secondary to external compression.

DIAGNOSTIC WORKUP & INITIAL MANAGEMENT

History and physical examination

- Complete history focusing primarily on the relevant cardiovascular history (e.g., recurrent pulmonary edema, history of kidney disease, previous imaging studies, intolerance to ACE inhibitors), surgical history, family history of aortic or renal artery disease, and medications
- Focus on the entire cardiovascular exam, because patients with abdominal vascular disease will likely have concurrent coronary artery, carotid artery, and lower extremity vascular disease
- In addition to auscultation of the abdominal bruit, the physical exam should include a cardiac exam, auscultation for a carotid bruit, examination of all four extremity pulses, and blood pressure measurements in both arms (to exclude subclavian stenosis)
- If suspect a vascular mass, carefully examine the liver, spleen, and regional lymph nodes

Initial diagnostic workup

- Duplex ultrasound is an excellent noninvasive tool to screen for abdominal aortic disease, renal artery stenosis, liver metastases, and liver and spleen sizes
- Abdominal CT, MRI, or MRA will demonstrate the most likely abdominal etiologies and is useful to better delineate anatomic relationships
- Laboratory studies may include a lipid panel, CBC, serum chemistries, and liver function tests; include ESR if suspect an inflammatory process
- Conventional angiography remains the gold standard for diagnosing renal artery stenosis
  - Measurement of renal vein renin levels following a captopril challenge is diagnostic for renal artery stenosis but is no longer commonly used

Initial patient management

- Treat the underlying etiology
- Recognize that atherosclerosis of the abdominal vasculature is a marker for systemic atherosclerosis and that close attention to coronary and carotid artery disease is warranted to prevent MI and stroke
- Vascular surgery may be necessary for significant abdominal aortic disease
- Angioplasty and stenting of severe renal artery stenosis may be an endovascular option for selected patients
- Nephrology consultation may be needed to help manage renal failure and dialysis
- Treat hypertension with ACE inhibitors cautiously if renal artery stenosis is present (particularly in those with bilateral renal artery stenosis), because renal failure can result

DIFFERENTIAL DIAGNOSIS

Vascular etiologies
- Abdominal aortic aneurysm or stenosis
- Arteriovenous malformation
- Renal artery stenosis
- Celiac artery stenosis
- Superior or inferior mesenteric artery stenosis
- Hepatic venous hum
  - A high-pitched, continuous murmur that decreases with forced held expiration
- Cruveilhier-Baumgarten murmur
  - A high-pitched, venous hum of portal hypertension that becomes louder with forced expiration
- Turbulence of the splenic artery
- Takayasu's arteritis

Liver etiologies
- Hepatocellular carcinoma (hepatoma)
- Cirrhosis
- Liver hemangioma

Other
- Tricuspid regurgitation
- Abdominal friction rub from serositis
  - Associated with hepatoma, cholangiocarcinoma, liver metastases, and inflammatory processes

Abdominal Distension

INTRODUCTION

A prominent "potbelly" contour is normal in infants and young children. Pathologic enlargement of the abdomen is a fairly common complaint that can result from reduced tone of the abdominal wall musculature or increased content (gas, liquid, or solid). The complaint should be evaluated carefully and systematically to rule out serious and life-threatening diagnoses and to evaluate for mundane diagnoses, such as swallowing air or overeating, without embarking on unnecessary testing. Acute onset of abdominal distention is a sign that should be taken seriously, especially when accompanied by other worrisome symptoms (e.g., bilious vomiting) or signs (e.g., rebound tenderness, evidence of GI bleeding).

DIAGNOSTIC WORKUP & INITIAL MANAGEMENT

History and physical examination

- History should include onset, duration, last bowel movement, associated symptoms (e.g., weight gain, bloating, flatus, reflux, diarrhea, pain, constipation), constitutional symptoms (e.g., fever), last menstrual period, and sexual history
- Physical exam should include a full abdominal exam, including palpation for hernias and masses, assessment for signs of cirrhosis and portal hypertension, abdominal tenderness, fluid wave, pelvic exam in women, and rectal exam

Initial diagnostic workup

- Initial laboratory testing may include CBC, stool cultures, workup for liver disease (liver function tests, hepatitis panel, liver biopsy), and pregnancy testing
- Biopsy may be indicated for masses and suspected tumors
- Plain-film (flat and upright) abdominal radiographs may reveal bowel obstruction (distended proximal bowel loops with air-fluid levels), constipation, air swallowing, or paralytic ileus
- Abdominal and pelvic CT may reveal pancreatic pseudocyst, ovarian masses, cirrhosis, and/or aneurysm
- Abdominal and pelvic ultrasound may reveal ovarian mass, ascites, liver disease, and/or pregnancy
- Paracentesis is diagnostic for spontaneous bacterial peritonitis and malignant ascites and may provide symptomatic relief
- Colonoscopy or sigmoidoscopy may be indicated to rule out organic colorectal pathology

Initial patient management

- Identify, treat, or refer based on underlying causes
- Nasogastric tube decompression and bowel rest may be indicated (e.g., bowel obstruction, pancreatitis)
- Laxatives for constipation
- Antibiotics for spontaneous bacterial peritonitis
- Treat underlying liver diseases, and manage complications
- For distention from swallowing air, awareness can lead to self-control: Eat slowly; avoid carbonated drinks, chewing gum or sucking on candies, drinking through a straw, or sipping hot drinks
- Change diet or reduce milk intake for malabsorption syndromes
- Irritable bowel syndrome is treated with increased dietary fiber, stress reduction, and antidepressants
- Oncology referral for masses when appropriate
- Surgical referral for hernias when appropriate

DIFFERENTIAL DIAGNOSIS

Mechanical intestinal obstruction
- Adhesions from previous surgery
- Neoplasm
- Hernia
- Crohn's disease
- Abscess
- Volvulus
- Intussusception
- Fecal impaction

Functional intestinal obstruction
- Paralytic ileus (e.g., postsurgical, sepsis)
- Postabdominal surgery
- Electrolyte abnormalities (e.g., hypokalemia, hyponatremia, hypomagnesemia, uremia)
- Drugs (e.g., narcotics, α- and β-blockers, anticholinergics, psychotropic agents)
- Lower lobe pneumonia
- Sepsis
- Retroperitoneal hemorrhage
- Vertebral compression fracture
- Spontaneous bacterial peritonitis
- Intestinal perforation
- Gastroparesis
- Toxic megacolon
- Dysmotility/colonic pseudo-obstruction (Ogilvie's syndrome)

Renal enlargement
- Hydronephrosis
- Ureteropelvic junction syndrome
- Bladder distension
- Polycystic kidneys

Ascites
- Portal hypertension (e.g., cirrhosis)
- Congestive heart failure
- Nephrotic syndrome
- Hypoalbuminemia (e.g., malnutrition, liver failure)
- Metastatic cancer (e.g., colon, ovarian)

Hepatomegaly
- Congestive heart failure
- Amyloidosis
- Budd-Chiari syndrome
- Glycogen storage disease

Other
- Tumors (e.g., ovarian cancer) or cysts (e.g., pancreatic pseudocyst)
- Splenomegaly
- Functional gas/constipation
- Overeating, obesity
- Lactose intolerance
- Air swallowing (nervous habit)
- Irritable bowel syndrome
- Leukemia
- Lymphoma
- Abdominal aneurysm
- Pregnancy
- Abdominal trauma with intra-abdominal bleeding
- Abdominal compartment syndrome

Abdominal Guarding

INTRODUCTION

Abdominal guarding refers to muscular rigidity of the abdomen upon palpation. It may be involuntary or voluntary. Involuntary guarding may be an early sign of peritonitis and may require emergent intervention. The examiner may try to limit voluntary guarding during the physical exam by having the patient bend both knees and/or rest the head on a pillow and then asking him or her to voluntarily relax the abdominal muscles.

DIAGNOSTIC WORKUP & INITIAL MANAGEMENT

History and physical examination

- Evaluate onset, duration, and associated symptoms (e.g., pain, vomiting, fever, anorexia, dysuria, vaginal discharge, diarrhea, constipation)
  - Note similarity to past episodes and factors that aggravate or alleviate the pain
  - Peritoneal signs may be masked in elderly, alcoholic, and immunocompromised patients
- Obtain a brief history of the current complaint; review medical/surgical history
- Perform a focused physical exam
  - Assess vital signs, including pulse oximetry and fingerstick blood glucose level
  - Note bowel sounds, abdominal tenderness, rebound, distension, and masses
  - If the patient is thought to have a "surgical" abdomen (i.e., peritoneal signs, such as severe or rebound tenderness), call for a surgical consultation immediately
  - Examine the patient for jaundice or scleral icterus
  - All patients require a rectal exam, and all female patients require a pelvic exam
  - Hypotension may be due to sepsis, vomiting, diarrhea, blood loss, or "3rd-spacing"

Initial workup and management

- Hemodynamically unstable patients require IV fluids and emergent surgical consult
- Place a nasogastric tube in cases of small bowel obstruction or persistent vomiting
- Distinguish serious etiologies and those requiring acute surgical intervention
  - Life-threatening causes include ruptured AAA, perforated viscus, intestinal obstruction, ectopic pregnancy, mesenteric ischemia, and myocardial ischemia
  - In general, patients who present with extremely severe pain of acute onset require prompt surgical evaluation and consideration of CT or ultrasound
- Initial tests should include CBC, electrolytes, liver function tests, amylase/lipase, lactate level (to evaluate for mesenteric ischemia), urinalysis, and cultures
- Females of reproductive age require a rapid urine pregnancy test
- Imaging studies may be necessary to establish a diagnosis:
  - Plain-film (flat and upright) abdominal and upright chest radiographs may reveal obstruction or perforation (free air)
  - Ultrasound if suspect biliary disease, aortic aneurysm, ectopic pregnancy, or peritoneal fluid
  - CT if suspect appendicitis, obstruction, mesenteric ischemia, or diverticulitis
- Symptomatic treatment of emesis (e.g., promethazine, metoclopramide), if present
- Treat pain as necessary: Narcotics for severe pain; NSAIDs (e.g., IV ketorolac) for colicky pain (especially renal); proton pump inhibitors, H_2-blockers, or antacids for burning epigastric pain; anticholinergics (e.g., Donnatal) or antispasmodics (e.g., dicyclomine) for intestinal cramping
- Administer broad-spectrum antibiotics (e.g., piperacillin-tazobactam) for suspected intra-abdominal infections (to cover gram-negatives and anaerobes) or perforated viscus

DIFFERENTIAL DIAGNOSIS

Emergent or life-threatening etiologies

Ruptured abdominal aortic aneurysm (AAA)
- Severe, colicky back, abdominal, or flank pain; a pulsatile abdominal mass may be present
- Immediate intervention is critical: Clinical suspicion of a ruptured or leaking AAA (via a bedside ultrasound that identifies an aneurysm) is sufficient to proceed to surgery

Perforated viscus
- Presents with severe abdominal pain
- Upright chest radiograph showing "free air" is usually sufficient for diagnosis (if not, CT scan)

Appendicitis
- The most common abdominal surgical emergency; presentation is often vague epigastric or periumbilical pain that migrates to the right lower quadrant (McBurney's point) over 24 hours
- A presentation of pain before emesis has nearly 100% sensitivity for appendicitis
- Emergent appendectomy is generally required, because rupture can occur within 24 hours

Pancreatitis
- Steady, severe epigastric pain, often 1–4 hours after a large meal or alcohol intake
- Pain may radiate to the back and is sometimes relieved by leaning forward
- Severe cases may present with peritonitis (guarding, rebound tenderness, fever) and shock

Small bowel obstruction
- The most common causes are adhesions, hernias, and tumors; others include foreign bodies (e.g., gallstone ileus), inflammation (e.g., Crohn's disease), and volvulus
- "3rd-spacing," hypotension, sepsis, strangulation, bowel ischemia, or perforation may occur
- Surgery is indicated for complete obstructions or signs of strangulation

Acute mesenteric ischemia
- Results from sudden occlusion of a mesenteric artery or thrombosis of mesenteric veins
- Arterial occlusion most commonly results from a cardiac embolism (e.g., atrial fibrillation); venous thrombosis most commonly results from hypercoagulable states (e.g., myeloproliferative disorder) or low blood flow states (e.g., heart failure)

Others
- Ectopic pregnancy
- Nonabdominal etiologies (e.g., MI, atypical angina, pericarditis)
- Pneumoperitoneum secondary to trauma
- Hepatic or splenic contusion or laceration

Less immediately threatening etiologies
- Cholecystitis
- Diverticulitis
- Abdominal wall strain/injury
- Pelvic inflammatory disease
- Nephrolithiasis
- Peptic ulcer disease or GERD
- Anxiety
- Malingering
- Spontaneous bacterial peritonitis
- Ovarian cyst
- Urinary tract infection/pyelonephritis
- Herpes zoster
- Insect toxins (e.g., black widow spider)
- Abscess (e.g., iliopsoas)
- Incarcerated hernia
- Abdominal migraine
- Intussusception
- Volvulus
- Dyspepsia

Abdominal Masses

INTRODUCTION

Many disease processes, including malignancies, infections, bowel obstruction, and organomegaly, present with abdominal masses. The most serious and dramatic etiology is an abdominal aortic aneurysm, which is responsible for 15,000 deaths per year. More frequently, abdominal masses result from constipation and other nonemergent etiologies. Most abdominal masses develop slowly, and even the patient may be unaware of their presence. Thus, many abdominal masses are discovered on routine physical examination. The location of the mass and its characteristics on palpation (e.g., firmness, texture, tenderness) provide clues to the etiology.

DIAGNOSTIC WORKUP & INITIAL MANAGEMENT

History and physical examination
- Note associated symptoms, especially fever, changes in bowel habits, diarrhea, abdominal pain, weight change, anorexia, urinary symptoms, and rectal bleeding
- Perform complete abdominal and pelvic examinations to localize areas of tenderness

Initial diagnostic workup
- Initial laboratory studies may include CBC, electrolytes, BUN and creatinine, liver function tests, urinalysis, and pregnancy testing
- Tumor markers (e.g., carcinoembryonic antigen, CA-125), blood cultures, and toxicology screen may be indicated
- Plain-film radiography may reveal constipation, obstruction, or free intraperitoneal air
- Abdominal CT with IV and oral contrast will evaluate for abscess, bowel pathology, neoplasm, and hepatosplenomegaly
- Barium enema may reveal abnormal bowel (either intraluminal mass or extrinsic compression of bowel) in cases of malignancy
- Colonoscopy to assess the lumen of the colon and rectum may be indicated
- Laparoscopy allows direct visualization of the intra-abdominal cavity in selected cases
- Paracentesis with fluid evaluation may be indicated in cases of ascites detected on exam, CT, or ultrasound

Initial patient management
- Immediate attention to life-threatening causes (e.g., ruptured abdominal aortic aneurysm)
- Most cases of abdominal masses are treatable once the etiology is identified
- Many malignant and benign masses (e.g., fibroids, hernia) require surgical intervention
- Infectious causes require antibiotics and may require operative intervention (e.g., abscess drainage)
- Constipation is typically treated with laxatives, enemas, and increased dietary fiber and fluids; manual disimpaction is reserved for fecal impaction; discontinue offending medications (e.g., narcotics)
- Gastroenterology and/or surgery consultation may be indicated

DIFFERENTIAL DIAGNOSIS

Constipation/inability to pass stool
- Most commonly results from dehydration and/or low dietary fiber intake
- Hirschsprung's disease
- Medications (e.g., narcotics, opiates, anticholinergics)
- Ogilvie's syndrome (colonic pseudo-obstruction)

Ascites
- Malignancy
- Nephrotic syndrome
- Liver disease
- Congestive heart failure

Large or small bowel obstruction
- Adhesions from previous surgery
- Neoplasms (extraluminal or intraluminal)
- Hernias
- Crohn's disease
- Abscess
- Volvulus
- Intussusception (rare in adults)
- Colonic pseudo-obstruction (Ogilvie's syndrome)
- Ileus (e.g., postsurgery, electrolyte abnormalities, drugs, sepsis)

Soft tissue mass
- Tumor (e.g., ovarian, uterine, bowel, liver)
- Uterine fibroids
- Lipoma
- Hernia
- Pyloric stenosis (primarily in infants)
- Pregnancy
- Massive lymphadenopathy (e.g., lymphoma)
- Organomegaly (e.g., hepatomegaly, splenomegaly)
- Infection (intra-abdominal or tubo-ovarian abscess)
- Abdominal aortic aneurysm

Cyst
- Mesenteric cysts
- Hydatid cyst
  - Caused by the larval form of *Echinococcus granulosus*
  - Typically found in the livers of patients with a history of travel to tropical areas
- Dermoid cyst

Palpable gallbladder (Courvoisier's sign)
- Common bile duct obstruction

Abdominal Pain, Lower Quadrants

INTRODUCTION

Lower abdominal pain is a common complaint that must be evaluated carefully and systematically to reach the appropriate diagnosis in a timely manner. All diagnoses must be considered, with the most emergent etiologies ruled out first, followed by a careful evaluation and treatment for the most common diagnoses. Abdominal pain in the lower quadrants is often associated with the distal intestinal tract, but nonabdominal causes, such as genitourinary or pelvic etiologies, must also be considered. Elderly patients and those with significant comorbid illnesses may benefit from early surgical consultation and thoughtful coordination of medical and surgical care.

DIAGNOSTIC WORKUP & INITIAL MANAGEMENT

History and physical examination

- Evaluate the nature, location, radiation, intensity, and quality of the pain
  - Diffuse, crampy, colicky pain that occurs in waves implies distension or contraction of a hollow abdominal organ (e.g., intestine, stomach); constant, localized pain suggests inflammation (e.g., appendicitis, diverticulitis, cholecystitis)
  - Note similarity to past episodes and factors that aggravate or alleviate the pain
  - Peritoneal signs may be masked in elderly, alcoholic, and immunocompromised patients
- Associated symptoms may include nausea, vomiting, fever, anorexia, weight loss, melena, hematochezia, change in caliber of stool, diarrhea, constipation, and dysuria; in women, ask about menstrual cycles, vaginal bleeding, unusual vaginal discharge
- Obtain a brief history of the current complaint, and review the medical and surgical history
- Perform a focused physical exam
  - Assess vital signs, including pulse oximetry and fingerstick blood glucose level
  - Note bowel sounds, abdominal tenderness, rebound, guarding, distension, masses
  - If the patient is thought to have a "surgical" abdomen (i.e., peritoneal signs, such as severe or rebound tenderness), call for a surgical consultation immediately
  - Examine the patient for jaundice and scleral icterus
  - Perform a rectal exam and pelvic exam in women
  - Hypotension may be due to sepsis, vomiting, diarrhea, blood loss, or "3rd-spacing"

Initial workup and management

- Initial tests may include CBC, electrolytes, liver function tests, amylase and lipase, lactate level (to evaluate for mesenteric ischemia), urinalysis, and cultures
- Imaging studies may be necessary to establish a diagnosis
  - Plain-film (flat and upright) abdominal and upright chest radiography may reveal obstruction or perforation (free air)
  - US if suspect biliary disease, aortic aneurysm, ectopic pregnancy, or peritoneal fluid
  - CT if suspect appendicitis, urolithiasis, obstruction, mesenteric ischemia, or diverticulitis
- Evaluation of cardiac and pulmonary etiologies may require ECG and cardiac enzymes
- Consider endocervical gonorrhea and chlamydia cultures in sexually active females; females of reproductive age may be tested for pregnancy
- Symptomatic treatment of emesis (e.g., promethazine, metoclopramide, ondansetron)
- Treat pain as necessary: Narcotics for severe pain; NSAIDs (e.g., IV ketorolac) for colicky pain (especially renal); proton pump inhibitors, H_2-blockers, or antacids for burning epigastric pain; anticholinergics (e.g., Donnatal) or antispasmodics (e.g., dicyclomine) for cramping
- Place nasogastric tube for obstruction or persistent vomiting
- Broad-spectrum antibiotics if suspect a perforated viscus or intra-abdominal infection
- Stool studies for bacteria, ova/parasites, *Giardia,* and *C. difficile* if diarrhea.
- Consider colonoscopy if initial tests are unrevealing

DIFFERENTIAL DIAGNOSIS

Right lower quadrant
- Appendicitis
- Diverticulitis
- Salpingitis/pelvic inflammatory disease
- Endometritis
- Endometriosis
- Ectopic pregnancy
- Hemorrhage or rupture of ovarian cyst
- Nephrolithiasis
- Intussusception
- Strangulated hernia
- Cecal volvulus
- Inflammatory bowel disease
- Pyelonephritis
- Cholecystitis
- Colitis (e.g., infectious, ischemic, medication-induced, inflammatory bowel disease)

Pelvic/hypogastric region
- Cystitis
- Salpingitis/pelvic inflammatory disease
- Ectopic pregnancy
- Diverticulitis
- Strangulated hernia
- Endometriosis
- Appendicitis
- Ovarian cyst
- Ovarian torsion
- Testicular torsion
- Bladder distension
- Nephrolithiasis
- Prostatitis
- Malignancy
- Abdominal aortic aneurysm

Left lower quadrant
- Diverticulitis
- Intestinal obstruction
- Colitis (e.g., infectious, ischemic, medication-induced, inflammatory bowel disease)
- Strangulated hernia
- Inflammatory bowel disease
- Gastroenteritis
- Pyelonephritis
- Nephrolithiasis
- Mesenteric lymphadenitis or thrombosis
- Aortic aneurysm
- Volvulus
- Salpingitis/pelvic inflammatory disease

Abdominal Pain, Upper Quadrants

INTRODUCTION

Upper abdominal pain is a common presenting symptom. A complete differential diagnosis should be developed based on the organs of the upper abdomen in addition to the associated history and physical examination. Gallbladder disease and peptic ulcer disease are two of the most common causes of upper abdominal pain. Be sure to consider nonabdominal etiologies in the differential of abdominal pain (e.g., pulmonary embolus, pneumonia, myocardial ischemia).

DIAGNOSTIC WORKUP & INITIAL MANAGEMENT

History and physical examination

- Evaluate the nature, location, radiation, intensity, and quality of the pain
  - Diffuse, crampy, colicky pain that occurs in waves implies distension or contraction of a hollow abdominal organ (e.g., intestine, stomach); constant, localized pain suggests inflammation (e.g., appendicitis, diverticulitis, cholecystitis)
  - Note similarity to past episodes and factors that aggravate or alleviate the pain
  - Peritoneal signs may be masked in elderly, alcoholic, and immunocompromised patients
- Associated symptoms may include nausea, vomiting, fever, chest pain, cough, anorexia, dysuria, vaginal discharge, diarrhea, or constipation
- Obtain a brief history of the current complaint, and review the medical and surgical history
- Perform a focused physical exam
  - Assess vital signs, including pulse oximetry and fingerstick blood glucose level
  - Note bowel sounds, abdominal tenderness, rebound, guarding, distension, and masses
  - If the patient is thought to have a "surgical" abdomen (i.e., peritoneal signs, such as severe or rebound tenderness), call for a surgical consultation immediately
  - Examine the patient for jaundice and scleral icterus
  - All patients require a rectal exam, and all female patients require a pelvic exam
  - Hypotension may be due to sepsis, vomiting, diarrhea, blood loss, or "3rd-spacing"

Initial workup and management

- Initial tests may include CBC, electrolytes, liver function tests, amylase and lipase, lactate level (to evaluate for mesenteric ischemia), urinalysis, and cultures
- Females of reproductive age may be tested for pregnancy
- Imaging studies may be necessary to establish a diagnosis
  - Plain-film abdominal radiographs may reveal obstruction or perforation (free air)
  - US if suspect biliary disease, aortic aneurysm, ectopic pregnancy, or peritoneal fluid
  - CT if suspect appendicitis, urolithiasis, obstruction, mesenteric ischemia, or diverticulitis
  - Consider MRCP if suspect biliary disease and ultrasound is unrevealing
- Evaluation of cardiac and pulmonary etiologies may require ECG and cardiac enzymes
- Consider endocervical gonorrhea and chlamydia cultures in sexually active females
- Consider upper GI endoscopy if the patient has alarm symptoms: dysphagia, weight loss, hematemesis, black or bloody stools, chest pain, choking, persistent vomiting, anemia
- Symptomatic treatment of emesis (e.g., promethazine, metoclopramide, odansetron)
- Treat pain as necessary: Narcotics for severe pain, NSAIDs (e.g., IV ketorolac) for colicky pain (especially renal), H2-blockers or antacids for burning epigastric pain, anticholinergics (e.g., Donnatal) or antispasmodics (e.g., dicyclomine) for intestinal cramping
- Place nasogastric tube for obstruction or persistent vomiting
- Give broad-spectrum antibiotics if suspect perforated viscus or intra-abdominal infection
- Gastroenterology or surgery consultation may be indicated

DIFFERENTIAL DIAGNOSIS

Right upper quadrant pain

- Cholecystitis
- Fatty liver or nonalcoholic steatohepatitis (NASH)
- Congested liver (e.g., secondary to heart failure)
- Cholangitis
- Hepatitis
- Gastritis or pancreatitis
- Pneumonia
- Fitz-Hugh-Curtis syndrome (gonococcal perihepatitis secondary to pelvic inflammatory disease)
- Cholelithiasis
- Sphincter of Oddi dysfunction
- Nephrolithiasis
- Appendicitis

Epigastric pain

- Gastritis
- Peptic ulcer disease
- Pancreatitis
- Gastroenteritis
- Intestinal obstruction
- Myocardial infarction
- Aortic aneurysm
- Pancreatic cancer

Left upper quadrant pain

- Peptic ulcer disease
- Gastritis
- GERD
- Splenic infarct
- Pulmonary embolism
- Pancreatitis
- Acute splenomegaly (e.g., mononucleosis)
- Left lower lobe pneumonia
- Nephrolithiasis

Nonfocal pain

- Early appendicitis
- Herpes
- Sickle cell crisis
- Irritable bowel
- Mesenteric ischemia
- Peritonitis
- Pleurisy
- Uremia
- Lead poisoning
- Porphyria
- Toxin ingestion

Abdominal Pain with Rebound Tenderness

INTRODUCTION

In evaluating an acute abdomen, rebound tenderness is one of the most important signs of peritonitis. It is elicited by pressing deeply on the abdomen and then suddenly releasing pressure, which stretches the peritoneum and causes increased abdominal pain. Guarding and rebound often indicate that immediate surgical evaluation is necessary, and delayed diagnosis and intervention may be life threatening.

DIAGNOSTIC WORKUP & INITIAL MANAGEMENT

- Distinguish etiologies requiring emergent or urgent surgical intervention (e.g., ruptured aortic aneurysm, perforated viscus [e.g., diverticulitis, peptic ulcer], appendicitis, intestinal obstruction, ischemic bowel, ruptured ectopic pregnancy) from nonemergent causes (e.g., renal colic, pelvic inflammatory disease, pancreatitis)

History and physical examination
- Assess the nature, location, onset, duration, and intensity of pain; similarity to past episodes; aggravating and alleviating factors; associated symptoms (e.g., nausea, vomiting, constipation or diarrhea, anorexia, dysuria, hematuria); guarding; bowel sounds; distension; presence of a mass; blood on rectal exam; and cervical or adnexal tenderness
  - Crampy, colicky pain that occurs in waves implies distension of a hollow viscus (e.g., renal colic, intestinal obstruction)
  - Constant, localized pain implies inflammation and direct irritation of the peritoneum (e.g., appendicitis, diverticulitis, cholecystitis)
- Hypotension and shock may occur
- Children, elderly patients, and immunocompromised patients may have atypical presentations

Initial diagnostic workup
- Initial laboratory testing includes CBC, electrolytes, BUN and creatinine, liver function tests, amylase and lipase, urinalysis, and pregnancy test
- Plain-film abdominal radiography may reveal obstruction, perforation (free air), or other pathology
- Ultrasound is a quick, inexpensive test for biliary tract disease, abdominal aortic aneurysm (AAA), ectopic pregnancy, or peritoneal fluid
- Abdominal CT will often establish the diagnosis for appendicitis, aortic aneurysm, and diverticulitis
- Diagnostic peritoneal lavage was previously used to assess for suspected trauma, bowel perforation, or peritonitis; however, it is no longer used today

Initial patient management
- Hemodynamically unstable patients require immediate resuscitation, including volume replacement with IV fluids and/or blood transfusion
- In general, patients who present with extremely severe pain of immediate onset require surgical intervention
- Evidence of hemorrhage (e.g., ruptured aortic aneurysm, ruptured ectopic pregnancy) or early sepsis (e.g., perforated diverticulitis, perforated bowel) may represent a life-threatening emergency that requires urgent surgical intervention
- Place a nasogastric tube for obstruction or persistent vomiting
- Administer broad-spectrum, empiric antibiotics if suspect a perforated viscus or intra-abdominal infection
- Direct treatment toward the underlying condition

DIFFERENTIAL DIAGNOSIS

Emergent, life-threatening etiologies

Ruptured abdominal aortic aneurysm
- Severe, colicky back, abdominal, or flank pain; a pulsatile abdominal mass may be present
- Immediate intervention is critical: Clinical suspicion of a ruptured or leaking AAA (via a bedside ultrasound that identifies an aneurysm) is sufficient to proceed to surgery

Perforated viscus (e.g., perforated duodenal ulcer, perforated diverticulum)
- Presents with severe abdominal pain
- Upright chest radiograph showing "free air" is usually sufficient for diagnosis (if not, CT scan)

Appendicitis
- The most common abdominal surgical emergency; presentation is often vague epigastric or periumbilical pain that migrates to the right lower quadrant (McBurney's point) over 24 hours
- A presentation of pain before emesis has nearly 100% sensitivity for appendicitis
- Emergent appendectomy is generally required because rupture can occur within 24 hours

Pancreatitis
- Steady, severe epigastric pain, often 1–4 hours after a large meal or alcohol intake
- Pain may radiate to the back and is sometimes relieved by leaning forward
- Severe cases may present with peritonitis (guarding, rebound tenderness, fever) and shock

Small bowel obstruction
- The most common causes are adhesions, hernias, and tumors; other causes include foreign bodies (e.g., gallstone ileus), inflammation (e.g., Crohn's disease), and volvulus
- "3rd-spacing," hypotension, sepsis, strangulation, bowel ischemia, or perforation may occur
- Surgery is indicated for complete obstructions or signs of strangulation

Acute mesenteric ischemia
- Results from sudden occlusion of a mesenteric artery or thrombosis of mesenteric veins
- Arterial occlusion is most commonly caused by a cardiac embolism (e.g., atrial fibrillation); venous thrombosis is most commonly caused by hypercoagulable states (e.g., myeloproliferative disorder) or low blood flow states (e.g., heart failure)

Ruptured ectopic pregnancy

Less immediately threatening etiologies
- Cholecystitis
- Gastroenteritis
- Gastritis
- Biliary or renal colic
- Bacterial peritonitis
- Intra-abdominal or pelvic abscess
- Colitis
- Urinary tract infection or pyelonephritis
- Sickle cell crisis
- Nonabdominal causes of pain that mimic an acute abdomen are numerous and may include MI, atypical angina, pericarditis, pneumonia, pulmonary embolus, and pelvic pathology (e.g., pelvic inflammatory disease, ovarian torsion, ovarian cyst rupture, tubo-ovarian abscess)

Acne

INTRODUCTION

Acne, the most common of all skin disorders, is an inflammatory disease of pilosebaceous follicles. It affects 17 million people in the United States, including 85% of adolescents and young adults. A genetic predisposition exists, but the pathogenesis is multifactorial and includes excess sebum secretion and retention under androgen stimulus, overgrowth of *Propionibacterium acnes* bacteria, hyperproliferation of epithelial cells causing obstruction of the pilosebaceous follicles, and inflammation. Obstruction of the pilosebaceous follicle leads to retention of sebum, which is an ideal medium for growth of *P. acnes* bacteria, and may result in rupture of the follicle. Both of these consequences lead to the typical inflammatory reaction of acne. Cosmetic agents and hair pomades may worsen acne.

DIAGNOSTIC WORKUP & INITIAL MANAGEMENT

History and physical examination

- Acne is a clinical diagnosis
- Examination should include the face, chest, and back
- Comedones are the hallmark: Open comedones ("blackheads") are follicles with dilated, black orifices; closed comedones ("whiteheads") are white papules without surrounding erythema
- Assess for severe acne: inflammatory papules, pustules, cysts, nodules, scars, and pits
- Document the number of comedones, inflammatory lesions, scars, and cysts
- Assess acne severity (mild, moderate, or severe) based on the number, size, and extent of lesions as well as on the presence or absence of scarring

Initial diagnostic workup

- Patients with evidence of virilization should have total testosterone, DHEA-S, FSH, and LH levels evaluated to assess for polycystic ovarian syndrome or adrenal tumors
- Clinical findings of Cushing's disease should prompt evaluation with 24-hour urine cortisol or salivary cortisol testing
- If acne remains recalcitrant to therapy, consider skin cultures to rule out gram-negative organisms or *Pityrosporum folliculitis*
- Bacterial culture may be necessary to rule out folliculitis

Initial patient management

- Patient education: Dispel common myths (e.g., acne is not caused by dirt), counsel against behaviors that may worsen acne (e.g., picking at lesions, using oil-containing cosmetics/moisturizers), and assess the level of psychologic distress
- Instruct patients to use mild cleansers and noncomedogenic moisturizers with sunscreen and to avoid excessive irritation or scrubbing of the face
- Topical therapies include benzoyl peroxide, antibiotics, retinoids, and salicylic acid
- Gentle comedone extraction may be performed with a comedone extractor
- Intralesional steroids may transiently decrease inflammation in severe cysts or nodules
- Systemic therapies include oral antibiotics (e.g., tetracycline, erythromycin, ampicillin) and hormonal therapy (e.g., oral contraceptives with low androgenic potential, spironolactone)
- Isotretinoin (Accutane) may be used with caution for severe cystic acne unresponsive to conventional therapy
  - Highly teratogenic and absolutely contraindicated in pregnancy; patients should be warned to use appropriate contraception, and they must submit formal consent
  - May be associated with an increased risk of suicide in adolescents
- Dermatologist referral is warranted for severe acne, refractory disease despite appropriate therapy, isotretinoin treatment, and management of acne scars
- Other treatments may include dermabrasion, peels, and laser treatments for acne scars

DIFFERENTIAL DIAGNOSIS

Acne vulgaris
- Characterized by severity type:
  - (I) Comedonal acne: Open ("whitehead") and closed ("blackhead") comedones without inflammatory lesions
  - (II) Mild inflammatory acne: Inflammatory papules and comedones
  - (III) Moderate inflammatory acne: Comedones, inflammatory papules, and pustules
  - (IV) Nodulocystic acne: Inflammatory lesions, large nodules >5 mm in diameter, with or without scarring
- May be secondary to or exacerbated by medications (e.g., corticosteroids, phenytoin, lithium, isoniazid) and polycystic ovarian syndrome

Acne rosacea
- Papules and pustules in the middle third of the face, telangiectasia, flushing, and erythema, but an absence of comedones
- Often worsened by ingestion of hot beverages or alcohol, exposure to sunlight, or prescription of vasodilating medications

Miliaria ("heat rash")
- Burning, pruritic vesicles, papules, or pustules on covered areas, usually the trunk and intertriginous areas

Folliculitis
- Gram-negative folliculitis results from *Klebsiella*, *Enterobacter*, and *Escherichia coli*; may develop during antibiotic treatment of acne
- Fungal folliculitis may result from *Pityrosporum* or *Malassezia*; does not respond to traditional acne therapy

Acne conglobata
- The most severe form of acne
- Presents with deep nodules, cysts, ulcers, abscesses, sinus tracks, and scars
- Causes severe scarring and keloid formation if untreated

Acne fulminans
- A severely destructive form of acne that presents with ulcerations, fever, and arthralgias

Pyoderma faciale
- Affects only adult women
- Presents with severe cysts and sinus tracks

Hidradenitis suppurativa
- Presents with pustules and cysts, often draining and very painful
- Primarily occurs in the axilla and groin

Other
- Perioral dermatitis
- Syringomas
- Cellulitis
- Herpes zoster
- Adenoma sebaceum
- Multiple trichoepitheliomas
- Erythema infectiosum

Alopecia

INTRODUCTION

Loss of hair is termed *effluvium,* and the resulting condition is alopecia. It may represent a significant loss or absence of hair affecting the scalp or other hair-bearing part of the body. Human hair follicles have three distinct growth phases: anagen (active), catagen (regressive), and telogen (resting). In healthy individuals, 50–100 hairs are lost daily, and 25% of hairs must be shed before thinning becomes apparent. Alopecia is characterized as scarring (cicatricial) or nonscarring. Nonscarring alopecia is more common and is differentiated by the absence of visible inflammation of the involved skin. Scarring alopecias are caused by several dermatologic conditions that also affect glabrous (nonhairy) skin. Scarring hair loss can be difficult to diagnose correctly and is a challenge to manage.

DIAGNOSTIC WORKUP & INITIAL MANAGEMENT

History and physical examination

- Note history of the hair loss (duration, tenderness, pruritus), past medical history (e.g., lupus, sarcoidosis, internal malignancies), medications used, stressful events (e.g., febrile illness, surgery, shock, diet, injury, emotional stress), and family history
- Evaluate for scarring (loss of hair follicles, ablation of the follicular orifice), hair loss elsewhere on the body (lichen planopilaris, some autoimmune diseases, and some lymphomas may manifest with scarring alopecia not limited to the scalp), and rashes or plaques on any part of the body (e.g., scleroderma and sarcoidosis often have skin findings beyond the scalp)
- Examine the scalp for inflammation, atrophy, and scales; "salt and pepper" appearance may occur in tinea capitis
- Examine the hair root and shaft: "exclamation point" hairs (the hair shaft narrows just near the follicle) are pathognomonic for alopecia areata; telogen hairs have a club-shaped tip; hair is broken in various lengths in trichotillomania or child abuse
- Subcutaneous masses, scalp bogginess, and cervical lymphadenopathy suggest infection

Initial diagnostic workup

- Trichogram (forcible hair pluck) to evaluate hair phase: normally, 80%–90% of hairs are in anagen phase (translucent hair shaft and deeply pigmented matrix); in androgenetic alopecia and telogen effluvium, telogen hairs (large bulb, transparent hair shaft) are increased
- Perform a 4-mm punch biopsy of an affected area; if any redness or scale, include that area in the biopsy so that the primary pathologic process can be examined
- Laboratory testing may include free and total testosterone, DHEA-S, prolactin, thyroid function tests, iron studies, RPR, CBC, metabolic panel, ESR, and ANA
- Obtain viral and bacterial cultures of any pustules
- Scrape any scaly areas for KOH prep to rule out tinea capitis

Initial patient management

- Once an area of scarring alopecia has developed, hair will not likely regrow in that area; the goal is to make the diagnosis and begin treatment to avoid further hair loss
- Treat the inciting causes of scarring alopecia (e.g., folliculitis, SLE, ingrown follicles)
- Wigs and/or hair transplants may be used
- Androgenetic alopecia: Oral finasteride is currently approved for men only; visible results take 3–4 months; topical minoxidil prevents further loss and may provide regrowth within 4–12 months; in women, use antiandrogens (e.g., spironolactone, cimetidine) if adrenal androgens are increased
- Telogen effluvium: Reassure that recovery is the norm
- Anagen effluvium: Withdraw drug or treat illness
- Alopecia areata: Superpotent topical steroids, intralesional steroid injections, cyclosporine, glucocorticoids, psoralen plus UV-A light
- Tinea capitus or kerion: Oral antifungals

DIFFERENTIAL DIAGNOSIS

Nonscarring alopecia

Androgenetic alopecia (male or female pattern baldness)
- Presents as gradually thinning hair at the hairline or vertex in men or widening of the part in women

Telogen effluvium (telogen = resting hair)
- Partial alopecia noted 3 months after a stressful event; usually reversible
- Diffuse thinning may occur following pregnancy, crash diets, change in birth control pills, stress, medications (e.g., ACE inhibitors, β-blockers, CNS agents)

Anagen effluvium (anagen = growing hair)
- Sudden, rapid, pronounced loss of growing hairs caused by disruption of the anagen phase
- Usually caused by antineoplastic agents (e.g., folic acid and purine antagonists, alkylating agents, alkaloids), irradiation, or intoxication (e.g., lead, thallium, arsenic, bismuth, warfarin)

Alopecia areata
- Sudden loss of hair in localized, rounded patches
- May be associated with autoimmune disease (e.g., vitiligo, endocrine)
- May be associated with Scotch plaid nails (transverse and longitudinal pitting rows)
- Ophiasis alopecia starts at the posterior occiput and extends anteriorly
- Other forms show loss of all scalp hair (alopecia totalis) or body hair (alopecia universalis)

Trauma
- Traction (e.g., trichotillomania [pulling hair out], tight braiding, ponytails)
- Pressure (e.g., prolonged bed rest, especially in infants)

Metabolic
- Thyroid disease

Hair shaft anomalies
- Monilethrix
- Trichothiodystrophy
- Pili torti

Other
- Seborrheic dermatitis
- Thyroid disease
- Congenital triangular alopecia
- Tinea capitis

Scarring (cicatricial) alopecia

Dermatologic-related disorders
- Lichen planus, lichen planopilaris
- Discoid lupus erythematosus
- Acrodermatitis enteropathica
- Sarcoidosis, amyloidosis
- Scleroderma/morphea
- Acne keloidalis
- Dissecting cellulitis
- Pseudopelade of Brocq (may be primary or secondary to inflammatory diseases)

Infectious
- Prolonged scalp infections, tuberculosis, syphilis, herpes zoster
- Extensive tinea capitis (*Trichophyton tonsurans, Microsporum canis*) or kerion
- Pseudofolliculitis barbae (inflammatory response to ingrown beard and/or neck hairs)

Other
- Folliculitis decalvans (occurs in beard or scalp due to merging of pustular hair follicles)
- Various neoplasms (e.g., lymphoma)

Amenorrhea

INTRODUCTION

Amenorrhea, the complete absence of menses, can be transient, intermittent, or permanent (and is normal in prepubertal, pregnant, and postmenopausal women). It may result from dysfunction of the hypothalamus, pituitary, ovaries, or outflow tract (uterus or vagina). Primary amenorrhea is defined as the absence of menarche by age 16; secondary amenorrhea (more common than primary amenorrhea) is defined as the absence of menses in women previously menstruating for at least three cycles or 6 months. Differentiate amenorrhea from oligomenorrhea, in which menses are less frequent than normal.

DIAGNOSTIC WORKUP & INITIAL MANAGEMENT

History and physical examination

- Note the timing and course of amenorrhea
- Note the presence of symptoms of pregnancy (e.g., nausea, vomiting, breast tenderness)
- Note weight changes and dietary history, and calculate BMI; assess for eating disorders
- Note presence of stressors, depression, and fatigue
- Assess for headache or visual field defects
- Note development of secondary sexual characteristics
- Note heat or cold intolerance
- Menstrual history, medical and surgical history, and review of medications
- Note history of radiation exposure
- Perform a detailed physical exam, including Tanner staging and pelvic exam
- Assess for signs of outflow tract abnormalities, including imperforate hymen (hematocele) and transverse vaginal septum
- Assess for hirsutism, acne, acanthosis nigricans, and galactorrhea

Initial workup and management

- All patients require a pregnancy test; *any woman with amenorrhea should be considered pregnant until proven otherwise*
- Anatomic abnormalities should be excluded before performing an endocrine evaluation
  - Pelvic ultrasound will evaluate for the presence or absence of Mullerian structures
- Endocrine evaluation may include LH, FSH, estradiol, testosterone, prolactin, TSH, 17-hydroxyprogesterone, and DHEA-S levels
  - Elevated gonadotropins (FSH and LH) suggest ovarian failure
  - Low FSH and LH suggest a hypothalamic (e.g., hypothalamic amenorrhea) or pituitary disorder (e.g., congenital GnRH deficiency)
  - Elevated DHEA-S suggests adrenal hyperplasia or tumor
- Diagnostic administration of medroxyprogesterone acetate ("progesterone challenge test") may be used
  - Withdrawal bleeding within 2–7 days confirms the presence of endogenous estrogen, appropriate endometrial response, and an intact outflow tract, and suggests a diagnosis of anovulation
- Head MRI or CT is indicated if primary hypogonadotropic hypogonadism, elevated prolactin, visual field defects, or headaches are present
- If the uterus and/or breasts are absent, order a karyotype analysis followed by testosterone and serum FSH levels

DIFFERENTIAL DIAGNOSIS

Secondary amenorrhea
- Pregnancy
- Lactation
- Hypothyroidism
- Polycystic ovarian syndrome
  - May present with peripubertal onset of menstrual irregularities with hyperandrogenism (acne and hirsutism) and obesity
  - Associated with an elevated LH:FSH ratio
- Functional hypothalamic amenorrhea
  - May result from stress, eating disorders, weight loss, or excessive exercise
- Prolactinoma or hyperprolactinemia
  - May present with galactorrhea, virilization, gynecomastia, headache, and diplopia
  - May occur secondary to medications (e.g., oral contraceptives, phenothiazines) or a pituitary adenoma
- Anatomic abnormalities (e.g., Asherman's syndrome, cervical stenosis)
- Ovarian dysfunction or premature ovarian failure
- Behavioral disorder (e.g., anorexia nervosa, excessive exercise)
- Sheehan's syndrome (postpartum pituitary apoplexy)

Primary amenorrhea
- Constitutional delay of puberty
- Outflow tract disorders
  - Asherman's syndrome
  - Cervical stenosis
  - Transverse vaginal septum
  - Imperforate hymen
  - Agenesis of the uterus or vagina
  - Mullerian agenesis (Mayer-Rokitansky-Hauser syndrome): Agenesis of the fallopian tubes, uterus, and vagina
- Complete androgen insensitivity syndrome
  - An X-linked recessive disorder (46,XY) resulting in resistance to testosterone because of a defect in the androgen receptor

Less common etiologies
- Turner's syndrome (46,XO)
- Ovarian failure (e.g., autoimmune oophoritis, chemotherapy or radiation injury)
- 5α-reductase deficiency
- 17α-hydroxylase deficiency
- Craniopharyngioma
- Hypopituitarism
- Congenital GnRH deficiency (Kallman's syndrome if associated with anosmia)
- Cushing's syndrome
- Savage's syndrome (gonadotropin-resistant ovary syndrome)
- Swyer's syndrome (XY gonadal dysgenesis)
- Kallmann's syndrome (a genetic disease that usually affects males; in women, it is associated with lack of FSH and LH and no pubertal development)
- Trauma

Amnesia

INTRODUCTION

Amnesia is an inability to remember previous events and to process new information despite a normal level of consciousness. The memory center in the brain is housed in the temporal lobes; thus, the development of true amnesia requires pathology of both temporal lobes. The most common cause of transient amnesia is acute head trauma with concussion. Alzheimer's disease is the most common nontransient cause of amnesia. Anterograde amnesia is defined as an inability to remember events that follow the onset of the amnesia, whereas retrograde amnesia is defined as an inability to remember events that occurred before the onset of the amnesia.

DIAGNOSTIC WORKUP & INITIAL MANAGEMENT

History and physical examination
- Assess level of consciousness: Alert and interactive, drowsy (falls asleep easily but responds to voice), stupor (does not respond to voice but awakes to painful stimuli), or comatose (no response to pain or voice)
- Assess orientation to person (identify self), place (identify location, city, country), time (identify year, month, day, date), and situation
- Assess memory: Recent memory is tested by asking the patient to immediately repeat several digits or items; recent memory can also be tested by presenting several unrelated words or items and then, several minutes later, asking the patient to recite them; observe whether the patient looks to a spouse or other caregiver for answers
- Assess attention span and concentration by asking the patient to spell "WORLD" backward or to list the days of the week forward and then backward
- Assess behavior and mood by observing dress and appearance, alertness, irritability or agitation, attentiveness, interpersonal skills, and appropriateness of expressions to questions
- Complete neurologic and head examinations
- Life-threatening head trauma and CNS infection should be considered initially in patients with altered mental status and amnesia

Initial diagnostic workup
- Initial laboratory testing may include CBC, electrolytes, glucose, calcium, magnesium, phosphorus, coagulation studies, and serum and urine toxicology screens
- Lumbar puncture and CSF analysis should be considered early if suspect a CNS infection
  - Test for opening pressure, appearance (e.g., clear, cloudy, bloody), protein, glucose, CSF:serum glucose ratio, Gram's stain, culture
  - Cryptococcal antigen and acid-fast bacilli smear and culture if in endemic area or HIV positive
  - If lumbar puncture is delayed by need for imaging (e.g., head CT to rule out increased intracranial pressure), administer empiric antibiotics immediately
- Head CT without contrast may be needed to exclude bleeding in cases of head trauma and may also identify structural lesions
- Head MRI with diffusion-weighted imaging is more sensitive for diagnosing stroke, tumor, and the subtle white matter changes associated with vascular disease
- EEG to rule out seizure disorder

Initial patient management
- Immediate attention to airway, breathing, and circulation
- Prompt treatment of suspected infections and trauma
- Surgical intervention may be necessary to evacuate space-occupying traumatic lesions
- Concussions are treated symptomatically; patients should refrain from contact sports
- Control elevated intracranial pressure with head elevation, moderate hyperventilation, mannitol administration, and/or surgical drainage

DIFFERENTIAL DIAGNOSIS

Head trauma (e.g., concussion, hemorrhage)
- Usually results in transient retrograde and anterograde amnesia

Dementia
- Alzheimer's disease is the most common cause of chronic amnesia
- Refer to the *Dementia* entry for other etiologies

Infection
- Herpes simplex encephalitis is a particularly common cause of infectious amnesia, because it has a predilection for the temporal lobes

Seizure disorders
- Retrograde amnesia is most common after a generalized tonic-clonic seizure during the postictal period
- Some complex partial seizure foci (particularly temporal lobe epilepsy) can also produce "blank" periods of memory

Toxicologic insults
- Binge alcohol consumption
- Benzodiazepine use (e.g., the "date rape" drug flunitrazepam, also known as Rohypnol)

Psychogenic causes
- Relatively common
- Typified by a patient who claims to forget his or her name or shows significant impairment of very old memories
- Should be a diagnosis of exclusion

Wernicke-Korsakoff syndrome
- Symmetric hemorrhagic necrosis with neuronal damage, demyelination, and astrocytosis in bilateral thalamus, cerebellar vermis, and periaqueductal gray matter of the midbrain because of thiamine deficiency, most commonly in alcoholics
- Results in truncal ataxia, ophthalmoplegia, and short-term memory loss

Transient global amnesia
- A rare, transient, ischemic attack–like condition of proposed vascular etiology
- Causes abrupt onset of short-term memory loss lasting minutes to hours
- Typically occurs in patients older than 50 years
- Can be seen in patients with migraines or seizures

Anosmia

INTRODUCTION

More than 2 million people in the United States (1%–2% of the population) suffer from anosmia, an absent sense of smell. Temporary anosmia may result from any condition that irritates the nasal mucosa to cause swelling and obstruction of the nasal passages and sinuses. Permanent anosmia is commonly associated with damage and destruction of the olfactory neuroepithelium or a part of the olfactory nerve.

DIAGNOSTIC WORKUP & INITIAL MANAGEMENT

History and physical examination

- Assess onset and duration, associated symptoms (e.g., allergic symptoms), recent head trauma, exposures (particularly to intranasal zinc), medications, and past medical and surgical history
  - Rhinitis and sinusitis may be associated with chronic nasal congestion, rhinorrhea, postnasal drip, pale or boggy nasal mucosa, sinus swelling and tenderness, and headaches
  - Upper or lower respiratory symptoms and renal involvement suggest Wegener's granulomatosis
- Include a complete head and neck exam and a full neurologic exam
  - Enlarged nasal turbinates suggest sinusitis (turbinates are pale and boggy in chronic allergic sinusitis and erythematous in nonallergic sinusitis)
  - Assess for septal disease (midline granuloma) and polyps

Initial diagnostic workup

- Several types of smell tests are available:
  - Olfactory threshold and odor identification test
  - University of Pennsylvania scratch and sniff test
  - Alcohol sniff test
- Initial laboratory testing may include CBC, electrolytes, glucose, BUN and creatinine, calcium, ESR, thyroid profile, liver function tests, and vitamin B_{12} level
- Blood and/or urine toxicology screen if suspect drug use or poisoning
- Nasal discharge testing for β-transferrin in CSF rhinorrhea of posttraumatic patients
- Allergy testing may be indicated
- Head CT may be indicated to evaluate skull base, brain, nasal cavity, and sinuses
- MRI may be indicated to evaluate brain and soft facial tissues
- Antibodies to Ro/SSA and LA/SSB are positive in Sjogren's syndrome

Initial patient management

- Temporary anosmia because of nasal and/or sinus disease is usually successfully treated medically with systemic and/or intranasal corticosteroids, antibiotics if coexisting bacterial infection is present, antihistamines and avoidance measures if an allergic component exists, or decongestants and/or saline lavage for nasal congestion
  - Polypectomy and sinus surgery may be necessary if initial therapy is ineffective
- No cure is available for permanent anosmia (e.g., from postviral infections, trauma, congenital disorders); however, regeneration of neural elements may occur over a period of days to years
- Anosmia caused by CNS and endocrine diseases requires treatment of the underlying illness
- Vitamin and mineral supplementation in cases of deficiency

DIFFERENTIAL DIAGNOSIS

Nasal and sinus disease
- The most common cause of anosmia
- Allergic or vasomotor rhinitis and sinusitis result in temporary anosmia
- Intranasal polyposis may result in obstruction of nasal passages with temporary anosmia

Head or facial trauma
- Probably the second most common cause of anosmia
- May result in permanent anosmia
- CNS rhinorrhea may occur

Post-upper respiratory viral infection
- Accounts for 20%–30% of cases of anosmia

Iatrogenic
- Amphetamines
- Certain antibiotics (e.g., amikacin, doxycycline, amoxicillin, clarithromycin)
- Nasal steroids
- Antithyroid agents
- Radiation

Poisoning
- Chemical pollutants
- Heavy metals (e.g., lead)
- Volatile organic compounds (e.g., acetone, acrylates, butyl acetate, carbon disulfide)
- Inorganic compounds (e.g., vanadium, chromates, cadmium)

Illicit drugs
- Intranasal cocaine

Granulomatous disease with destruction of the olfactory nerve
- Wegener's granulomatosis
- Sarcoidosis

CNS disorders
- Alzheimer's disease
- Parkinson's disease
- Anxiety disorders

Neoplasms
- Meningioma of the olfactory groove
- Nasal cavity tumors
- Brain tumors

Endocrine disorders
- Diabetes mellitus
- Hypothyroidism
- Adrenal insufficiency

Congenital disorders
- Kallman's syndrome
- Turner's syndrome

Vitamin deficiencies
- Malnutrition
- Vitamin B_{12} deficiency (pernicious anemia)
- Niacin deficiency (pellagra)
- Zinc deficiency

Sjogren's syndrome

Anxiety

INTRODUCTION

Anxiety includes symptoms of physiologic arousal (e.g., autonomic hyperactivity, increased motor tension) and psychologic arousal (e.g., excessive worry, increased vigilance). It may present as a primary psychiatric condition or secondary to a broad variety of medical and psychiatric diseases. It is hypothesized that pathologic anxiety results from disturbances in the cerebral cortex, specifically the limbic system (hypothalamus, septum, hippocampus, amygdala, cingulate), other neural bodies, and the connections between these structures. The major neuroendocrine mediators of anxiety disorders are norepinephrine and serotonin. Anxiety disorders are the most common mental illness in the United States, affecting nearly 15% of adults. Most anxiety disorders begin in childhood, adolescence, or early adulthood.

DIAGNOSTIC WORKUP & INITIAL MANAGEMENT

History and physical examination

- Complete medical and psychiatric history, including a detailed history of onset, duration, and type of anxiety symptoms as well as specific events, stressors, or medical illnesses that produce anxiety
- Complete drug and medication history, including caffeine, alcohol, over-the-counter preparations, herbals, illicit drugs, and prescription drugs
- Physical exam should be directed toward ruling out organic medical diseases that may present with anxiety, including cardiovascular, pulmonary, endocrine, and neurologic disorders
- A complete psychiatric examination is indicated for all patients (e.g., appearance, sleep evaluation, mini-mental status exam, affect)

Initial diagnostic workup

- No laboratory or imaging tests are indicated except those that assess for underlying medical disorders (e.g., thyroid function tests, ECG, urine catecholamines, toxicology screen)
- DSM-IV criteria are used to determine the specific psychiatric disorders; the anxiety disorders include generalized anxiety disorder (GAD), panic disorder with or without agoraphobia, obsessive-compulsive disorder (OCD), post-traumatic stress disorder (PTSD), acute stress disorder, social phobia, and specific phobias (e.g., agoraphobia)

Initial patient management

- Early treatment improves prognosis and limits social and occupational impairment
- Discontinue (or decrease to a reasonable level) caffeine-containing products (e.g., coffee, tea, cola, chocolate)
- Consider the need for psychiatric evaluation
- Cognitive behavioral therapy, interpersonal, or psychodynamic therapy may be helpful
- Benzodiazepines may be used for rapid control of panic attacks, acute situational anxiety disorder, and adjustment disorder when the duration of pharmacotherapy is anticipated to be 6 weeks or less (use with caution because of abuse potential)
- Certain anxiety disorders may be treated with specific antianxiety drugs
  - GAD: venlafaxine, buspirone, paroxetine
  - Social phobia: paroxetine
  - OCD: fluoxetine, sertraline, paroxetine, fluvoxamine
  - PTSD: sertraline
- Consider inpatient care if suicide is a risk or detoxification is needed for comorbid substance dependence
- Prognosis for recovery depends on the specific disorder, severity of symptoms, and specific causes of the anxiety
- Complications of anxiety disorders include sedative abuse, substance abuse, depression, occupational impairment, and marital and familial difficulties

DIFFERENTIAL DIAGNOSIS

Generalized anxiety disorder
- Excessive worry associated with at least three symptoms, including restlessness or an edgy feeling, fatigue, difficulty concentrating, irritability, muscle tension, or sleep disturbance
- The most common anxiety disorder in primary care

Panic disorder
- A chronic, relapsing form of anxiety characterized by recurrent panic attacks (episodes of severe anxiety with associated physical symptoms) followed by persistent anticipatory anxiety (fear of recurrence), fear of the implications of the attacks, or change in behavior because of the attack (usually avoidance); somatic symptoms are often present (e.g., tachycardia)
- Etiologies may include genetic and biochemical factors, a deficit of the inhibitory neurotransmitter GABA, and/or overabundance of sympathetic or serotonin activity in the locus ceruleus
- May be a learned response from internal physical cues
- Often associated with depression and agoraphobia

Depression
- Anxiety often presents in a mixed state with depression

Medications
- Bronchodilators, steroids, antidepressants, and antihypertensives are often implicated
- Substance use, including drugs (e.g., alcohol, caffeine, cocaine, cannabis)
- Drug or medication withdrawal (e.g., alcohol, heroin, benzodiazepines)

Obssessive-compulsive disorder
- Obsessions are persistent ideas, images, or impulses that generate anxiety
- Compulsions are intentional, repetitive behaviors or mental acts aimed at reducing the distress of obsessions

Anxiety disorder caused by a general medical condition
- Cardiovascular etiologies include coronary artery disease, acute coronary syndrome, angina, arrhythmias, congestive heart failure, mitral valve prolapse
- Respiratory etiologies include asthma, COPD, and pulmonary embolism
- Endocrine etiologies include hyper- or hypothyroidism, hypoglycemia, and Cushing's syndrome
- Neurological etiologies include Parkinson's disease and epilepsy
- Numerous cancers

Pheochromocytoma
- An adrenal tumor that usually presents with hypertension and increased heart rate and sometimes with a fright reaction of sweating, headache, and pale facial appearance

Parkinson's disease
- Parkinson's tremor presents at rest and usually in one hand (as opposed to the more generalized essential tremor that occurs in cases of anxiety)
- May be exacerbated by anxiety

Other
- PTSD
- Acute stress disorder
- Social anxiety disorder
- Specific phobia
- Bipolar disorder (especially manic stage)
- Conversion disorder (a somatoform disorder in which psychological stress is unconsciously transformed into physical symptoms, such as visual loss, focal neurologic deficits, or pseudoseizures

Aphasia

INTRODUCTION

Aphasia refers to the inability to produce and/or comprehend spoken language, despite preservation of the mechanical and visual means to do so. Thus, facial weakness, oropharyngeal paresis, or primary disturbances of vision and hearing do not constitute aphasia. Usually, aphasia reflects damage to portions or all of the speech areas in the dominant hemisphere. To localize the lesion within the cerebrum, aphasias are generally separated into receptive (Wernicke's aphasia) or expressive (Broca's aphasia) types. Further subgroups include anomic, conduction, transcortical sensory, and transcortical motor. Loss of reading comprehension (inability to read and comprehend printed words) frequently accompanies aphasia.

DIAGNOSTIC WORKUP & INITIAL MANAGEMENT

History and physical examination
- Complete medical, neurologic, psychiatric, and medication history
- Exam should include a comprehensive neurologic exam, cardiovascular exam, and head and neck exam
- Assess language by evaluating spontaneity and fluency of speech, reading and writing ability, comprehension of conversation, and ability to follow commands

Initial diagnostic workup
- The cornerstone of diagnosis is cerebral imaging; MRI has the highest sensitivity and specificity
- Initial laboratory tests include CBC, electrolytes, BUN and creatinine, calcium, glucose, RPR to test for syphilis, and vitamin B_{12} level
- Consider toxicology screen
- Echocardiography (transesophageal echocardiogram is best) and blood cultures may be indicated to diagnose endocarditis
- CSF analysis and EEG to diagnose viral encephalitis versus status epilepticus
- Psychometric testing for dementia
- Normal brain imaging with or without associated psychiatric signs may suggest status epilepticus, hypoglycemia, or a dissociative state

Initial patient management
- Speech therapy is useful to help maintain motivation to improve language function and to avoid depression from communication impairment
- Treat the underlying etiology as necessary
- Embolic stroke from a cardiac source is sometimes treated with anticoagulation; however, if secondary to endocarditis, do not initiate anticoagulation because of an increased risk of hemorrhage; instead, treat with antibiotics
- Thrombotic stroke is generally treated with antiplatelet therapy (e.g., aspirin, clopidogrel) and risk factor reduction (e.g., lipid and hypertension therapy)
- Viral encephalitis may be treated with IV acyclovir for 10–14 days
- Acetylcholinesterase inhibitors are of variable effectiveness in Alzheimer's disease
- Status epilepticus requires immediate IV lorazepam and anticonvulsants
- Correct underlying metabolic disturbances (e.g., hypoglycemia, electrolyte abnormalities)
- Oral or IV benzodiazepines may "break the spell" of a dissociative state; electroconvulsive therapy may be necessary

DIFFERENTIAL DIAGNOSIS

Stroke
- The most common cause of aphasia
- Sudden onset suggests cerebral embolization from a cardiac source (e.g., endocarditis, atrial fibrillation) or a carotid artery source
- A stuttering onset suggests in situ arterial thrombosis

Less common etiologies
- Alzheimer's dementia
- Sensorineural hearing loss
- Dysarthria (impaired mechanics of speech, such as motor weakness of the tongue or lips)
- Postconcussion syndrome
- Rasmussen's encephalitis
- Nonconvulsive status epilepticus
- Dissociative state
- Subdural hematoma
- Trauma
- Severe hypoglycemia
- Sedative-hypnotic drug intoxication
- Herpes encephalitis
- Tertiary syphilis

Types of aphasia

Receptive, fluent (Wernicke's) aphasia
- Inability to name objects, follow written or spoken commands, and repeat
- Verbal (semantic, neologistic) errors are abundant; however, speech is fluent
- Patients are verbose (words sound normal) but make little sense, and answers are not related to the questions asked
- Localized to the dominant posterior superior temporal lobe (superior temporal gyrus)
- Comprehension is impaired

Expressive, nonfluent (Broca's) aphasia
- Stuttering, nonfluent speech with literal (phonemic) errors; however, comprehension is preserved
- Patients use few words, become easily frustrated, and use frequent paraphasic errors (e.g., referring to a watch as a "time")
- Localized to the inferior lateral dominant frontal lobe, particularly the operculum (the region where the frontal and temporal lobes join)
- Often associated with mild contralateral hemiparesis

Anomic aphasia
- Isolated inability to name simple objects
- Localized to the angular gyrus; commonly seen in patients with dementia

Conduction aphasia
- Comprehension and repetition are impaired
- Localized to the arcuate fasciculus, a white matter band connecting Wernicke's area to Broca's area

Transcortical sensory aphasia
- Similar to Wernicke's aphasia but with preserved repetition (ask the patient to repeat "no ifs, ands, or buts"); localized to the superior posterior temporal lobe

Transcortical motor aphasia
- Similar to Broca's aphasia but with preserved repetition and echolalia (aimlessly repeating other's spoken words); localized to medial dominant frontal lobe

Global aphasia
- Represents lesions that involve both Broca's and Wernicke's areas
- Patients are unable to comprehend language or speak fluently and are often mute

Ataxia and Gait Abnormalities

INTRODUCTION

Disorders of gait may arise from problems virtually anywhere in the nervous or musculoskeletal system. Observation of gait is an important part of the neurologic examination. Gait abnormalities are described as slapping, steppage, or mixed. A slapping gait presents with a tendency to slap the feet firmly against the ground to improve proprioceptive input. A steppage gait, as seen in patients with foot drop, involves carefully lifting the foot to prevent it from catching and tripping the patient. Ataxia is defined as gross incoordination of muscle movements and can involve multiple areas of the body. Eye movements, upper or lower extremities, and even speech can be referred to as ataxic. Ataxia results from dysfunction of the cerebellum or its connections. It can present as an acute or chronic, progressive disorder

DIAGNOSTIC WORKUP & INITIAL MANAGEMENT

History and physical examination

- Note history of injury (acute vs. chronic), progression, episodicity, events leading to onset of gait problems (recent illness, intoxication, drug or toxin ingestion, trauma), previous episodes, associated symptoms (e.g., headache, papilledema, myoclonus, retinopathy), and family history
- Give careful attention not only to the type of gait disturbance but also to associated findings on neurologic exam (e.g., symmetric distal sensory loss and hyporeflexia suggest a peripheral neuropathy; circumducting gait with hemiparesis, hemisensory loss, and ipsilateral hyperreflexia suggest a cerebral lesion)
- Perform a complete neurologic exam, including cranial nerves, cerebellar function, ophthalmologic and nystagmus exam, reflexes, and proprioceptive sense
- Perform a complete gait exam, including posture, station, ambulation, and ability to stand from a seated position
- Posture is analyzed for telltale discrepancies:
  - Patients with unstable posture may have cerebellar, basal ganglia, or labyrinthine disease
  - Excessively erect posture is associated with progressive supranuclear palsy
  - "Stooped" (universal flexion) posture is associated with Parkinson's disease
  - Exaggerated lumbar lordosis is associated with proximal lower extremity weakness (e.g., muscular dystrophy)
  - Wide-based posture is often associated with cerebellar dysfunction
- Station refers to positioning of the body during erect stance (test with eyes opened/closed):
  - Swaying with eyes opened indicates disorder of vestibular or cerebellovestibular system (e.g., ataxic gait)
  - Swaying with eyes closed (Romberg sign) indicates dysfunction of large-fiber peripheral nerves in the lower extremities or posterior columns
  - Inability to stand on one foot suggests cerebellar, basal ganglia, or labyrinthine disease

Initial workup and management

- Initial laboratory testing may include CBC, chemistries, toxicology screen and alcohol level, vitamin B_{12} and folate levels, ESR, and anticonvulsant levels (especially phenytoin)
- Neuroimaging (CT or MRI) may be indicated
- Lumbar puncture may be indicated to assess for infection or multiple sclerosis
- EMG and nerve conduction studies may help diagnose neuropathy or myopathy
- DNA testing is available for inherited neuropathies (e.g., Charcot-Marie-Tooth syndrome) and many of the spinocerebellar ataxias
- If the etiology of a gait abnormality is uncertain, a full gait analysis by a specially trained physical therapist, podiatrist, orthopedic surgeon, or neurologist is often indicated
- Specific symptomatic measures to improve gait stability and efficiency may clearly improve functional abilities, including assistive devices (e.g., canes, walkers, wheelchairs), orthotics (e.g., ankle-foot orthoses for foot drop), and physical therapy
- Treat underlying disorders as appropriate

DIFFERENTIAL DIAGNOSIS

Peripheral neuropathy (sensory and/or motor)
- Diabetes mellitus
- Monoclonal gammopathy
- Alcoholic neuropathy
- Vasculitic neuropathy
- Nutritional causes (e.g., vitamin B_{12}, thiamine, or biotinidase deficiency)
- Medication-induced neuropathy
- Miller-Fischer variant of Guillain-Barré syndrome

Mononeuropathy or radiculopathy affecting the lower extremities
- For example, a peroneal neuropathy or L5 radiculopathy causing a unilateral steppage gait

Myelopathy
- Patients with bilateral lower extremity weakness and hypertonicity secondary to a spinal cord lesion may exhibit a spastic gait with stiffness of both legs

Myopathy
- Waddling gait may occur with weakness of the trunk, hip, or proximal lower extremity muscles

Brainstem or cortical lesions (e.g., multiple sclerosis, stroke)
- Most commonly result in a hemiparetic gait with circumduction of the weak leg

Cerebellar lesions
- Result in ataxia, which tends to be wide-based, irregular, and staggering
- Cerebellar hemorrhage or ischemia

Inherited neuropathies
- Charcot-Marie-Tooth disease
- Friedreich's ataxia
- Dejerine-Sottas neuropathy
- Roussy-Levy syndrome

Intoxication or medication-induced
- Alcohol
- Medications include sedatives, phenytoin, carbamazepine, and antihistamines

Infectious
- Postinfectious cerebellitis (varicella, Epstein-Barr virus, mumps, *Legionella,* hepatitis A)
- Encephalitis or meningitis
- Acute disseminated encephalomyelitis
- Neurosyphilis
- Cerebellar abscess
- Labyrinthitis

Parkinsonism
- Stooped posture, decreased arm swing, and shuffling (taking many small steps)

Other
- Orthopedic issues affecting the foot, ankle, leg, knee, or hip
- GALOP syndrome (gait disorder, autoantibodies, late-age onset, polyneuropathy)
- Posterior fossa tumor (e.g., medulloblastoma, glioma)
- Spinocerebellar ataxia
- Hereditary spastic paraparesis
- Hysterical gait
- Normal pressure hydrocephalus
- Opsoclonus/myoclonus syndrome
- Ataxia-telangiectasia syndrome
- Basilar migraine
- Postconcussion
- Seizure
- Hartnup disease
- Refsum disease
- Episodic ataxia type I or II
- Conversion disorder
- Arnold-Chiari or Dandy-Walker malformation
- Metabolic disorders (e.g., urea cycle disorder)
- Sphingolipidoses
- Mitochondrial disease
- Celiac disease with cerebellar calcification

Aura

INTRODUCTION

A subjective sensory phenomenon that may involve any of the five senses, such as visual auras (often described as flashing lights, zig-zag lines, or scotoma), sensory auras (usually paresthesias), or auditory auras. Other auras may be described as dream-like sensations, déjà vu, or odd odors. The type of symptom may be related to the brain area involved. For example, visual aura suggests occipital lobe pathology.

DIAGNOSTIC WORKUP & INITIAL MANAGEMENT

History and physical examination

- Assess type of aura (any of five senses)
- Note associated activities and triggers (e.g., stress, medications, exertion, trauma, foods) and post-aura symptoms (e.g., headache, loss of consciousness, seizure)
- Note personal or family history of seizures or migraines
- Review past medical history for head injury, stroke, dementia, intracranial infection, and alcohol or drug abuse
- Full head, neck, and neurologic exam (look for one-sided features that suggest pathology on the opposite side of the brain)
- Examine for trauma following loss of consciousness

Initial diagnostic testing

- Initial tests may include glucose, electrolytes, calcium, magnesium, CBC, BUN and creatinine, and toxicology screen
- EEG may be indicated if seizure activity is suspected (provocative EEG with triggers gives higher yield); however, a normal EEG does not rule out epilepsy, and an abnormal EEG may be seen in migraines in addition to seizures
- Consider MRI to rule out cerebral pathology
- Urgent CT may be indicated if a physiologic seizure or trauma is involved (not indicated in patients with migraine and normal neurologic exam unless the pattern of migraine has changed)

Initial patient management

- Assess for serious underlying conditions, and treat accordingly
- Eliminate any potentially causative medications, including over-the-counter and alternative/complementary medications
- Educate patients about their condition, and have them try to identify triggers; if necessary, have patients keep a log of aura frequency and timing
- Migraine headache: Avoid triggers, and treat with serotonin agonists (e.g., sumatriptan), NSAIDs, and/or ergotamines; in patients who experience more than one migraine weekly, consider prophylactic medications (e.g., β-blockers, calcium channel blockers, tricyclic antidepressants, anticonvulsants)
- In patients with a first seizure, treatment is determined by weighing the risks and benefits of medical treatment versus observation; consider withholding treatment in low-risk patients until a second seizure occurs, because the majority of patients have only one lifetime seizure
  - If drug treatment is initiated, monotherapy is always preferred
  - For most seizures, valproate, carbamazepine, and phenytoin are the initial choices
  - Older antiepileptic drugs (e.g., carbamazepine, phenobarbital, valproate) are as effective as newer drugs (e.g., gabapentin, lamotrigine, topiramate, oxcarbazine); newer drugs may have fewer side effects and easier dosing and may not require frequent monitoring

DIFFERENTIAL DIAGNOSIS

Epilepsy
- Epilepsy is defined as two or more unprovoked seizures
- Patients with one seizure have a 20% chance of a recurrent seizure within 1 year in the absence of focal brain lesions; after two seizures, the risk increases to 85%
- 1% of the population is diagnosed with epilepsy (10% of the population will have a single, unprovoked seizure during their lifetime)

Migraine with aura
- Migraine headache usually follows aura within 60 minutes and lasts 4–72 hours; however, aura may occur without a headache
- May be associated with a prodrome (mood changes, insomnia, nausea), visual or sensory aura, photophobia, phonophobia, nausea, and numbness
- Rarely, migrainous infarction may occur

Partial seizure
- 60% of patients with focal seizures have an accompanying aura
- Aura symptoms are associated with the brain area in which they originate (e.g., occipital lobe seizure results in seeing lights)
- Aura is more likely to precede simple partial seizures

Generalized seizure
- Rarely, tonic-clonic (grand mal) seizure and absence (petit mal) seizure may be associated with an aura

Pituitary adenoma
- Pituitary adenoma or other underlying cerebral pathology may predispose to migraines, seizures, or altered sensations (taste, smell)

Hallucinations
- Not actually an aura

Physiologic nonepileptic seizures
- Usually results from an underlying physiologic cause (e.g., fever, hypoglycemia, hypo- or hyperthyroidism, renal failure, cerebral anoxia)

Babinski Sign

INTRODUCTION

Babinski sign is elicited by gently stroking the lateral sole of the foot with a slightly blunted object (e.g., cotton-tip swab) and drawing the stimulus slightly medially across the metatarsal area. A positive response has two components: dorsiflexion of the great toe, and slight abduction (fanning) of the remaining toes. A positive sign represents disinhibition of the normal spinal reflex because of damage to descending inhibitory pathways from the brain or spinal cord. A positive Babinski sign, however, is normal in neonates because of immaturity in the myelination of these pathways.

DIAGNOSTIC WORKUP & INITIAL MANAGEMENT

History and physical examination

- Complete history and neurologic exam
- A variety of conditions that affect the spinal cord and brain result in a positive Babinski sign; differential diagnosis depends on localization of signs
- In cases of unilateral positive Babinski sign, the lesion may be in any portion of the brain or spinal cord
- Bilateral Babinski signs suggest a spinal cord lesion in awake patients or a brain lesion in patients with persisting delirium
- In patients with increased reflexes in the arms and an exaggerated finger-flexor response, the lesion probably is localized to the cervical spinal cord or brain

Initial diagnostic workup

- Brain and spinal cord imaging are the most sensitive and specific identifiers of pathologies resulting in Babinski sign
- Patients with suspected stroke may undergo carotid Doppler ultrasound, MRA of cerebral and carotid arteries, echocardiography, and lipid and coagulability profile
- Potential tumors may require PET scan for diagnosis
- EEG if suspect seizure activity
- Lumbar puncture and blood and CSF cultures for suspected encephalitis or cerebritis
- MRI or CT of the brain and spinal cord in cases of suspected stroke

DIFFERENTIAL DIAGNOSIS

- False positive (e.g., toe withdrawal, previous podiatric surgery resulting in the appearance of chronic upgoing toe)
- Stroke is the most common cause
  - Ischemic infarction: Usually occurs in the cerebral gray matter but may also occur in the subcortical white matter or brainstem corticospinal tracts
  - Cerebral hemorrhage: Secondary to cerebral infarction, primary hypertensive bleeding (usually in the putamen, internal capsule, or brainstem), or coagulopathy (e.g., excessive anticoagulation, trauma, surgery, tumor)
- Spinal cord infarction
  - Occurs in the thoracic region due to poor collateral circulation, cardiogenic embolism, or ischemia secondary to surgical clamping during aneurysm surgery
- Spinal cord hemorrhage
  - Results from trauma, tumor, arteriovenous malformation, or excessive anticoagulation
- Postictal state
- Brain abscess
- Viral encephalitis
- Embolism from bacterial endocarditis
- Meningitis or cerebritis
- Cerebral palsy
- Multiple sclerosis
- Cerebral aneurysm
- Venous sinus thrombosis
- Arteriovenous malformation
- Cavernous malformation
- Severe metabolic disturbance (e.g., hepatic, renal, or hypoxemic processes)
- Sedative-hypnotic drug intoxication
- Post–cardiac arrest state
- Degenerative brain and spinal cord disease (e.g., Alzheimer's disease, Parkinson's disease, Friedreich's ataxia)
- Neuronal storage diseases (e.g., ceroid lipofuscinosis, gangliosidoses, sialidoses)
- Post-seizure
- Congenital or idiopathic

Bell's Palsy and Facial Paralysis

INTRODUCTION

Bell's palsy is a unilateral facial paralysis or weakness caused by edema and compression of the facial nerve (cranial nerve VII). It is the most common cause of facial nerve (fascicular) paralysis. Most patients recover completely, but more than 8,000 people yearly in the U.S. are left with facial weakness. One must differentiate supranuclear (central) from nuclear (peripheral) facial palsy. Supranuclear palsy primarily involves the lower part of the face, and emotional responses may be intact (e.g., the patient may not be able to show you his teeth but will smile to a joke). Nuclear palsy affects all ipsilateral muscles of facial expression, resulting in paralysis of the entire ipsilateral side (e.g., mouth is pulled to the normal side and may droop on the affected side, facial creases are effaced, eyelid may not close).

DIAGNOSTIC WORKUP & INITIAL MANAGEMENT

History and physical examination

- Complete history, including onset, duration, characteristics, associated symptoms (e.g., retroauricular pain, tingling, loss of taste, visual changes, fever, headache, nausea/vomiting)
- Associated neurologic deficits may occur (e.g., weakness of the arm or leg, aphasia) due to involvement of surrounding brain areas in a vascular event
- Depending on the site of interruption, the patient may have hyperacusis, loss of taste over the unilateral anterior two-thirds of the tongue, deafness, tinnitus, dizziness, or associated brainstem signs
- Assess for herpetic lesions in the pharynx or external auditory canal
- Assess the 8th cranial nerve, because it courses very close to the facial nerve
- Perform complete head, neck, and neurologic exams
- Attempt to distinguish central palsy from peripheral palsy: sparing of the forehead muscles suggests central palsy

Initial diagnostic workup

- Bell's palsy is a clinical diagnosis; reserve testing for atypical presentations or slowly resolving cases
- Initial laboratory testing may include CBC, glucose, ESR, and Lyme titer
- In cases of supranuclear palsy, a workup for stroke, demyelinating processes and/or tumors may be indicated; this may include head CT, MRI, or CSF studies
- In general, peripheral palsies do not warrant immediate tests
- EMG and nerve conduction studies of the facial nerve may be useful for prognostic purposes in patients with complete loss of function
- Lumbar puncture is not necessary unless suspect Lyme disease or Guillain-Barré syndrome
- Lyme antibody titer is only indicated if other clinical features of Lyme disease are present (e.g., arthralgias, characteristic rash)

Initial patient management

- Early use of corticosteroids and acyclovir may lead to improved facial function outcomes; it will relieve the retroauricular pain, but it is uncertain if it helps to improve the facial palsy
- Eye protection is necessary, including lubricating drops during the day and eye ointment and patch at night
- Gentle massage of the face is recommended
- Electrical stimulation has not been shown to have benefit
- Surgical decompression is not beneficial and not recommended
- 80% of patients recover within 2–3 weeks; 10% may take up to a year to recover; 10% of cases do not recover and develop synkinesis of face (contracture of muscles)
  - Poor prognostic factors include age over 60, hypertension, diabetes, pregnancy, pain other than in the ear, impairment in taste, complete facial weakness, or no recovery by 3 weeks

DIFFERENTIAL DIAGNOSIS

Bell's palsy (idiopathic facial palsy of the lower motor neuron)
- The most common cause of facial nerve paralysis

Stroke
- Whereas Bell's palsy involves the entire face with inability to close the eye completely, strokes primarily affect the lower part of the face

Lyme disease
- Can present with single or multiple cranial neuropathies

Tumors that invade the temporal bone
- Cholesteatoma
- Carotid body tumor

Ramsay-Hunt syndrome (herpes zoster)
- Herpes zoster eruption in the pharynx and external auditory canal
- May also affect the 8th cranial nerve

Acoustic neuroma
- May compress the facial nerve

Pontine lesions
- May occur secondary to infarcts, demyelinating processes, or tumors
- May be associated with signs of brainstem involvement

Facial diplegia or bilateral facial palsy
- Guillain-Barré syndrome (associated with ascending areflexic motor paralysis)
- Heerfordt's syndrome (a form of sarcoidosis; also known as uveoparotid fever)
- Hemifacial spasm

Melkersson-Rosenthal syndrome
- Recurrent facial palsy, labial edema, and tongue plication

Other etiologies
- Diabetic neuropathy
- Leprosy
- Ectatic basilar artery and compression of the facial nerve
- Hysterical facial contractures, including blepharospasm
- Multiple sclerosis

Bleeding (Excessive)

INTRODUCTION

Bleeding is abnormal if it occurs spontaneously (without a precipitating cause), if it is excessive, or if it does not stop promptly with compression. Causes of abnormal bleeding are divided into vascular disorders (structural abnormalities of the blood vessels), platelet disorders (decreased number of platelets or dysfunctional platelets), and coagulation factor disorders.

DIAGNOSTIC WORKUP & INITIAL MANAGEMENT

- In cases of acute, excessive blood loss, emergent intervention may be indicated:
  - Assess airway, breathing, and circulation
  - Provide supplemental oxygen, rapid IV hydration, hemostasis (usually with direct pressure), and transfusion if bleeding is brisk and/or hemodynamic compromise occurs
  - Remove offending medications (e.g., heparin) if appropriate

History and physical examination

- Ask about personal and family history of bleeding, including tendency to bleed upon minor trauma, postsurgical bleeding, menorrhagia, and tooth extractions
- Ask about medications, including over-the-counter and herbal remedies
- Perform a complete physical exam, including rectal exam and stool guaiac testing for occult GI bleeding
- Assess joints for hemarthrosis

Initial workup and management

- Initial laboratory tests include CBC with peripheral smear, platelet count, urinalysis (for hematuria), and coagulation studies; coagulation studies include:
  - Prothrombin time (PT) evaluates the extrinsic coagulation pathway: coagulation factors X, VII, V, II, and I
  - Partial thromboplastin time (PTT) evaluates the intrinsic coagulation pathway: coagulation factors XII, XI, IX, VIII, V, II, and I
  - Thrombin time measures the ability of thrombin to transform fibrinogen into fibrin
  - Bleeding time evaluates platelet function and capillary integrity
- Additional tests may be indicated, including:
  - Fibrinogen assay
  - Urea clot lysis test (evaluates factor XIII deficiency)
  - Mixing studies (determines the presence of an anticoagulant in the blood)
  - Specific factor assays
  - Platelet adhesion and aggregation tests (to evaluate platelet function)
  - Bone marrow aspirate (to evaluate platelet production and rule out leukemia)
- Consider hematology consultation

DIFFERENTIAL DIAGNOSIS

Drug etiologies

Antiplatelet drugs
- Cyclooxygenase inhibitors (e.g., NSAIDs, aspirin)
- Phosphodiesterase III inhibitors (e.g., colostazol)
- Glycoprotein IIb/IIIa inhibitors (e.g., abciximab)
- Adenosine reuptake inhibitors (e.g., dipyridimole)
- ADP inhibitors (e.g., clopidogrel, ticlopidine)

Anticoagulants
- Heparin
- Low-molecular-weight heparin (e.g., enoxaparin)
- Fondaparinux
- Warfarin
- Lepirudin

Thrombolytic therapy drugs
- t-PA
- Recombinant (genetically engineered) t-PA
- Streptokinase
- Urokinase
- Tenecteplase

Other drugs
- Alcohol
- Steroids
- Chemotherapy
- Dietary supplements (e.g., fish oil, ginkgo biloba, garlic, ginger)

Nondrug etiologies
- Senile purpura
- Uremia
- Liver disease (e.g., cirrhosis)
- HIV infection
  - Platelets decrease in number because of infection of megakaryocytes
- Severe vitamin K deficiency
- Disseminated intravascular coogulation (DIC)
- Henoch-Schönlein purpura
- Von Willebrand's disease
- Hemophilia
- Idiopathic thrombocytopenic purpura
- Heparin-induced thrombocytopenia
- Myelodysplasia
- Thrombotic thrombocytopenic purpura–hemolytic uremic syndrome (TTP–HUS)
- Leukemia
- Aplastic anemia
- Hereditary hemorrhagic telangiectasia
- Ehlers-Danlos syndrome
- Bernard-Soulier syndrome
- Arteriovenous malformation
- Pancytopenia
- Isolated coagulation factor deficiency
- Nutrition deficiencies (e.g., vitamins C, K, B)
- Trauma (accidental or abuse)

Blurred Vision

INTRODUCTION

Blurred vision is one of the most common ophthalmologic symptoms. It may be caused by any alteration of the optical surfaces (e.g., cornea), the media through which incident light traverses (e.g., cataract, vitreous hemorrhage), or neural processing (retina or optic nerve). History and physical examination will usually lead to a reasonable differential diagnosis. Treatment aims to restore the ideal refractive and transparent media and surfaces of the eye. Most commonly, blurred vision results from a refractive error that can be corrected with glasses, but more serious pathology must not be missed. Refer also to the *Vision Loss* entry.

DIAGNOSTIC WORKUP & INITIAL MANAGEMENT

History and physical examination

- Review the onset and progression (sudden vs. gradual, transient vs. prolonged) and duration (minutes, days, or months) of symptoms
- Note whether bilateral or unilateral, near versus far vision
- Note associated symptoms (e.g., headache, seizure activity or change in level of consciousness, stroke-like symptoms, fever, irritated or dry eyes, floaters, flashing lights)
- Assess past medical history (e.g., diabetes, eye or head trauma, cataracts), family history, exposures, and medications
- Complete ophthalmologic exam, including best corrected visual acuity using Snellen chart or near card, slit-lamp exam, and dilated fundus exam
  - Improvement of vision with pinhole test suggests a refractive error or mild media opacity
- Neurologic and head and neck exam

Initial diagnostic workup

- Initial laboratory tests may include fasting (or random) blood glucose (with a repeat glucose and Hb_{A1c} if glucose is initially elevated), CBC, and coagulation studies (PT, PTT)
- Further studies may be warranted depending on suspicions and underlying diseases
- EEG if suspect a seizure disorder

Initial patient management

- Consider ophthalmology referral
- Glasses or contact lenses for refractive errors
- Treat underlying pathology if possible (e.g., correct hyperglycemia, cataract surgery)
- Lubrication for dry eyes
- Ocular media opacity requires medical or surgical correction
- Retinal detachment requires surgical repair
- Hyperviscosity should be treated appropriately (e.g., aspirin, discontinue cigarettes)
- Antiseizure prophylaxis for seizure disorders

DIFFERENTIAL DIAGNOSIS

Disorders of the lens or extraocular muscles

- Refractive error (blurred far vision)
- Presbyopia (blurred near vision with good distance vision) from loss of lens elasticity or curvature or loss of ciliary muscle function
- Cataract
- Dry eye/poor tear film
- Extraocular muscle paralysis (diplopia may be misinterpreted as blurred vision; however, this will clear upon covering either eye)

Conjunctivitis

- May be infectious, toxic (topical medications, cosmetics, preservatives), allergic (hay fever, allergens), or immunogenic (e.g., Graves disease, rheumatoid arthritis, Sjogren's syndrome, SLE, Wegener's granulomatosis, relapsing polychondritis, polyarteritis nodosa)

Macular/retinal disease

- Age-related macular degeneration
- Diabetic retinopathy
- Retinal detachment
- Macular edema
- Central serous chorioretinopathy
- Retinitis pigmentosa

Ocular media opacity

- Corneal edema (decreased deturgescent capacity or increased intraocular pressure)
- Uveitis (anterior or posterior)
- Hyphema
- Cataract
- Vitreous hemorrhage
- Mass lesion

Corneal irregularity or abrasion

Disease of the optic nerve, optic chiasm, optic radiations, or visual cortex

Acute angle-closure glaucoma

CNS

- Migraine
- Ischemic stroke
- Intracerebral hemorrhage
- Compressive mass lesion (pituitary adenoma, aneurysm, meningioma, craniopharyngioma)
- Head trauma
- Seizure disorder/postictal phenomenon

Hyperglycemia

- Poorly controlled diabetes mellitus
- Medication effects

Medication or drug side effects

- Anticholinergics, antihypertensives, psychotropics
- Cyclosporine
- Amphetamine abuse

Vascular disease

- Retinal artery or vein occlusion
- Hyperviscosity/hypercoagulation
- Carotid stenosis
- Temporal arteritis

Other

- Myasthenia gravis
- Carbon dioxide narcosis
- Prolonged hypotension or hypertension
- Botulism
- Tobacco or alcohol amblyopia

Bowel Sounds, Decreased

INTRODUCTION

Decreased bowel sounds can be as innocent as a hungry patient anticipating his or her next meal or as ominous as an impending abdominal catastrophe necessitating emergent laparotomy. The sensitivity and specificity of the auscultation of bowel sounds, however, are quite low, differ subjectively by clinician, and vary from one moment to the next. Rule of thumb: Before declaring a complete absence of bowel sounds, auscultate for a minimum of 5 minutes ("if you didn't hear them, you didn't listen long enough").

DIAGNOSTIC WORKUP & INITIAL MANAGEMENT

History and physical examination

- Characterize any pain
- Patients with peritonitis will appear very ill and have abdominal tenderness, rebound, and guarding
- Auscultate before palpation
  - The length of auscultation is more important than the area of auscultation, because bowel sounds radiate throughout the abdomen (thus, it is not necessary to auscultate each quadrant)
- Physical exam should include a rectal exam

Initial diagnostic workup

- Initial laboratory testing includes CBC, electrolytes, glucose, BUN and creatinine, calcium, liver function tests, amylase, lipase, and urinalysis
- Imaging studies may include x-rays, CT, and ultrasound
  - Flat and upright radiographs may reveal rupture (free air) or obstruction (dilated proximal loops of bowel with air-fluid levels); thoracic and/or lumbar radiographs may reveal spinal fractures
  - Abdominal CT gives more anatomic detail and may better differentiate ileus from obstruction
  - Ultrasound is useful to diagnose gynecologic disorders
- Differentiate postoperative ileus from obstruction
  - Some degree of ileus is expected following laparotomy (3–5 days); prolonged ileus should be investigated
  - Both can cause nausea and vomiting, constipation or obstipation, distension, tenderness, and tympany
  - A transition point or lack of gas in the rectum may suggest an obstruction

Initial patient management

- Although treatment decisions should rarely (if ever) be made based on bowel sounds, serial assessment may be a useful sign of a patient's clinical evolution
- Ileus is treated conservatively by bowel rest (no oral intake), IV hydration, and nasogastric decompression (for nausea and vomiting)
  - Correct electrolyte abnormalities as necessary
  - Discontinue constipating drugs (especially narcotics)
  - Prokinetic drugs (e.g., metoclopramide, erythromycin) have mixed results but are often used
  - Encourage ambulation
  - Decreased nasogastric output, "normal" bowel sounds, passage of flatus, improved radiographs, or hunger may indicate readiness to begin oral intake
- Peritonitis generally requires emergent surgical intervention; treatment is directed at the specific underlying diagnosis

DIFFERENTIAL DIAGNOSIS

Benign etiologies
- Normal variant: 5–30 bowel sounds per minute is typical; however, several minutes may elapse without any sounds
- Failure to auscultate long enough
- Hunger (may also result in increased bowel sounds)
- Inappropriate auscultation immediately following abdominal palpation or percussion (always listen for bowel sounds before palpating the abdomen)

Complete bowel obstruction
- While complete bowel obstruction presents without bowel sounds, partial bowel obstructions often have increased bowel sounds

Intestinal ischemia
- Often occurs in older patients with existing cardiovascular or cerebrovascular disease

Adynamic ileus
- Postabdominal surgery
- Electrolyte abnormalities (e.g., hypokalemia, hyponatremia, hypomagnesemia, uremia)
- Drugs (e.g., narcotics, α- and β-blockers, anticholinergics, psychotropic agents)
- Lower lobe pneumonia
- Sepsis
- Retroperitoneal hemorrhage
- Vertebral compression fracture
- Colonic pseudo-obstruction (Ogilvie's syndrome)

Peritonitis
- Acute appendicitis (or ruptured appendix)
- Perforated gastric ulcer
- Perforated diverticulum or diverticulitis
- Ruptured ectopic pregnancy
- Ruptured abdominal aortic aneurysm
- Pancreatitis
- Pelvic inflammatory disease
- Infected peritonitis
- Solid organ injury (e.g., following trauma)

Less common etiologies
- Diabetic coma
- Hypoparathyroidism
- Rib fractures
- MI
- Spinal injury
- Perforated gallbladder
- Black widow spider bite

Bowel Sounds, Increased

INTRODUCTION

Normal bowel sounds are intermittent, low- to medium-pitched gurgles interspersed with occasional high-pitched, tinkling metallic sounds heard every 10–30 seconds. In acute intestinal obstruction (usually of the small bowel), bowel sounds are markedly increased. High-frequency, low-pitched gurgles (borborygmi) that often rise to a high-pitched crescendo that coincides with colicky abdominal pain is pathognomonic of small bowel obstruction. This represents bouts of peristaltic activity in an attempt to "overcome" the obstruction. Despite extensive efforts to evaluate and classify bowel sounds using auscultation and advanced technology, many physicians believe that meaningful interpretation of bowel sounds remains clinically futile and contributes little to clinical decision making.

DIAGNOSTIC WORKUP & INITIAL MANAGEMENT

History and physical examination

- Assess vital signs for evidence of fever and dehydration
- Note associated symptoms, medical history, surgical history, travel history, recent trauma or illness, and medications
- Bowel sounds should be auscultated before palpation
- Hyperactive, high-pitched "tinkles" or "rushes" ("cathedral" sounds) often occur with bowel obstructions
- Mechanical bowel obstruction may present with distension, hiccups, nausea and vomiting, crampy abdominal pain or spasms, constipation, or watery diarrhea
- Abdominal exam should include all hernia orifices and evaluate for signs of incarceration and strangulation
- Physical exam should include a rectal exam

Initial diagnostic workup

- Initial laboratory testing may include CBC, electrolytes, BUN and creatinine, glucose, calcium, liver function tests, amylase, lipase, and urinalysis
- Flat and upright (or decubitus) abdominal radiographs are helpful to diagnose obstructions
- Abdominal CT is the most useful test and may demonstrate the etiology
- Ultrasound or upper GI radiographic series may be indicated if suspect obstruction
- Enteroclysis is helpful to determine the level and degree of obstruction

Initial patient management

- Aggressive fluid and electrolyte replacement
- Complete bowel obstruction with signs of strangulation (e.g., fever, leukocytosis, peritonitis) requires emergent operative intervention
- Highly selected patients with complete obstruction and no peritonitis may be managed conservatively for a short period of time but risk development of strangulation
- Partial small bowel obstructions can usually be managed conservatively by nasogastric decompression, bowel rest (no oral intake), and IV fluids
- Serial evaluations are required to detect progression to complete obstruction
- Treatment is aimed at the underlying cause in nonsurgical cases

DIFFERENTIAL DIAGNOSIS

Benign etiologies
- Variation of normal (5–30 sounds per minute)
- Recent meal or premeal
- Borborygmi ("stomach growling"): loud, rumbling, and gushing sounds caused by movement of large amounts of fluid and air
- Air swallowing

Mechanical bowel obstruction
- Adhesions from previous surgery are the most common cause of bowel obstructions (60% of cases)
- Neoplasms (20%): May be extra- or intraluminal
- Hernias (10%): May be external (inguinal, femoral, ventral) or internal (diaphragmatic, congenital, mesenteric defects)
- Crohn's disease (5%)
- Abscess
- Volvulus
- Intussusception (rare in adults)
- Colonic pseudo-obstruction (Ogilvie's syndrome)

Diarrhea
- Acute gastroenteritis
- Malabsorption syndrome
- Lactase deficiency
- Infection

Other etiologies
- Drugs (prokinetic agents, such as metoclopramide or erythromycin)
- "Succussion splash": A large collection of stagnant air and fluid in the distal stomach secondary to a gastric outlet obstruction, gastroparesis, or recent large meal may be auscultated while vigorously shaking the patient
- Gallstone ileus
- Peutz-Jeghers syndrome: polypoid hamartoma of the bowel resulting in intussusception
- Foreign body
- Carcinoid syndrome
- Hiatal hernia

Etiologies in children
- Hypertrophic pyloric stenosis
- Congenital small bowel obstruction (e.g., malrotation with or without volvulus, duodenal atresia or stenosis, jejunal or ileal atresia or stenosis, annular pancreas, intestinal duplication, intra-abdominal hernia, meconium ileus)
- Acquired small bowel obstruction (e.g., intussusception, incarcerated inguinal hernia, postsurgical adhesions, duodenal hematoma, ascariasis, Crohn's disease, superior mesenteric artery syndrome)
- Colonic obstruction (e.g., Hirschsprung's disease, small left colon syndrome, adhesions, fibrosing colonopathy, Chagas' disease)
- Acute gastroenteritis
- Early peritonitis
- Intestinal pseudo-obstruction

Breast Masses

INTRODUCTION

Although breast lumps are anxiety-provoking to patients and warrant evaluation because of the risk of cancer, most breast lumps and other breast complaints are of benign origin. Multiple methods are available to differentiate benign from malignant breast lesions, including clinical examination, mammography, ultrasound, fine-needle aspiration, and needle-core or open-breast biopsy. Most breast masses should be examined radiographically, and solid lesions require biopsy to rule out malignancy. Though rare, breast cancer does occur in males.

DIAGNOSTIC WORKUP & INITIAL MANAGEMENT

History and physical examination

- Collect historical information to establish baseline risk, including age, menstrual status, parity, family history, previous biopsy results, and exogenous hormone use
- Clinical breast exam should document approximate size, site, mobility, and shape of the mass as well as associated skin retraction, erythema, or adenopathy
  - Indirect evidence supports the effectiveness of clinical breast exam: sensitivity, 40%–69%; specificity, 86%–99%
  - Normal physiologic nodularity ("fibrocystic disease") can be difficult to distinguish from a discrete mass; it is less likely to have clear borders, is often cordlike, and may change with the menstrual cycle
  - Benign features include smooth, well-demarcated, and mobile lesions
  - Malignant features include hard, irregular, fixed lesions; bloody nipple discharge; nipple retraction; and skin dimpling or peau d'orange rash

Initial workup and management

- Diagnostic evaluation depends on age
  - Age < 35 years: Ultrasound to determine cystic versus solid lesion (cysts may be aspirated)
  - Age > 35 years: Perform diagnostic bilateral mammography first; if lesion is benign-appearing or not seen, ultrasound is warranted to determine cystic versus solid
- Mammogram is often the first test ordered but may not be helpful in younger patients because of higher breast density
  - Findings suggestive of malignancy include increased density, irregular margins, spiculation, and irregular microcalcifications
- Ultrasound is used as an adjunct to delineate masses that cannot be seen on a mammogram, to determine whether a lesion is solid or cystic, and if age < 35 years
- MRI may be considered for indeterminate mammogram or ultrasound
- Biopsy of masses, nonpalpable lesions, or suspicious calcifications on mammogram may be indicated
  - Fine-needle aspiration extracts cells for cytologic exam to assess benign from malignant
  - Needle-core biopsy of solid lesions or complex cysts extracts tissue and provides a definitive diagnosis
  - Excisional biopsy is definitive and may be curative if the full lesion is removed
- Perform a cytologic exam of any nipple discharge

Follow-up

- Frequent follow up (every 3–6 months) if an exam is particularly difficult in order to maintain familiarity and confirm stability
- Cystic masses require follow up 4–6 weeks after aspiration to ensure no reaccumulation; recheck every 6 months thereafter, and perform biopsy if the cyst recurs
- Enlarging masses require surgical excision, even if benign

DIFFERENTIAL DIAGNOSIS

Fibroadenoma
- The most common cause of a unilateral discrete breast mass in young women
- A painless, mobile mass; may be bilateral and/or multiple
- Growth is stimulated by exogenous estrogen or progesterone, lactation, and pregnancy
- Common in women with "fibrocystic changes" of the breast
- A benign lesion; requires surgical excision for diagnosis and treatment, but patient has no increased risk for malignancy after excision

Cystic disease
- Gross cystic disease is found in ~7% of adult women in the United States, most frequently during the fourth decade and perimenopause
- Arise from dilatation or obstruction of the collecting ducts
- May be painful and may vary in size with menses

Intraductal papilloma
- Associated with nipple discharge

Normal physiologic nodularity
- Often incorrectly called fibrocystic disease
- Found in more than 60% of adult women in the United States
- May be treated by reducing dietary caffeine or fat intake, wearing well-fitted bras, aspiration of large or painful cysts, and medical therapies (e.g., danazol, oral contraceptives) for pain relief

Breast cancer
- The most common cause of a discrete breast mass in women > 50 years
- Types include infiltrating ductal (most common), infiltrating lobular, and medullary carcinoma
- Increased risk with advancing age and with obesity, infertility, nulliparity or late first pregnancy (after age 30 years), early menarche or late menopause, uterine cancer, history of breast cancer in a first-degree relative (up to 10-fold increased risk), *BRCA* gene mutation, hormone therapy use, and postradiation
  - In 75% of women with breast cancer, advanced age is their only apparent risk factor
- Often presents with a nontender mass, nipple discharge, or (occasionally) nipple bleeding

Galactocele
- Presents during or shortly after breast-feeding
- Needle aspiration is usually curative
- If fluid is bloody or mass does not disappear, an excisional biopsy is required

Breast abscess
- Commonly caused by *Staphylococcus aureus* or *Streptococcus*
- Usually presents as a painful, nonmobile mass with rapid onset
- Associated with mastitis
- May be associated with overlying blanching erythema, fevers, and chills

Other
- Gynecomastia
- Cystosarcoma phylloides
- Mammary duct ectasia
- Fat necrosis
- Cystic mastitis
- Lymphoma
- Lipoma
- Intramammary node
- Metastatic disease to the breast (e.g., carcinoid, gastric adenocarcinoma)
- Myoid hamartoma
- Trauma
- Radial scar

Breast Pain and Discharge

INTRODUCTION

Breast pain (mastalgia) is a common complaint. Pain and tenderness may be normal during early pregnancy and before menses. Breast discharge, however, is rarely normal except in pregnant or lactating women, and it generally requires a full workup.

DIAGNOSTIC WORKUP & INITIAL MANAGEMENT

History and physical examination

- History should include duration and pattern of pain and/or discharge, past medical history, family history of breast or gynecologic cancer, and menstrual and pregnancy history
- Breast exam should be performed 7–9 days after menstrual flow
  - Fibrocystic areas are usually slightly irregular, mobile, bilateral, and commonly in the upper outer quadrant; compression causes tenderness
  - Breast cancer may be solitary, irregular, or stellate and is usually hard, nontender, and sometimes fixed to the underlying chest wall; not clearly delineated from surrounding tissue; may be associated with lymphadenopathy
  - Mastitis presents with inflamed, edematous, erythematous, indurated, and tender areas; associated with axillary lymphadenopathy
  - Nipple discharge is suspicious for cancer if it is bloody or serosanguinous; oral contraceptives, estrogens, or elevated prolactin levels may result in clear, serous, or milky discharge

Initial workup and management

- Diagnostic mammogram is indicated in patients > 30 years who present with a solitary or dominant mass or asymmetric thickening
  - Compare with previous mammograms, if possible
  - Breast tissue in patients < 30–35 years may be too dense for accurate mammographic results
- Ultrasound is used as an adjunct to mammography to delineate masses that cannot be seen on mammogram, to determine whether a lesion is solid or cystic, and in younger patients
- Biopsy of masses, nonpalpable lesions, or suspicious calcifications on mammogram may be indicated
  - Fine-needle aspiration extracts cells for cytologic exam to assess benign from malignant
  - Needle-core biopsy of solid lesions or complex cysts extracts tissue and provides a definitive diagnosis
  - Excisional biopsy is definitive and may be curative if the full lesion is removed
- Perform a cytologic exam of any suspicious nipple discharge
- Ductogram and/or galactogram may be indicated to localize a ductal abnormality in preparation for biopsy during the evaluation of patients with nipple discharge
- Endocrine evaluation may include prolactin, TSH, FSH, and LH levels

DIFFERENTIAL DIAGNOSIS

Breast pain

- Normal physiologic nodularity ("fibrocystic change")
  - The most common benign breast condition
  - Clinically present in 60% of women; histologically present in 90% of women
- Mastitis
  - Associated with lactation
  - Treat with warm compresses and antibiotics to cover *S. aureus* and *Streptococcus* (e.g., cephalexin); may require IV antibiotics and/or drainage if abscess develops
  - Consider inflammatory breast cancer if no response after 5 days of treatment in a non-lactating female
- Extramammary causes of pain
  - Cervical radiculitis
  - Costochondritis
  - Herpes zoster
  - Angina
- Breast cancer
  - Women have a 1 in 9 risk of developing breast cancer in their lifetime
- Cyst
- Breast abscess
- Unilateral or bilateral gynecomastia
- Phylloides tumor
- Intraductal papilloma
- Fat necrosis
- Trauma
- Fibroadenoma
- Lipoma
- Pregnancy

Breast discharge

- Duct ectasia (dilated mammary duct)
- Galactorrhea
- Mondor's disease (thrombophlebitis of superficial chest wall veins)
- Chronic nipple stimulation
- Pregnancy
- Hypothyroidism
- Sarcoidosis
- SLE
- Cirrhosis or other hepatic disease
- Breast cancer
- Intraductal papilloma
- Normal physiologic nodularity ("fibrocystic change")
- Medications (e.g., phenothiazines, metoclopramide, tricyclic antidepressants, reserpine, opiates, cimetidine, androgens)
- Hypothalamic and pituitary abnormalities
  - Prolactinoma
  - Acromegaly
  - Empty sella syndrome
- Pseudocyesis (presence of pregnancy symptoms without conception)

Cardiomegaly

INTRODUCTION

Cardiomegaly is the enlargement of the heart above normal size. When looking at a chest radiograph, one must assess size using a posteroanterior view, because the heart may appear falsely enlarged on an anteroposterior view. When true cardiomegaly is present, further evaluation by echocardiography or other definitive testing is often indicated to identify the cause of the enlargement and to help guide treatment.

DIAGNOSTIC WORKUP & INITIAL MANAGEMENT

History and physical examination

- Assess onset, duration, and characteristics of present illness, if any
- Associated symptoms may include fatigue, dyspnea, chest pain, palpitations, dizziness, or syncope
- Assess medical and surgical history, family history of heart disease or sudden death, social history (including habitual use of alcohol or recreational drugs), and medications

Initial diagnostic workup

- Chest radiography and ECG may suggest enlargement of the heart
- Transthoracic echocardiogram is often indicated to evaluate for valvular and pericardial disease, chamber size, wall motion abnormalities, and ventricular function
- Stress testing and/or cardiac catheterization is indicated if suspect coronary artery disease (e.g., left ventricular or regional wall motion abnormality on echocardiogram, angina)
- Laboratory studies may include CBC, ESR, serum chemistries, cardiac biomarkers, and TSH
- Blood cultures and viral studies are indicated in some cases if suspect infection
- Consider ANA, rheumatoid factor, and screening for pheochromocytoma (urinary metanephrines and vanillylmandelic acid) and hemochromatosis (iron studies) in selected patients
- Fat-pad biopsy may be indicated if suspect amyloidosis
- Endomyocardial biopsy may be necessary in some cases

Initial patient management

- Treat the underlying cause
- Discontinue offending drugs
- Administer supplemental oxygen, antiarrythmics, diuretics, anti-ischemic therapy, inotropes, or vasodilators as indicated for symptomatic relief
- Consider cardiology consultation
- Cardiac catheterization and pulmonary artery catheterization may be necessary in some cases to guide therapy
- Implantation of a defibrillator may also be indicated in some cases
- Ventricular assist devices and, possibly, heart transplantation may be necessary in end-stage symptomatic heart failure refractory to medical treatment

DIFFERENTIAL DIAGNOSIS

- Normal "athletic" heart
- Congestive heart failure
- Ischemic heart disease
- Chronic hypertension with left ventricular hypertrophy
- Valvular disease (primarily mitral regurgitation, aortic stenosis, aortic regurgitation)
- Hypertrophic cardiomyopathy
- Congenital heart disorders (e.g., atrial septal defect, ventricular septal defect, patent ductus arteriosus, coarctation of the aorta, Ebstein's anomaly, tetralogy of Fallot)
- Idiopathic cardiomyopathy
- Alcoholic cardiomyopathy
- Lung disease leading to right-sided chamber enlargement (e.g., pulmonary embolus, COPD, cor pulmonale, primary pulmonary hypertension)
- Subacute bacterial endocarditis
- Myocarditis
- Renal failure (risk of pericardial effusion)
- Anemia
- Scleroderma
- SLE
- Sickle cell disease
- Marfan's syndrome
- Pregnancy
- Drugs (numerous drugs are cardiotoxic)
- Postradiation
- Mediastinal mass
- Kyphoscoliosis
- Rheumatoid arthritis
- Infiltrative diseases (e.g., amyloidosis, hemochromatosis, atrial myxoma, endocardial fibroelastosis, Fabry's disease, Hurler's syndrome, Pompe's disease)
- Pericardial fat pad
- Carcinoid syndrome
- Acromegaly
- Hyper- or hypoparathyroidism
- Severe cases of hypocalcemia, hypomagnesemia, and/or hypophosphatemia

Carotid Bruits

INTRODUCTION

A carotid bruit is a blowing sound or murmur over the carotid artery and is best heard with the bell of the stethoscope. It is usually associated with carotid stenosis secondary to atherosclerosis. It may imply an increased risk of stroke, depending on the degree of stenosis and history of transient ischemic attack symptoms.

DIAGNOSTIC WORKUP & INITIAL MANAGEMENT

History and physical examination

- Attention to symptoms, patient history, family history, cardiovascular risk factors, and medications
- Note previous symptoms of transient ischemic attack or stroke
- Significant carotid stenosis may present with amaurosis fugax, which is often described as a "shade coming down over the eye" contralateral to the stenosis
- Complete cardiovascular and neurologic exams
- The pitch of the bruit increases as stenosis worsens but may become silent when full occlusion occurs

Initial diagnostic workup

- Laboratory evaluation may include lipid panel, CBC, glucose, electrolytes, homocysteine level (an independent risk factor for stroke), vitamin B_{12} and folate levels, TSH, and ESR
- Carotid duplex ultrasound will evaluate the degree of stenosis
- MRA, CT angiography, or arteriography may be indicated to better evaluate symptomatic stenosis that may require surgery

Initial patient management

- A patient with symptomatic stenosis (presence of stroke-like symptoms in the appropriate distribution) and ≥70% carotid stenosis confirmed by duplex ultrasound should strongly consider carotid endarterectomy or carotid artery stenting
- Symptomatic patients with 50%–69% stenosis have greater benefit from surgery than from a medical approach, although less benefit than those with >70% stenosis
- Asymptomatic patients and those who cannot tolerate surgery should begin aspirin (60–325 mg/day) and/or antiplatelet therapy (e.g., clopidogrel)
- Smoking and alcohol cessation
- Treat hypertension, diabetes, and hyperlipidemia
- Carotid angioplasty is currently under study
- Treat underlying diseases as appropriate

DIFFERENTIAL DIAGNOSIS

Internal carotid artery stenosis
- While atherosclerosis is the most common cause of carotid stenosis, traumatic dissection is an important cause of carotid disease in the young

External carotid artery stenosis
- Can present with a high-pitched bruit but without internal carotid artery stenosis
- Treatment is unnecessary

Normal (non-stenotic), yet tortuous, carotid arteries
- Usually evident on imaging

Heart murmur with radiation to the neck (e.g., aortic stenosis)
- Can be differentiated from focal carotid bruits by listening to the entire length of the carotid:
  - Focal bruit from arterial stenosis will have a focal, high-pitched bruit
  - Aortic stenosis will have an equivalent bruit along the entire carotid without focality

Excessive compression of the stethoscope over the neck vessels
- Results in deformity of the vessel wall, turbulence to blood flow, and an audible sound

Hyperthyroidism
- Results in hyperdynamic circulation, tachycardia, and hypertension

Takayasu's arteritis
- Decreased pulses and bruits may occur over the abdominal aorta, carotid arteries, brachial arteries, and subclavian arteries

Fisher's contralateral systolic bruit
- Heard over the carotid bifurcation, eyeball, and/or skull on the unaffected side due to increased flow, as the "silent" side is completely occluded

Chest Pain

INTRODUCTION

The goal in addressing chest pain is to quickly and accurately diagnose and treat emergent cases while minimizing unnecessary testing and hospitalization for benign etiologies. Though most often benign (e.g., GERD, musculoskeletal pain), there are 5 primary etiologies of acute, life-threatening chest pain: aortic dissection, MI, esophageal rupture, tension pneumothorax, and pulmonary embolism. Improvement with antacids does not rule out a cardiac etiology, and improvement with nitroglycerin does not definitively diagnose cardiac ischemia. Further, a "normal" ECG does not eliminate the possibility of acute MI (e.g., left circumflex artery occlusion may be electrically silent). Women and elderly may have atypical symptoms.

DIAGNOSTIC WORKUP & INITIAL MANAGEMENT

- Obtain vital signs, including pulse oximetry and blood pressure in both arms
- Establish the patient's resuscitation status to determine appropriate interventions
- Administer supplemental oxygen, and ensure IV access ($\geq$ 18-gauge IV)

History and physical examination

- Note characteristics of the pain (e.g., dull, pressure-like, burning, sharp, tearing), location, radiation, duration, frequency, aggravating factors (e.g., exertion, deep respiration, supine position, palpation), alleviating factors (e.g., immobility, leaning forward), and associated symptoms (e.g., diaphoresis, lightheadedness, nausea, dyspnea)
- Note cardiac history and risk factors, including age (men > 45 years; women > 55 years), history of heart disease, diabetes mellitus, hypertension, hyperlipidemia, tobacco use, obesity, sedentary lifestyle, and family history of premature heart disease; note recent long plane or car rides, trauma, or invasive procedures (e.g., central line, catheterization, upper GI endoscopy, transesophageal echocardiogram, surgery)

Initial diagnostic workup

- 12-lead ECG, cardiac monitoring, and chest radiography are usually indicated
- Laboratory testing may include CBC, chemistries, cardiac enzymes, coagulation studies, liver function tests, amylase, and lipase
- Chest CT with contrast if suspect aortic dissection or PE; if contraindicated (e.g., renal insufficiency, dye allergy), V/Q scan (to assess for PE) or MRI, MRA, or transesophageal echocardiogram (to assess for aortic dissection) may be diagnostic
- Consider abdominal CT or ultrasound if suspect abdominal pathology
- Echocardiography may be indicated to evaluate for left ventricular dysfunction, pericardial effusion, aortic dissection, or right ventricular dysfunction due to PE
- Consider measuring B-type natriuretic peptide (BNP)
  - If low (< 8 pg/ml), congestive heart failure is unlikely
  - Elevated BNP may occur in several conditions (e.g., acute coronary syndrome, chronic renal failure, PE) in addition to congestive heart failure

Initial patient management

- Administer aspirin (160–325 mg) if suspect acute coronary syndrome
- Give sublingual nitroglycerin if systolic blood pressure > 100 mm Hg; avoid if sildenafil was recently used; use with extreme caution in those with right ventricular infarction, severe aortic stenosis, and hypertrophic cardiomyopathy
- Administer metoprolol if suspect acute coronary syndrome or aortic dissection; however, avoid if bradycardic, hypotensive, wheezing from COPD, or in heart failure
- Consider IV heparin or enoxaprin for MI or PE once aortic dissection is ruled out

DIFFERENTIAL DIAGNOSIS

Cardiovascular etiologies
- Myocardial ischemia or MI
- Unstable angina
- Pulmonary embolus
- Pericarditis
- Arrhythmias
- Congestive heart failure
- Mitral valve prolapse
- Aortic stenosis
- Aortic dissection
- Cardiac tamponade

Pulmonary etiologies
- Pneumonia
- COPD
- Asthma
- Tension pneumothorax
- Hemothorax
- Empyema
- Pneumomediastinum
- Lung cancer

Gastrointestinal etiologies
- Esophagitis
- GERD
- Gastritis
- Peptic ulcer disease
- Perforated ulcer
- Esophageal spasm
- Pancreatitis
- Esophageal rupture
- Pneumoperitoneum
- Cholecystitis
- Hepatitis
- Peritonitis

Musculoskeletal etiologies
- Muscle strain or spasm
- Intercostal muscle spasm
- Costochondritis
- Trauma (e.g., rib fracture)

Less common etiologies
- Varicella zoster (shingles)
- Cancer (e.g., lymphoma, liver cancer)
- Panic disorder
- Tietze's syndrome
- Pott's disease (tuberculosis of the spine)
- Xyphodynia

Chorea

INTRODUCTION

Chorea (Greek for "dance") refers to brief, irregular, nonrhythmic, abrupt, jerking movements that are involuntary and often possess a writhing quality. They often flow from one part of the body to the other. Chorea is often accompanied by athetosis, a disorder of slow, writhing, involuntary movements. These movement disorders are thought to result from dysfunction of the basal ganglia. They often interfere with the ability to complete daily activities. A characteristic feature is an inability to maintain voluntary sustained contractions. When chorea is proximal and of large amplitude, it is called ballismus.

DIAGNOSTIC WORKUP & INITIAL MANAGEMENT

History and physical examination

- Complete history and physical exam, including neurologic exam, medication use, illicit drugs, carbon monoxide exposure, and family history of chorea or unexplained psychiatric disorders
- Huntington's disease may present with psychiatric symptoms (e.g., depression) before other manifestations; onset of symptoms typically occurs in the fourth and fifth decades of life
- The appearance of Kayser-Fleischer rings in the cornea on slit-lamp exam is diagnostic for Wilson's disease

Initial diagnostic workup

- Neuroimaging (CT or MRI) to rule out mass lesions and Huntington's disease (cerebral/basal ganglion atrophy)
- Genetic testing for Huntington's disease
- Echocardiography to diagnose carditis
- Throat culture or serology (ASO) for streptococcal infection
- Low level of serum ceruloplasmin and elevated 24-hour urine copper in Wilson's disease
- Thyroid function tests to rule out hyperthyroidism
- ANA to rule out SLE
- In cases of neuroacanthocytosis, acanthocytes appear on the peripheral blood smear with clinical symptoms of chorea, dystonia, and tics
- Clinical diagnosis is sufficient for Sydenham's chorea (associated with rheumatic fever)
- Confirm absence of pregnancy in women

DIFFERENTIAL DIAGNOSIS

Huntington's disease (chronic progressive hereditary chorea)
- Autosomal dominant transmission
- Associated with psychiatric symptoms and progressive dementia
- Caudate atrophy on neuroimaging studies
- Marker on chromosome 4

Sydenham's chorea
- Symptoms follow febrile illness (20%–30% of cases are associated with group A streptococci)
- Seen in cases of rheumatic fever

Chorea gravidarum
- Develops during the first 4–5 months of pregnancy and resolves following delivery

Drug-induced
- Levodopa
- Stimulants
- Anticonvulsants
- Antidepressants
- Neuroleptics
- Oral contraceptives

Wilson's disease
- An autosomal recessive disorder resulting in abnormal copper metabolism
- Associated with hepatic dysfunction, dystonia, and dysarthria

Benign hereditary chorea
- An autosomal dominant disorder with onset before age 5 years
- Symptoms are nonprogressive

Neuroacanthocytosis
- Etiology is unknown
- Characterized by chorea and deformed erythrocytes

Dentatorubropallidoluysian atrophy
- Most common in Japan
- Characterized by chorea, ataxia, epilepsy, and dementia

Other
- SLE or antiphospholipid antibody syndrome
- AIDS
- Hyperthyroidism
- Stroke
- Neoplasm
- Postcardiac surgery
- Familial paroxysmal choreathetosis
- Encephalitis
- Postinfectious
- Hallervorden-Spatz syndrome
- Fahr's disease
- Lesch-Nyhan syndrome
- Ataxia-telangiectasia syndrome
- Abetalipoproteinemia
- Kernicterus

Chronic Pain

INTRODUCTION

Chronic pain is often underestimated by physicians and overestimated by patients and their families. It is defined as pain that persists beyond the recognized time for the body to heal. Although acute pain serves a physiologic purpose, protecting the body from further injury or disease, persistence of the pain can become a disease state in itself. Pain is categorized as diffuse or regional, depending on the symptom distribution. Be aware of the high rate of psychiatric comorbidities that exist with these conditions.

DIAGNOSTIC WORKUP & INITIAL MANAGEMENT

History and physical examination

- History of symptoms should include onset, location, character (burning, sharp, or dull), intensity, duration, radiation, aggravating and alleviating factors, and associated symptoms; assess how the symptoms affect the patient's life
- Take a detailed medical and surgical history, and inquire about any previous evaluations and treatments
- Physical exam should include a comprehensive assessment of each region where the symptoms are described, including all affected joints and soft tissue regions; body regions and joints above and below the area in pain should be thoroughly examined
- Complete mental status exam, including affect, mood, ideation, and insight
- Comprehensive review of systems, including travel, exercise, and social issues

Initial diagnostic workup

- Lab testing is dictated by the distribution of symptoms and associated organ systems
- General screening tests include CBC, BUN and creatinine, electrolytes, glucose, calcium, vitamin D, TSH, and urinalysis
- Consider ESR or CRP to assess for inflammatory conditions
- For muscular complaints, consider CPK to assess for myopathies
- Imaging may be helpful if targeted to specific conditions (e.g., plain-film radiography or CT for bony abnormalities or radiculopathy, MRI for soft tissue mass or neural lesions, bone scan for reflex sympathetic dystrophy)
- Consider EMG for neuropathic symptoms (burning or tingling)

Initial patient management

- NSAIDs and acetaminophen, combined or in alternating doses, are often used, especially for inflammatory disorders; tramadol is often used as a bridge between NSAIDs and narcotics
- Narcotics are usually reserved as adjuvant therapy after conservative measures have failed; patient and physician concern for addiction is a common barrier to use
- Tricyclic antidepressants and anticonvulsants are useful for neuropathic pain
- Low-dose tricyclics and SSRIs may be effective for fibromyalgia
- Spinal delivery of pain medications may be useful for radicular pain and reflex sympathetic dystrophy
- Physical and occupational therapy is often very useful in a variety of conditions, especially reflex sympathetic dystrophy, low back pain, and fibromyalgia
- Alternative therapies may be useful as primary treatment or adjuvant therapy
- Psychiatric evaluation may be indicated for potential primary psychiatric conditions and comorbidities
- Consider referral to a pain specialist

DIFFERENTIAL DIAGNOSIS

Headache
- Migraine headache
- Cluster headache
- Tension headache
- Cervical radiculopathy
- Temporomandibular joint syndrome (TMJ)
- Medication withdrawal headaches
- Rebound headaches

Low back pain
- Myofascial pain
- Lumbar radiculopathy
- Spinal stenosis
- Facet syndrome

Musculoskeletal pain
- Soft-tissue injury
- Repetitive strain syndromes
- Myofascial pain syndrome
- Fibromyalgia
- Chronic fatigue syndrome
- Polymyositis
- Rheumatoid arthritis
- Osteoarthritis
- Polymalagia rheumatica
- Systemic lupus erythematosus (SLE)
- Viral syndrome
- Lyme disease
- Metabolic myopathy
- Myelopathy
- Endocrinopathies (e.g., hypothyroidism, hyperthyroidism, corticosteroid excess)

Neuropathic pain
- Diabetic neuropathy
- Postherpetic neuralgia
- Cervical radiculopathy
- Reflex sympathetic dystrophy (chronic regional pain syndrome)
- Phantom limb
- Postoperative thoracotomy

Paraneoplastic and cancer pain syndromes
- Bony pain secondary to metastasis
- Visceral pain secondary to mass effects
- Postradiation neuritis or mucositis

Pelvic/abdominal pain
- Endometriosis
- Fibroids
- Irritable bowel syndrome
- Interstitial cystitis

Psychiatric
- Depression
- Anxiety
- Somatization
- Physical, sexual, and/or emotional abuse
- Malingering/drug seeking

Constipation

INTRODUCTION

Constipation is the most common digestive complaint in the U.S. (2.5 million physician visits annually). Successful defecation depends on normal colonic motility (peristalsis), rectal function, and coordination of the pelvic floor muscles and anal sphincters. Peristalsis is regulated by neuronal excitation coupled with inhibition of contraction, which is mediated by the enteric nervous system and interstitial cells of Cajal. Rectal function includes adaptation to increasing volumes of distension. The pelvic floor muscles and anal sphincters receive parasympathetic innervation from the sacral nerves. Constipation can be difficult to assess. A common definition is <3 stools/wk; however, patient descriptions often include a myriad of complaints, including straining during defecation, hard stools, and a sensation of incomplete evacuation.

DIAGNOSTIC WORKUP & INITIAL MANAGEMENT

History and physical examination

- Note time of onset of constipation, amount of dietary fluid and fiber intake, and medications
- Note history of back trauma, neurologic problems, malignancy, and normal bowel patterns
- Risk factors include insufficient fluid intake, decreased mobility or inactivity, low calorie intake, diabetes, thyroid disease, neurologic disease, and medications (often polypharmacy), including NSAIDs, opioids, diuretics, antihypertensives, antidepressants, antispasmodics, anticonvulsants, aluminum antacids, and calcium and iron supplements
- Abdominal exam: Note surgical scars, palpate for masses (stool) and hepatosplenomegaly, check for hernias; however, exam results are often normal
- Rectal examination: Determine presence of stool, masses, hemorrhoids, fistulas, abscesses, or fissures; note resting and squeezing sphincter tone; when the patient bears down, relaxation of anal tone and perineal descents should be palpable

Initial diagnostic workup

- Initial laboratory testing may include CBC, electrolytes, BUN and creatinine, glucose, calcium, phosphate, thyroid function tests, and fecal occult blood testing
- Visualization of the colon will evaluate for anatomic lesions
  - Direct visualization by colonoscopy is preferable, especially for patients with hematochezia, heme-positive stools, anemia, weight loss, acute onset of symptoms, change in stool caliber, family history of colon cancer, or advanced age (> 50 years)
  - In patients < 50 years without alarming symptoms, a barium enema or flexible sigmoidoscopy may be considered as an alternative to colonoscopy
- Transit studies using radiopaque markers are useful to assess for delayed colonic transit
  - If the marker settles in the right colon, consider colonic inertia
  - If it settles in the sigmoid colon, consider outlet obstruction or pelvic floor dysfunction
- Defecography may be used to evaluate the pelvic floor muscles and assess for a rectocele (thick barium is introduced into the rectum; patient evacuates the barium under fluoroscopy)
- Anorectal manometry is valuable to assess for rectal sensation and compliance of internal and external anal sphincters, and it can rule out Hirschsprung's disease
- Consider a stool examination for ova and parasites

Initial patient management

- Correct identifiable causes (e.g., medications, metabolic or endocrine disorders)
- Initial management includes patient education and dietary modification to achieve a gradual increase in fiber (target of 25 g/day) and fluid intake
- A daily stool softener may be helpful (e.g., docusate sodium)
- Use laxatives as necessary: Saline laxatives (e.g., milk of magnesia) act as hyperosmolar agents; stimulant laxatives (e.g., bisacodyl, senna) increase intestinal motility
  - Consider hyperosmolar agents (e.g., lactulose, sorbitol, polyethylene glycol) if no response
- Biofeedback and relaxation training are useful for pelvic floor dysfunction

DIFFERENTIAL DIAGNOSIS

Functional constipation

- The Rome III criteria suggests functional constipation if ≥ 2 criteria are present for at least 3 months during the past 6 months:
  - Straining in more than one-fourth of defecations
  - Lumpy or hard stool in more than one-fourth of defecations
  - Sensation of incomplete evacuation in more than one-fourth of defecations
  - Sensation of anorectal obstruction/blockage in more than one-fourth of defecations
  - Manual maneuvers needed to facilitate more than one-fourth of defecations
  - < 3 defecations per week
  - Absence of loose stool and insufficient criteria for irritable bowel syndrome

Medications

- Narcotic analgesics
- Antihypertensives (e.g., calcium channel blockers)
- Tricyclic antidepressants
- Aluminum hydroxide or calcium antacids
- Iron supplements
- Anticholinergics
- Bismuth
- Cough suppressants
- Opioid analgesics
- Phenobarbital

Neurological dysfunction

- Diabetes mellitus
- Multiple sclerosis
- Myelomeningocele
- Hypotonia (e.g., Down's syndrome, myopathies, prune-belly syndrome)
- Cerebral palsy
- Hirschsprung's disease

Mechanical difficulties

- Colorectal cancer
- Hernia
- Diverticulitis
- Inflammatory bowel syndrome
- Adhesion
- Stricture
- Torsion
- Volvulus

Metabolic and endocrine disorders

- Hypothyroidism
- Hypercalcemia
- Hypokalemia
- Hyperparathyroidism
- Pregnancy
- Reduced steroid hormones during luteal and follicular phases of menstrual cycle

Other

- Chronic laxative abuse
- Inadequate dietary fiber or liquid intake
- Irritable bowel syndrome
- Celiac disease
- Cystic fibrosis
- Lead toxicity
- Structural abnormality (e.g., perianal fissure, anal stenosis, sacral teratoma, colonic stricture)

Cough, Nonproductive

INTRODUCTION

The initial history of cough should include an assessment for sputum production. Additional important clues to the etiology include history and physical examination findings, with particular attention to the characteristics of the cough, circumstances surrounding coughing episodes, and social details (e.g., history of smoking, farm work, allergen exposure). A persistent, nonproductive cough caused by ACE inhibitor use must not be overlooked, because it is both concerning and annoying to the patient and can be easily solved by adjusting the medication regimen.

DIAGNOSTIC WORKUP & INITIAL MANAGEMENT

History and physical examination
- Assess onset, duration, associated symptoms, medical history, family history, medications, and social history
- Note acute (<3 weeks) onset versus chronic (>8 weeks) or recurrent

Initial diagnostic workup
- Initial tests may include pulse oximetry, CBC, ESR, peak flow measurements, PPD, and eosinophil count
- Chest radiography and/or CT may be indicated if the patient has symptoms of concern (e.g., weight loss, hemoptysis, fever)
- Consider blood and sputum cultures if suspect infection
- If imaging is normal and empiric treatment for GERD does not resolve symptoms, consider upper GI tract endoscopy or esophageal pH monitoring
- Consider CT of the sinuses or nasolaryngoscopy to evaluate for sinusitis
- Consider bronchoscopy to identify subtle pulmonary causes
- Consider cardiac workup if pulmonary and GI evaluations are negative and a cardiac disorder is possible

Initial patient management
- Emergency management, including possible intubation, may be necessary if signs or symptoms of respiratory distress are present
- Discontinue smoking, causative medications (e.g., ACE inhibitors), and occupational exposures
- Treat the underlying cause rather than the cough itself; nonspecific agents (antitussives, expectorants, mucolytics) do not take the place of specific therapies
- An empiric therapeutic trial for asthma, GERD, postnasal drip, sinusitis, or bronchitis may be advisable
  - Postnasal drip: Antihistamines (e.g., diphenhydramine) plus decongestants (e.g., pseudoephedrine); add nasal steroid if no improvement within 1 week; add antibiotics if sinusitis is present
  - Cough-variant asthma: Remove allergens; treat with inhaled bronchodilators, inhaled steroids, leukotriene antagonists, and mast cell stabilizers as needed
  - GERD: Proton pump inhibitor for 1–2 months; antireflux measures
  - Chronic bronchitis or bronchiectasis: Smoking cessation, inhaled ipratropium and β-agonist, antibiotics, chest physiotherapy, postural drainage, expectorants
  - Postviral: Antihistamine plus decongestant; add β-agonist and inhaled or systemic steroids as needed
- Over-the-counter therapies are of little value

DIFFERENTIAL DIAGNOSIS

Smoker's cough
- The most common overall cause of cough

Postnasal drip
- The most common cause of chronic cough in nonsmokers
- Associated with chronic sinusitis, allergic rhinitis, and other upper airway disorders

GERD
- The second most common cause of chronic cough in nonsmokers

Asthma/reactive airway disease
- Classically presents with a triad of chronic cough, dyspnea, and wheezing; however, cough may be the only symptom

ACE inhibitor use
- Approximately 20% of patients on ACE inhibitors develop a dry cough
- May also result in rhinitis and upper respiratory tract symptoms
- Resolution may take days to weeks after withdrawal of the drug

Acute bronchitis
- Most commonly caused by viruses (e.g., influenza, adenovirus, rhinovirus, respiratory syncytial virus)
- Postviral bronchitis may last beyond 6 weeks

Pneumonia
- "Typical" pneumonia (e.g., *Streptococcus pneumoniae*, *Haemophilus influenzae*) is characterized by acute or subacute onset of fever, dyspnea, fatigue, pleuritic chest pain, and cough
- "Atypical" pneumonia (e.g., *Mycoplasma*, *Legionella*, *Chlamydia pneumoniae*, influenza and parainfluenza viruses) is characterized by more gradual onset, dry cough, headache, fatigue, and minimal lung signs

Aspirated foreign body
- Abrupt onset of unilateral wheezing or stridor, cough, and decreased breath sounds
- Leading cause of home accidental death in children younger than 6 years

Bronchiolitis obliterans organizing pneumonia
- Most commonly occurs following a viral infection or exposure

Other
- Lung cancer
- COPD (emphysematous variant)
- Sarcoidosis
- Congestive heart failure
- Aspiration
- Bronchiectasis (cough is usually productive but may be dry)
- Filarial disease

Cough, Productive

INTRODUCTION

Cough is the most common symptom for which patients visit primary care physicians. It is an important defense mechanism that protects the airway from aspiration of excessive secretions and foreign material. Cough is generally reflexive but can be initiated (and sometimes suppressed) voluntarily. Cough can be a symptom of a variety of underlying conditions. It is categorized as acute (lasting < 3 weeks) or chronic (lasting >8 weeks). Acute cough is most frequently a result of the common cold. Chronic cough is often simultaneously the result of more than one condition; the most common causes are postnasal drip syndrome, asthma, and GERD.

DIAGNOSTIC WORKUP & INITIAL MANAGEMENT

History and physical examination

- Assess the time course (i.e., acute vs. chronic) and quality (productive vs. dry; barking, honking, or brassy) of the cough
- Note general appearance (cyanosis or pallor)
- Note signs of respiratory distress (tachypnea or accessory muscle use)
- Pay attention to inciting factors (e.g., history of smoking, farm work, allergen exposure)

Initial diagnostic workup

- Culture and Gram's stain of the sputum are warranted in all but the most obvious cases of productive cough (e.g., upper respiratory infection)
  - Eosinophils suggest asthma or hypersensitivity reaction
  - Polymorphonuclear cells suggest acute infection
  - Routine or special cultures may be indicated based on likely pathogens
- Chest radiography may be indicated if symptoms are of concern
  - Infiltrates suggest pneumonia, pneumonitis, or tuberculosis
  - Bronchiectasis suggests cystic fibrosis, immunodeficiency, ciliary dyskinesia, chronic aspiration, or history of childhood pneumonia
  - Volume loss may indicate aspiration of a foreign body
  - Hyperinflation suggests asthma or COPD
  - Mediastinal lymphadenopathy suggests tuberculosis, fungal infection, or malignancy
- Further testing may include pulse oximetry, peak flow measurements, CBC, ESR, blood cultures, PPD, and acid-fast bacilli stain
- Consider pulmonary function tests with or without methacholine challenge
- Chest CT and/or sputum cytology may be indicated if the patient has symptoms of concern (e.g., weight loss, hemoptysis, fever)
- Consider CT of sinuses or nasolaryngoscopy to evaluate for sinusitis
- Consider bronchoscopy with possible bronchoalveolar lavage and/or biopsy to identify subtle pulmonary etiologies

Initial patient management

- Emergency management, including possible intubation, may be necessary if signs or symptoms of respiratory distress are present
- The key to success is ruling out serious causes and identifying the etiology
- Treat the underlying cause of cough rather than the cough itself
- Consider empiric treatment for postnasal drip (antihistamine, decongestant, nasal steroids)
- Smoking cessation counseling should be offered to all smokers
- Over-the-counter therapies are of little value; cough suppression medication should generally be avoided but may assist with sleep

DIFFERENTIAL DIAGNOSIS

Acute bronchitis

- Most commonly caused by viruses (e.g., influenza, adenovirus, rhinovirus, respiratory syncytial virus)
- Bacteria are much less common (e.g., *Streptococcus pneumoniae*, *Mycoplasma*, *Haemophilus influenzae*)

Pneumonia

- May be community acquired, hospital acquired, or aspiration
- "Typical" pneumonia (e.g., *S. pneumoniae*, *H. influenzae*) has acute or subacute onset of fever, dyspnea, fatigue, pleuritic chest pain, and productive cough
- "Atypical" pneumonia (e.g., *Mycoplasma*, *Legionella*, *Chlamydia*, *Pneumocystis carinii*, influenza and parainfluenza viruses) has more gradual onset, dry cough, headache, fatigue

Smoker's cough

- May be productive or nonproductive

Postnasal drip

- The most common cause of chronic cough in nonsmokers
- Associated with chronic sinusitis, allergic rhinitis, and other upper airway disorders

Congestive heart failure

- Associated with "frothy" sputum

Other

- Lung cancer
- Asthma with secondary infection
- COPD (chronic bronchitis component)
- Tuberculosis

Cyanosis

INTRODUCTION

Cyanosis is a bluish discoloration of the skin or mucous membranes that is caused by significantly decreased oxygenation of the blood. It may be generalized or confined to the periphery.

DIAGNOSTIC WORKUP & INITIAL MANAGEMENT

- Supplemental oxygen is generally indicated in patients with central cyanosis
  - Cyanosis and hypoxemia resulting from (most) lung diseases and carbon monoxide poisoning will quickly improve with oxygen administration
- Respiratory support with intubation and mechanical ventilation may be necessary
- Treat shock as necessary with IV fluids, vasopressors, and correction of underlying cause

History and physical examination

- Clubbing of the fingers or toes may indicate congenital heart disease or chronic pulmonary disease
- Blood pressure, capillary refill, and heart and lung exams are always indicated
- Pulses and neurologic function in all involved extremities must be evaluated in cases of peripheral cyanosis

Initial workup and management

- Initial laboratory testing includes pulse oximetry, arterial blood gas (to assess oxygenation and presence of methemoglobin or carboxyhemoglobin), CBC, electrolytes, BUN/creatinine, glucose, and ECG
- Chest radiography and/or CT to evaluate for lung pathology and heart size
- Echocardiography may be indicated to assess ventricular function and valves and to rule out structural abnormalities
- Consider pulmonary function tests
- Cardiac enzymes may be indicated to rule out MI
- Hemoglobin electrophoresis may be indicated to evaluate hemoglobin structure
- Pulmonary angiogram may be indicated to rule out arteriovenous fistula or massive pulmonary embolism
- For peripheral cyanosis isolated to one limb, arterial Doppler ultrasound studies or angiography may be indicated to rule out embolus

DIFFERENTIAL DIAGNOSIS

Central cyanosis (cyanosis of lips and mucous membranes)
Pulmonary disease
- Severe pneumonia
- Pulmonary edema
- Pulmonary arteriovenous fistula
- Tension pneumothorax
- Severe COPD or asthma
- Acute respiratory distress syndrome
- Lung cancer
- Obstruction (e.g., tracheal foreign body or stenosis)
- Exposure to high altitude
- Decreased respiration with oversedation
- Obstructive sleep apnea/obesity-hypoventilation syndrome

Congenital heart disease with shunting
- Tetralogy of Fallot
- Transposition of the great vessels (the most common cause of cyanotic heart disease in the immediate newborn period)
- Tricuspid atresia
- Truncus arteriosus

Cardiovascular disease
- Cardiogenic shock (e.g., massive MI)
- Severe valvular heart disease
- Cor pulmonale
- Massive pulmonary embolus

Abnormal hemoglobin
- Methemoglobinemia: Usually caused by drugs or chemicals (e.g., sulfa, dapsone, primaquine, naphthalene mothballs) or by genetic defects
- Hemoglobin Kansas
- Sickle cell disease

Toxins/poisons
- Carbon monoxide
- Nitroprusside
- Cyanide

Peripheral cyanosis (cyanosis of phalanges, earlobes, and nose)
Increased resistance to blood flow
- Raynaud's phenomenon
- Acrocyanosis
- Superior vena cava obstruction
- Venous hypertension
- Arterial embolism
- Exposure to cold air or water

Decreased cardiac output
- Shock
- Congestive heart failure
- Mitral stenosis

Increased blood viscosity
- Polycythemia vera

Decreased Breath Sounds

INTRODUCTION

Decreased breath sounds represent either decreased flow of air through the airway or decreased transmission of sound across the chest wall. Lung pathology is a common etiology; however, physical causes (e.g., obesity) can be less obvious. A careful history and thorough physical exam can differentiate potentially life-threatening processes that require emergent intervention from chronic and/or benign processes. Determining whether the decrease in breath sounds is an acute or chronic process and identifying accompanying symptoms and signs will narrow the differential diagnosis significantly.

DIAGNOSTIC WORKUP & INITIAL MANAGEMENT

History and physical examination

- History should include associated symptoms (e.g., fever, dyspnea, wheezing, chest pain) and a detailed medical, surgical, and exposure history
- Physical exam should include vital signs; examine the oral cavity and neck for evidence of a mass, foreign body, or tracheal deviation; inspect and palpate the chest wall to assess for symmetric movement; percuss and auscultate all chest fields for related abnormalities (e.g., rhonchi, wheezes, rales, rubs, egophony)

Initial diagnostic workup

- Initial laboratory testing may include CBC, pulse oximetry, arterial blood gas, and TSH
- Chest radiography is the initial imaging test
- Associate the area of decreased breath sounds to hyperlucency or increased opacity on chest radiograph
  - Tracheal shift to a side with a density and decreased breath sounds likely signifies atelectasis or endobronchial obstruction
  - Tracheal shift away from a side with hyperlucency and decreased breath sounds may indicate tension pneumothorax
- Lateral neck radiography may be indicated to rule out epiglottitis ("thumb sign")
- With evidence of external airway compression, chest and neck CT may be necessary for further evaluation
- Pulmonary function testing may be indicated

Initial patient management

- Closely monitor airway, breathing, and circulation
- Administer supplemental oxygen as needed
- Treat the underlying etiology (e.g., removal of a foreign body, bronchodilators, steroids)
- Emergent interventions may be necessary for patients in extremis (e.g., chest tube insertion)

DIFFERENTIAL DIAGNOSIS

Decreased airflow through respiratory tree

- Airway obstruction
  - Aspirated foreign body
  - Asthma
  - Bronchitis
  - Bronchiolitis
  - Croup
  - Epiglottitis
  - Neoplasm
  - Goiter
- Alveolar or interstitial processes
  - Pulmonary edema
  - Pneumonia
  - Pleurisy
- Decreased lung expansion
  - Atelectasis
  - COPD or emphysema
  - Bronchiectasis
  - Kyphosis or scoliosis
  - Increased abdominal girth (e.g., ascites, obesity, pregnancy)
- Pulmonary fibrosis
- Diaphragmatic paralysis
- Abdominal, chest wall, or pleuritic pain that prevents sufficient breathing

Obstructed transmission of sound

- Obesity
- Pleural effusion
- Pneumothorax, hemothorax, or chylothorax
- Pleural thickening
- Large pulmonary embolus

Less common etiologies

- Cystic fibrosis
- Alveolar hemorrhage
- Bronchiolitis obliterans organizing pneumonia (BOOP)
- Pneumonectomy (postsurgical)
- Systemic lupus erythematosus (SLE)
- Vocal cord paralysis
- Vocal cord dyskinesia
- Poor inspiratory efforts
- Psychogenic

Delirium

INTRODUCTION

Delirium is an acute confusional state caused by a disturbance in global cortical function, further defined as the inability to maintain a coherent stream of thought or action. Features include disturbance of consciousness, change in cognition, fluctuations of symptoms, and evidence that it results from an underlying medical condition. Arousal is maintained by the reticular activating system and the cerebral cortex; unconsciousness occurs when both cerebral hemispheres are depressed or the reticular activating system is dysfunctional. Acetylcholine is the most important neurotransmitter involved in consciousness, and conditions that decrease its synthesis may cause delirium. Of note, multiple etiologies may present simultaneously, and delirium is present in up to 30% of older hospitalized patients.

DIAGNOSTIC WORKUP & INITIAL MANAGEMENT

History and physical examination

- Begin with vital signs, including blood sugar level and oxygen saturation
- History should include evaluation of memory difficulties, disorientation, incoherent speech, and level of attention and a discussion with patients' family or caregivers
- Review the medication list and administration records thoroughly
- Physical exam should include state of hydration, infectious foci, and neurologic exam, with complete investigation into possible medical etiologies
- Pupils may suggest the diagnosis: pinpoint pupils (opiate use, pontine hemorrhage, or clonidine overdose); dilated pupils (sympathomimetic use); dilated, fixed pupils without extraocular movement (cerebral herniation); preserved pupillary reflex (metabolic cause); "doll's eyes" (eyes remain fixed when the head moves, indicating brainstem lesion)
- Note attentional tasks (spell "WORLD" or days of the week backward)
- Funduscopic exam is always indicated to evaluate for papilledema

Initial diagnostic workup

- Initial testing includes CBC, chemistries, BUN/creatinine, calcium, magnesium, phosphorus, coagulation studies, thyroid tests, and vitamin B_{12} and folate
- Depending on the patient's medical history, consider liver function tests, urinalysis and urine culture, urine toxicology screen, alcohol level, blood cultures, chest radiography, and ECG
- Pulse oximetry and/or arterial blood gas to screen for hypoxia and/or hypercarbia
- Consider drug or medication withdrawal (e.g., alcohol, benzodiazepines)
- If no obvious etiology is discovered, noncontrast head CT is indicated (sensitivity for subarachnoid hemorrhage is 98% if done within 12 hours of symptom onset)
  - Consider CT with contrast in patients with AIDS or underlying malignancy
- Lumbar puncture should be performed if suspect meningitis
  - Rule out increased intracranial pressure (via CT) before lumbar puncture
  - Risk of meningitis is less than 5% if no fever, headache, or neck stiffness
- EEG may reveal slowing of α rhythms and unusual slow-wave activity in delirium

Initial patient management

- Maintain airway, breathing (have a low threshold for intubation in obtunded patients), and circulation (IV fluids); delirium is often reversible if the underlying cause is corrected
- Restraints may be necessary for patients who pose a risk to themselves or hospital staff (medications for chemical sedation include benzodiazepines and antipsychotics; elderly patients are sensitive to anxiolytics and may exhibit paradoxic agitation)
- Administer naloxone (to reverse opiate overdose), thiamine, and glucose (administer thiamine before glucose to prevent Wernicke's encephalopathy)
- Administer activated charcoal via nasogastric tube if suspect a drug overdose
- Administer empiric antibiotics if suspect infection (e.g., meningitis); do not delay administration of antibiotics while awaiting results of lumbar puncture

DIFFERENTIAL DIAGNOSIS

Other causes of altered mental status
- Dementia (in contrast to delirium, arousal and alertness are preserved)
- Obtundation
- Confusion

Medical etiologies
- Underlying brain disorder (e.g., stroke) is the most common risk factor
- Infections (e.g., urinary tract infection, pneumonia, encephalitis, meningitis)
- Drug toxicity, including alcohol
- Drug withdrawal (especially benzodiazepines)
- Fluid, electrolyte, and metabolic disorders (e.g., hyponatremia, hypoglycemia, hypercalcemia, uremia, hypercarbia)
- Nutritional deficiency (e.g., thiamine deficiency)
- Congestive heart failure
- Postsurgery
- Hypoxia (multiple causes, including congestive heart failure)
- Cerebral ischemia (multiple causes)
- Hypo- or hyperthermia
- Head trauma (e.g., subarachnoid hemorrhage)
- Complex partial seizure disorder is associated with an alteration of awareness
- Medications are a frequent cause of altered mental status, particularly in hospitalized patients
  - Sedatives
  - Steroids
  - Antidepressants
  - Narcotics
  - Anticonvulsants
  - Antiarrhythmics
  - Anticholinergics
  - Antihistamines
  - Antiemetics
  - NSAIDs

Psychiatric etiologies
- Depression
- Psychotic illness
- "Sundowning" (behavioral deterioration occurs during evening hours; typically occurs in demented, institutionalized patients)

Delusions

INTRODUCTION

Delusions are firmly held, stable, but false beliefs that are not consistent with educational or cultural background and are not given up even in the face of contrary evidence. They are an essential feature of psychosis. Delusions take many forms, such as persecutory or grandiose ideas, thoughts of being controlled or of a partner's infidelity, ideas of reference (believing neutral external events have specific personal meaning), or religious beliefs. Distinguish delusions (fixed false beliefs) from hallucinations (alterations in sensorium).

DIAGNOSTIC WORKUP & INITIAL MANAGEMENT

History and physical examination

- Differentiate between psychotic syndromes and distinguish functional vs. organic disease
  - Acute medical illness may exacerbate psychosis; thus, rule out medical illness even in patients with a history of psychiatric disease
- Mental status examination is required, including suicidal ideation/plan
- Medical family, and social history may shed light on the diagnosis
- Consider interviewing family and/or friends
  - Obtain background information on the patient's previous level of functioning, if possible
- Drug and alcohol history and appropriate workup, if present
- Dementia assessment, including mini-mental status examination and appropriate workup, if present

Initial diagnostic workup

- Suspicion of medical illness based on vital signs, physical exam, or history should be evaluated thoroughly
- Obtain lab work as necessary, possibly including head CT, alcohol level, drug screen, electrolytes, CBC, thyroid function tests, liver function tests, BUN and creatinine, and tests of endocrine function

Initial patient management

- Treat underlying medical disorders, if present
- Antipsychotic medications may be used, depending on the degree of agitation and symptomatology: IV or intramuscular haloperidol, intramuscular risperidone, or droperidol
  - Antipsychotic medications are effective more for behavioral control, associated symptoms (e.g., hallucinations), and distress rather than complete elimination of delusions
  - Newer antipsychotics (e.g., risperidone, olanzapine, quetiapine) cause fewer dystonic side effects; however, may cause weight gain and diabetes
  - Side effects include arrhythmias (especially droperidol), dystonic reactions, akathisia, seizures, or neuroleptic malignant syndrome
  - If an acute dystonic reaction occurs secondary to antipsychotic use, stop the drug and administer IV or IM benztropine or diphenhydramine
- Benzodiazepines (e.g., midazolam) are effective sedatives, especially in the acutely intoxicated (e.g., alcohol, cocaine) or withdrawing patient
- Physical restraints are often required to manage violent patients
- Psychotherapy may provide structure and support but usually does not eliminate delusions
- Environmental support and safety management is necessary in impaired patients, severe chronic schizophrenia, and dementia

DIFFERENTIAL DIAGNOSIS

Schizophrenia
- Delusions are the key symptom
- Complex, disorganized, persecutory thoughts; ideas of reference; thoughts of being controlled
- Hallucinations (usually auditory)
- Catatonic or disorganized behavior
- Disorganized speech
- Minimum duration of 6 months
- Social and/or occupational dysfunction

Mania or bipolar disorder
- Delusions are usually grandiose
- Associated with frantic, ill-considered activity (e.g., hypersexuality, gambling, overspending), irritability, reduced sleep, and reduced appetite

Psychotic depression
- Delusions of guilt, worthlessness in context of depressed mood, loss of interest/pleasure (anhedonia), suicidal ideas/plans, and sleep/appetite disturbance

Other psychotic disorders
- Schizoaffective disorder
- Delusional disorder (patients have well-formed, specific, fixed delusions, such as of being loved, persecuted, or having a specific somatic abnormality, but these do not interfere with other areas of functioning)
- Schizophreniform disorder
- Brief psychotic disorder
- Postpartum psychosis

Delirium
- Temporary disorganized thought, fluctuating awareness, misperceptions, paranoid fears

Dementia
- Delusions often seen in context of global cognitive decline
- Delusions most commonly occur in cases of paranoid-type Alzheimer's disease

Medical conditions
- Endocrine disorders (e.g., thyroid or adrenal abnormalities)
- Liver or renal failure
- Neurologic (e.g., meningitis, hemorrhage, seizure, stroke, tumors)
- Hypoglycemia or electrolyte abnormalities
- Hypertensive emergency
- Trauma (e.g., intracerebral bleed, closed head injury)
- Hypoxia
- Infection (e.g., HIV infection, sepsis, UTI, pneumonia, meningitis, Lyme disease)
- Drugs (steroid use, therapeutics, drugs of abuse, withdrawal states)
- Deficiency states (e.g., vitamin B_{12}, thiamine, folate)

Other
- Chronic psychostimulant and alcohol abuse
- Illicit drugs (e.g., LSD, mescaline, phencyclidine, mushrooms, amphetamines)
- Hyperparathyroidism

Dementia

INTRODUCTION

Dementia is a syndrome in which focal brain regions undergo premature neuronal death, resulting in loss of function in multiple cognitive and emotional abilities. It affects 1% of the population by age 60. The prevalence then doubles every 5 years to affect 30%–50% by age 85. More than 50 illnesses may cause dementia; Alzheimer's disease is the most common cause (50%–60%), followed by vascular (multi-infarct) dementia (20%). Potentially treatable diagnoses (e.g., depression, chronic alcohol abuse) account for 5%–10%. Common findings include aphasia (language disorder of speech, comprehension, naming, reading, and writing), apraxia (inability to perform previously learned tasks, such as combing hair or "saluting the flag"), and agnosia (impaired recognition or comprehension of auditory, visual, and tactile stimuli).

DIAGNOSTIC WORKUP & INITIAL MANAGEMENT

History and physical examination
- Assess medical and neurologic history, family history, and risk factors
- Rule out underlying medical, neurologic, or psychiatric illnesses that may mimic symptoms of dementia; distinguish dementia from delirium (an acute, metabolically induced state of fluctuating consciousness) and depression
- Elicit medication history to identify drugs that may contribute to cognitive changes (e.g., analgesics, sedatives, anticholinergics, antihypertensives)
- Perform a mini-mental status examination
- Diagnostic criteria require memory impairment and abnormalities in at least one of the following areas: language, judgment, abstract thinking, praxis, executive function, and visual recognition

Initial diagnostic workup
- Laboratory testing may include CBC, electrolytes, renal and liver function tests, glucose, thyroid function tests, vitamin B_{12} and folate, screening for inflammatory and infectious causes, and toxicology screen; consider screening for syphilis, HIV, and Wilson's disease
- Head CT without contrast to rule out structural lesions (e.g., infarct, small vessel disease, malignancy, hydrocephalus, extracerebral fluid collection)
- EEG is not routinely used but may identify toxic and metabolic disorders or Creutzfeldt-Jakob disease
- Genetic testing may be indicated if family history suggests Alzheimer's disease (especially early-onset disease)
- CSF analysis may be indicated
- HIV and syphilis (RPR) testing in patients with known risk factors

Initial patient management
- Most cases of dementia have no cure; treatment is palliative
- Treat reversible causes (e.g., hypothyroidism, vitamin deficiency, cerebral vasculitis, depression, neurosyphilis, HIV infection) as necessary, and modify risk factors for stroke
- Eliminate unnecessary medications, especially with known CNS and anticholinergic effects
- Anticholinesterase inhibitors (e.g., donepezil, galantamine, rivastigmine) may initially slow the progression of Alzheimer's disease; NMDA-receptor antagonists (e.g., memantine) are now being used as well
- In select cases, antidepressants (avoid tricyclic antidepressants) and neuroleptics (e.g., seroquel, risperdal) may be tried
- Social support (e.g., structured environments; social services to assess safety of the home environment, nutrition, medication, and placement issues); counseling for caregivers may help
- Optimize blood pressure and control diabetes
- Involve neurology or neuropsychiatry early in the course of disease

DIFFERENTIAL DIAGNOSIS

Cortical etiologies
- Alzheimer's disease
- Amyotrophic lateral sclerosis dementia complex
- Pick's disease

Subcortical etiologies
- Parkinson's disease
- Multisystem atrophy
- Progressive supranuclear palsy
- Huntington's disease

Mixed etiologies
- Multi-infarct dementia
- Corticobasal degeneration
- Lewy body dementia
- Chronic alcohol abuse
- Prion diseases
- Chronic subdural hematoma
- Chronic hydrocephalus
- Paraneoplastic encephalitis
- Wilson's disease
- Dialysis dementia
- Postanoxic dementia

CNS infections
- HIV encephalitis
- Meningitis
- Herpes encephalitis
- Creutzfeldt-Jakob disease
- Cerebral abscess
- Neurosyphilis

Other
- Normal cognitive aging
- Delirium
- Depression (pseudodementia)
- Vitamin deficiency (e.g., vitamin B_{12}, thiamine)
- Medication effects
- Wernicke's encephalopathy (occurs with ataxia and ophthalmoplegia in alcoholism)
- Head trauma
- Hypothyroidism
- Cerebral vasculitis
- SLE (lupus cerebritis)
- Chronic hypoglycemia or hypocalcemia
- Uremic encephalopathy
- Multiple sclerosis
- Hydrocephalus

Diarrhea, Acute

INTRODUCTION

Acute diarrhea (<14 days) is an increased volume of bowel movements or > 3 stools (> 200 g) per day. Stool is typically nonformed or liquid, reflecting increased water content in the stool, secondary to decreased water absorption or increased water secretion. Thus, diarrhea results in water loss and dehydration. Five primary mechanisms result in acute diarrhea: an osmotic agent (laxatives, lactose) causing increased water retention in the intestinal lumen; increased intestinal mucosal secretion (cholera, enterotoxigenic *E. coli*); inflamed intestinal mucosa allowing seepage of blood, mucus, or protein into the bowel [inflammatory bowel disease (IBD), GI lymphoma, Whipple's disease]; abnormal motility [irritable bowel syndrome (IBS), "diabetic diarrhea," scleroderma]; or systemic disease (thyrotoxicosis, carcinoid syndrome].

DIAGNOSTIC WORKUP & INITIAL MANAGEMENT

History and physical examination

- Note recent ingestions, including oysters (*Vibrio*) and ground beef (enterohemorrhagic *E. coli*); new medications (e.g., antibiotics, antacids, antihypertensives); immune status; HIV risk factors; recent travel, including woodland exposure (*Giardia*); and sick contacts
- Pathologic area can usually be localized by symptomatology: small volume stools, increased fecal urgency or frequency, and tenesmus suggest rectosigmoid pathology; large volume stools (1 L/day) without tenesmus suggest small bowel pathology
- Osmotic diarrhea resolves with fasting; secretory diarrhea does not
- Invasive bacterial diarrhea usually causes bloody diarrhea 12–24 hours after ingestion, fever, abdominal pain, and tenesmus; *E. coli* causes watery diarrhea by 6 hours after ingestion
- Exam should include vital signs (with orthostatics), full abdominal exam, back exam, genital and rectal exams, skin exam (e.g., jaundice, turgor), and assessment for signs of dehydration (e.g., loss of jugular pulsations, dry mucous membranes, skin tenting, orthostasis)

Initial diagnostic workup

- Acute diarrhea is usually self-limited and in-depth microbial evaluation unnecessary
- Further evaluation if concerning signs are present (e.g., dehydration, bloody diarrhea, fever, severe pain) and if high-risk (e.g., elderly, immunocompromised, history of IBD)
- In general, stool cultures should be used sparingly based on clinical discretion, because the diagnostic yield of stool cultures is low and regular testing can be costly
- Tailor specific testing to clinical suspicion
  - Stool culture and Shiga toxin in cases of systemic illness
  - Fecal leukocytes (or fecal lactoferrin) if suspect inflammatory diarrhea
  - *C. difficile* toxin in hospitalized patients or recent antibiotic exposure; must be sent from 3 separate stools if ELISA antigen assay is used to achieve sensitivity > 90% (one sample is adequate with cytotoxicity assay); testing for other pathogens is usually of low yield except in elderly, HIV-positive, or neutropenic patients and in outbreaks
  - *Giardia* and Cryptospora testing in hikers and patients who drink well water
  - Microspora, *Isospora, Cryptospora,* and *M. avium* testing in HIV-positive patients
  - In cases of persistent diarrhea after exclusion of common infectious pathogens, consider IBD and refer for a flexible sigmoidoscopy or colonoscopy
- Initial laboratory studies may include CBC, electrolytes, BUN, creatinine, glucose, urinalysis, liver function tests, and hepatitis serologies; consider also HIV testing

Initial patient management

- Treatment is generally supportive, including fluid resuscitation and increased salt intake
- Antimotility agents (e.g., loperamide) may shorten the overall course of disease
- Antibiotics are indicated in some situations (*Shigella, Campylobacter,* "traveler's diarrhea," *C. difficile*) and in patients at risk for bacteremia-related complications
- Admit to hospital if severe dehydration, fever, or systemic disease (bloody purulent stool)

DIFFERENTIAL DIAGNOSIS

Infectious etiologies

Viral
- Acute (viral) gastroenteritis
- Rotavirus
- Norwalk virus
- Enterovirus

Bacterial
- Invasive: *Campylobacter, Salmonella, Shigella, Yersinia enterocolitica*
- Enterotoxigenic: *E. coli, Staphylococcus, Bacillus cereus*
- "Traveler's diarrhea" (*Shigella, Salmonella*, enterotoxigenic *E. coli, Campylobacter*)
- *Clostridium difficile* (pseudomembranous enterocolitis)
- *E. coli* O157:H7 (commonly associated with raw meat)

Protozoa
- *Giardia lamblia*

Opportunistic
- *Cryptospora*
- Microspora
- *Isospora belli*
- *M. avium*
- Cytomegalovirus

Noninfectious

- Lactose intolerance
- Irritable bowel syndrome (IBS)
- Inflammatory bowel syndrome (Crohn disease, ulcerative colitis)
- Toxins (e.g., shellfish, heavy metals, common medications)
- Fecal impaction
- Tube feeding
- Ischemic colitis
- Medications (e.g., laxatives, antibiotics, anticholinergics, chemotherapy, metformin)
- Malabsorption syndromes
- Vasculitis
- Neoplasia
- Appendicitis
- Adrenal insufficiency
- Hyperthyroidism
- HIV

Diarrhea, Chronic

INTRODUCTION

Chronic diarrhea is defined as decreased fecal consistency persisting for > 4 weeks. Stool is typically nonformed or liquid, reflecting increased water content in the stool, secondary to decreased water absorption or increased water secretion. Thus, diarrhea results in water loss and dehydration. Five primary mechanisms result in diarrhea: an osmotic agent (laxatives, lactose) causing increased water retention in the intestinal lumen; increased intestinal mucosal secretion (cholera, enterotoxigenic *E. coli*); inflamed intestinal mucosa allowing seepage of blood, mucus, or protein into the bowel [inflammatory bowel disease (IBD), GI lymphoma, Whipple's disease]; abnormal motility [irritable bowel syndrome (IBS), "diabetic diarrhea," scleroderma); or systemic disease (thyrotoxicosis, carcinoid syndrome].

DIAGNOSTIC WORKUP & INITIAL MANAGEMENT

History and physical examination

- History should include onset, duration, timing, volume, and appearance of bowel movements (e.g., bloody, mucusy, greasy, color, consistency), recent travel history, recent changes in medications or food intake, weight loss, whether the diarrhea persists during fasting, associated symptoms (e.g., abdominal pain, fever, vomiting, rashes, bloating, flatulence), and personal or family history of IBD
- Physical exam should include vital signs, including orthostatics, full abdominal exam, back exam, genital and rectal exams, skin exam (e.g., jaundice, turgor), and assessment for signs of dehydration (e.g., loss of jugular pulsations, dry mucous membranes, skin tenting, orthostasis)

Initial diagnostic workup

- Initial laboratory testing may include CBC, electrolytes, liver function tests, BUN and creatinine, calcium, glucose, urinalysis, TSH, CRP, ESR, stool for occult blood
- Stool examination is warranted in most cases:
  - Blood suggests an inflammatory process
  - White blood cells suggest an inflammatory or infectious process
  - 72-hour stool collection for fecal fat with Sudan stain will diagnose malabsorption or oil-containing laxatives
  - Stool electrolytes should be measured to calculate stool osmolality and osmotic gap to differentiate secretory from osmotic diarrhea
  - Stool culture (including culture for parasites) if suspect infectious etiology
  - Stool pH
- Measure *C. difficile* toxin in most cases, particularly patients in hospital or with recent antibiotic exposure; must be sent from 3 separate stools (if ELISA antigen assay is used) to achieve sensitivity $> 90\%$; 1 sample is adequate for cytotoxicity assay
- Endoscopy (flexible sigmoidoscopy or colonoscopy with biopsy) to diagnose colonic disease; esophagogastroduodenoscopy for small bowel biopsy
- Breath hydrogen test for lactose intolerance
- Abdominal CT, small bowel radiographic series, and/or barium enema may be indicated
- Consider HIV testing

Initial patient management

- Fluid resuscitation: oral, if possible, or IV (e.g., normal saline or lactated Ringer's solution)
- Nonspecific antidiarrheal agents (e.g., loperamide, codeine, tincture of opium) and fiber supplementation may be attempted initially
- Appropriate antibiotic therapy as necessary
- Treat underlying etiologies as necessary
- GI, oncology, and/or surgery consultations may be necessary, depending on the situation

DIFFERENTIAL DIAGNOSIS

Abnormal bowel motility
- Irritable bowel syndrome (IBS)
- Diabetic neuropathy (uncontrolled, explosive, postprandial diarrhea, usually seen in patients with neurologic dysfunction and uncontrolled blood sugar)
- Hyperthyroidism
- Postileal resection
- Scleroderma
- Carcinoid syndrome

Secretory diarrhea
- Bacterial gastroenteritis (e.g., cholera, enterotoxigenic *E. coli*)
- Bile acid malabsorption
- Colitis
- Hyperthyroidism
- Collagen vascular diseases (e.g., SLE, MCTD, scleroderma)
- Neuroendocrine tumors (e.g., VIPoma, gastrinoma, carcinoid, Zollinger-Ellison syndrome, pheochromocytoma)

Osmotic diarrhea
- Malabsorption syndromes (e.g., celiac sprue, nontropical sprue, Whipple's disease)
- Nonabsorbable substances (e.g., laxatives, lactose, magnesium, sorbitol, olestra)

Inflammatory diarrhea
- Inflammatory bowel disease (IBD)
- Behçet's syndrome
- Invasive bacterial disease (e.g., *Campylobacter jejuni*)
- Intestinal neoplasm (e.g., GI lymphoma)
- Whipple's disease (*Tropheryma whippelii*)

Dietary etiologies
- Lactose intolerance
- Fructose intolerance
- Zinc deficiency
- Trehalase deficiency (trehalose is the sugar found in mushrooms)
- Low-fat diet

Other etiologies
- Allergic enteritis (e.g., cow's milk, soy)
- Cystic fibrosis
- Immune deficiency (e.g., hypogammaglobulinemia)
- Sucrase-isomaltase deficiency
- Neuroblastoma
- Abetalipoproteinemia
- HIV disease
- Bacterial overgrowth

Diplopia

INTRODUCTION

Diplopia, or double vision, is a common ophthalmologic complaint. The double vision may be horizontal, vertical, or diagonal (oblique). It occurs secondary to paralysis, paresis, and/or restriction of the extraocular muscles. Most cases are binocular, resulting from misalignment of the eyes. True monocular diplopia is caused by very rare CNS lesions, but monocular diplopia is rarely a "true" diplopia. Rather, it is a "ghosting" or superposition of images. Note that diplopia may be the presenting symptom for life-threatening conditions, such as aneurysm or stroke. As a rule of thumb, an associated pupillary abnormality suggests more severe pathology.

DIAGNOSTIC WORKUP & INITIAL MANAGEMENT

History and physical examination

- Note onset, duration, associated symptoms (e.g., eye or orbit pain, headache, erythema), trauma, and past history (e.g., diabetes, hypertension, stroke, infections, thyroid disease)
- Complete neurologic and ocular exams
  - Note focal neurologic deficits, cranial nerve involvement, cerebellar signs, and symptoms of demyelination (e.g., abnormal Romberg)
  - Assess vision, pupil size and reaction, eye motility ductions and versions, ptosis, fundus exam (optic nerve edema or pallor), visual field defect, proptosis, and ice test (for myasthenia gravis)
  - A child who is noted to have a "lazy eye" or "crossed eyes" always merits full ophthalmologic evaluation

Initial diagnostic workup

- Ophthalmology consultation is usually warranted
- If suspect a CNS lesion, MRI is usually the test of choice
- If suspect orbital etiology (e.g., trauma, thyroid orbitopathy), CT is usually superior
- MRI or MRA is indicated immediately for 3rd nerve palsy with pupil involvement, age < 50 years (to rule out demyelinating disease), no improvement over 3 months, aberrant regeneration, or multiple cranial nerve or systemic neurologic involvement
- Lumbar puncture may be necessary (after head CT, in order to rule out increased intracranial pressure) if suspect infection or neoplasm
- Further testing may include Tensilon test and acetylcholinesterase-receptor antibodies to rule out myasthenia gravis, fasting blood glucose and Hb_{A1C} to rule out diabetes, ESR or CRP to rule out giant cell arteritis (urgent temporal artery biopsy if temporal arteritis is strongly suspect), thyroid function tests and orbital ultrasound or CT for Graves orbitopathy

Initial patient management

- Patch one eye (usually the involved eye) as necessary
  - In children < 10 years, avoid patching and monitor for amblyopia ("lazy eye")
- Document the magnitude of ocular deviation and/or diplopia to determine improvement or stability between exams (measured with prisms by ophthalmologist)
- Prisms may be included in glasses for small, stable deviations
- Strabismus surgery for symptomatic diplopia in primary and reading positions if deviation is stable for > 6 months, for manifest head tilt, or for improving appearance
- Treat the underlying etiology as appropriate

DIFFERENTIAL DIAGNOSIS

Binocular diplopia

Decompensated phoria (misalignment of the eyes)
- Esophoria (inward deviation of the eye)

Third nerve palsy (vertical and horizontal diplopia)
- Compressive lesions (especially if pupil is involved), including aneurysm, cavernous sinus or orbit tumor, pituitary apoplexy, and uncal herniation
- Ischemic microvascular disease (e.g., diabetes mellitus, hypertension)
- Midbrain infarct
- Giant cell arteritis
- Herpes zoster
- Leukemia
- Meningitis
- Subarachnoid hemorrhage
- Ophthalmoplegic migraine
- Trauma

Fourth nerve palsy (vertical diplopia)
- Trauma, ischemic microvascular disease, congenital, multiple sclerosis, and other causes as above

Sixth nerve palsy (horizontal diplopia)
- Ischemic microvascular disease, trauma, increased intracranial pressure (bilateral palsy), tumor, multiple sclerosis, postlumbar puncture, sarcoidosis, vasculitis, pontine infarct, and other causes as above
- The most common cause of elevated intracranial pressure–related diplopia

Orbital disease
- Graves orbitopathy
- Orbital inflammation
- Tumor

Other
- Cavernous sinus or superior orbital fissure syndrome (multiple cranial nerve involvement)
- Myasthenia gravis
- Trauma or postocular surgery
- Brown's syndrome (restriction of superior oblique tendon)
- Internuclear ophthalmoplegia (e.g., multiple sclerosis, stroke)
- Vertebrobasilar insufficiency (vertigo)
- Botulism

Monocular diplopia
- Refractive error (high astigmatism)
- Corneal opacity or irregularity
- Cataract
- Dislocated lens or lens implant
- Extrapupillary openings
- Macular disease
- Retinal detachment
- Nonphysiologic

Other
- Convergence spasm (hysteria)
- Drug intoxication, including alcohol
- Fibrosis of the superior recti may be seen in advanced years in the absence of other disease
- Structural lesions of the brainstem

Displaced PMI

INTRODUCTION

The point of maximal impulse (PMI) represents the apical impulse of the left ventricle transmitted to the anterior chest wall. It should be palpated routinely during cardiac examination. Normally, the PMI lies in the left midclavicular line between the fourth and fifth ribs and typically is about the size of a quarter. Displacement of the PMI gives clues to the presence of abnormalities of the heart and, when coupled with inspection and auscultation, assists in diagnosis.

DIAGNOSTIC WORKUP & INITIAL MANAGEMENT

History and physical examination

- Assess associated symptoms, past medical and cardiovascular history, and medications
  - Dyspnea suggests congestive heart failure, pleural effusion, pulmonary hypertension, or pneumothorax
  - Orthopnea and lower extremity edema suggest congestive heart failure
  - Chest pain may suggest coronary artery disease, pulmonary embolism, or aortic dissection
  - Decreased exercise tolerance may suggest congestive heart failure
- Physical exam should concentrate on the heart and lungs
  - Elevated jugular venous pressure suggests cardiac dysfunction, pulmonary hypertension, or tamponade; an associated murmur suggests valve disease (typically aortic stenosis or mitral regurgitation if systolic and aortic regurgitation or mitral stenosis if diastolic)
  - A loud pulmonic component of the second heart sound suggests pulmonary hypertension
  - Decreased breath sounds and dullness to percussion suggests pleural effusion
  - Hyperresonance to percussion and tracheal deviation suggests pneumothorax

Initial diagnostic workup

- Chest radiography is helpful in the diagnosis of congestive heart failure, pleural effusion, and pneumothorax
- Transthoracic echocardiography may be useful to assess overall ventricular size and function, valve function, pericardial disease, and indirectly, pulmonary artery pressure
- Chest CT, MRI, and/or transesophageal echocardiography may be indicated to assess for aortic aneurysm, aortic dissection, eccentric mitral regurgitation jet, and other cardiac pathology

Initial patient management

- Treat the underlying etiology
  - Left ventricular hypertrophy: Blood pressure control is the mainstay of therapy
  - Pneumothorax may require needle decompression, chest tube, or supplemental oxygen therapy
  - Pleural effusion may be treated with thoracentesis and diuretics if symptomatic
  - Congestive heart failure is treated with diuretics, vasodilators, inotropes, and relief of ischemia as indicated
  - Aortic aneurysm: Surgical correction if symptomatic, large (abdominal aneurysm >5 cm, thoracic aneurysm >6 cm), rapidly expanding (growth of >0.5 cm/year), or evidence of thrombotic or embolic complications

DIFFERENTIAL DIAGNOSIS

Left ventricular hypertrophy
- PMI is enlarged
- Most commonly results from chronic hypertension

Left ventricular enlargement
- PMI is displaced inferolaterally
- May result from valve disease or underlying cardiomyopathy

Right ventricular dilation
- PMI is laterally displaced
- May have an associated right ventricular heave

Right-sided tension pneumothorax
- PMI is laterally displaced

Massive pleural effusion
- PMI is laterally displaced

Left ventricular aneurysm
- PMI is inferolaterally displaced

Thoracic aortic aneurysm
- Exam may reveal pulsation at the right second intercostal space

Right ventricular hypertrophy
- Exam may reveal epigastric or subxyphoid pulsations and a right ventricular heave

Cardiac tamponade
- PMI is absent

Dizziness or Light-headedness

INTRODUCTION

Light-headedness is an extremely common symptom in clinical practice, usually resulting from decreased cerebral blood flow. The term is imprecise, however, and may include symptoms of dizziness, vertigo, presyncope, or disequilibrium. Dizziness can be better classified as one of the following: (1) vertigo (a false sensation of movement, such as spinning, rotating, or swaying, of the patient or the environment), (2) presyncope (a syndrome of light-headedness associated with a graying of vision, tinnitus, and expectation of syncope), (3) dysequilibrium (a sense of imbalance that typically occurs when walking), or (4) postural hypotension, cardiogenic factors, and defective vasopressors mechanisms, which are common in the elderly.

DIAGNOSTIC WORKUP & INITIAL MANAGEMENT

- Place the patient in a safe, recumbent position with legs raised above head level
- Assess vital signs, including blood pressure (with orthostatics), heart rate, respirations oxygen saturation, temperature, fingerstick glucose measurement; assess pain
- Differentiate the type of dizziness
- Make sure the patient is in a safe environment and not at risk of falling
- Calm the patient; many cases are benign and often relate to volume depletion or medication issues

History and physical examination

- A complete history and physical exam should include:
  - Signs of dehydration or volume depletion (e.g., bleeding, vomiting or diarrhea, poor oral intake, excessive diuresis, dry mucous membranes, decreased urine output)
  - Questions about excessive pressure on the neck, headaches, palpitations, history of heart disease, hearing loss
  - Cardiac auscultation, orthostatic blood pressures, and complete head and neck, gait, and neurologic exams
- Assess the chronology of symptoms (e.g., isolated vs. recurrent); note whether symptoms recur at a certain time of day
- Review medications, especially those recently administered
- Vertigo may be evaluated via several specific maneuvers
  - Dix-Hallpike maneuver: With the patient sitting, rapidly move him/her to a supine position with the head over the back of the table, and observe for nystagmus (type and duration); repeat with head facing to the left and right

Initial workup and management

- Labs may include CBC, electrolytes, calcium, glucose, BUN and creatinine, BNP, ESR, carbon monoxide level, pulse oximetry, and stool occult blood testing
- Further testing may include ECG, 24-hour ECG monitoring, echocardiography, hearing evaluation, head CT, EEG, MRI, and/or MRA
- Consider a cortisol level if suspect adrenal insufficiency
- Head CT if focal neurologic signs or suspicion for stroke; CT scan can be normal for 6–24 hours after the acute event if stroke is the etiology
- Hold potentially offending medications (e.g., antihypertensives, diuretics), if possible
- If concern for volume depletion, start IV fluids (many liters may be necessary, but be cautious if the patient has documented congestive heart failure or is on dialysis)
- If the patient appears to be losing volume because of diarrhea or vomiting, begin appropriate agents (e.g., antiemetics, antidiarrheal medications)
- If the patient is hypoglycemic, administer IV dextrose, assess closely for alleviation or persistence of symptoms, and review all administered medications
- Symptomatic therapy includes vestibular suppressants (e.g., prochlorperazine, meclazine)

DIFFERENTIAL DIAGNOSIS

Medications
- Antihypertensive and psychotropic medications can cause dizziness, especially in elderly patients
- Other medications include sildenafil, terazosin (especially the initial dose), phenytoin, oto-toxic drugs (e.g., gentamicin, streptomycin, neomycin, quinine, salicylates), and nitrates
- Withdrawal of SSRIs can cause dizziness

Postural hypotension
- A common cause of dizziness in elderly and hospitalized patients
- Evaluate for orthostasis (dizziness, tachycardia, and hypotension that occur when moving from supine to standing); this is especially likely if these symptoms abate on recumbency
- Unstable vasomotor reflexes can cause orthostasis, especially in elderly, diabetic, and alcoholic patients

Cardiogenic etiologies
- Arrhythmias (e.g., atrial fibrillation, complete heart block, supraventricular tachycardia)
- Sick sinus syndrome may result in bradycardia, recurrent palpitations, and syncope
- Wolff-Parkinson-White syndrome may result in palpitations and intermittent tachycardia
- Mitral valve prolapse, aortic stenosis, and hypertrophic cardiomyopathy can cause dizziness, particularly during exercise
- Congestive heart failure

Hypoglycemia
- Often associated with diaphoresis, tachycardia, and trembling
- If the patient is diabetic, evaluate for recent insulin administration and last meal
- Consider administering IV dextrose solution or a high-carbohydrate snack

Stroke or transient ischemic attack
- Stroke may have associated symptoms of slurred speech, diplopia, paresthesias, nystag-mus, motor dysfunction, ataxia, and facial asymmetry
- Subclavian steal syndrome symptoms occur with movement of the arms; patients may have decreased left carotid pulse, bruit, or decreased blood pressure in left arm

Hyperventilation or psychogenic etiologies
- A diagnosis of exclusion, unless there is a documented history
- Emotional stress may be a trigger for symptoms, which may include paresthesias around the mouth or fingertips
- Not related to movement or postural changes
- May be relieved by rebreathing into a paper bag

Vertigo
- Generally a recurrent cause of dizziness-like symptoms; acute onset may occur in cases of vertebrobasilar stroke or labyrinthitis
- Causes include benign positional vertigo and Ménière's disease (associated with tinnitus)
- May have associated nausea and vomiting

Other
- Syncope
- Primary CNS dysfunction not associated with decreased blood flow (e.g., migraine, seizure, labyrinthine disease or labyrinthitis, acoustic neuroma, multiple sclerosis, brainstem tumor)
- Severe electrolyte disturbance
- Elevated intracranial pressure
- Panic attack
- Ictal aura
- Allergic reaction
- Post-concussion syndrome
- Carbon monoxide poisoning
- Tabes dorsalis
- Friedreich's ataxia

Dry Skin (Xerosis)

INTRODUCTION

Xerosis, or dry skin, is extraordinarily common and nearly always benign. It is most common on the legs but can affect the entire skin surface. Dry skin has a low level of sebum and can be prone to sensitivity. A significant decrease in free fatty acids in the stratum corneum results in transepidermal water loss up to 75 times that of healthy skin. The outer keratin layers require 10%–20% water concentration to maintain their integrity. Excess water loss from the epidermis results in dehydration of the stratum corneum and cell shrinkage. Mild xerosis can cause impaired skin barrier function and allow irritants and allergens to affect the skin more easily. Multiple etiologic factors may coexist, including environmental, nutritional, and physiologic factors, as well as preexisting disease. Xerosis may be intensely pruritic without an apparent rash.

DIAGNOSTIC WORKUP & INITIAL MANAGEMENT

History and physical examination

- A complete history should be taken, including social, family, environmental, and exposure history, as well as past medical history and medications
  - Note frequency of bathing, showering, and cleansing, and the soaps/cleansers used
  - Note the types of skin lubricants used and method and frequency of application
  - Dietary history may be revealing (e.g., fatty acid deficiency)
  - Note types of clothing worn (wool may cause irritation)
  - Patients may complain of tightness, chapping, and flaking of the skin, especially in cold temperatures or after bathing
- Perform a focused exam, including thyroid and complete skin exams
  - May be generalized or local (commonly on anterior shins, extensor arms, and flanks)
  - The skin may have a parched look because of its inability to retain moisture; erythema, scaling, and cracking are signs of extremely dehydrated skin
  - Excoriations may be present because of excessive rubbing or scratching

Initial diagnostic workup

- If xerosis is severe, of acute onset, or associated with intractable pruritus or other systemic symptoms, consider CBC, thyroid function tests, BUN and creatine, and liver function tests
- Consider HIV testing in at-risk patients with severe xerosis, especially of recent onset
- If conservative therapy fails, consider age-appropriate malignancy screening

Initial patient management

- Simple measures (e.g., daily emollient use) can make a big difference in patients' lives
- During bathing, use lukewarm water (hot water can dry out the skin), and limit bathing to no more than 15 minutes once a day to avoid stripping the skin of its natural oils
- Avoid harsh soaps that may dry out the skin, including deodorant soaps; use nondetergent, neutral-pH products (e.g., Dove, Oil of Olay Sensitive Skin, Cetaphil, Aquaphor) or liquid skin cleansers containing petrolatum
- Avoid vigorous use of a washcloths during cleansing; when towel drying, blot or pat rather than rubbing the skin dry
- Apply oil-based moisturizing emollients (e.g., petroleum jelly ointment, Aquaphor) or creams (e.g., Eucerin, Cetaphil) twice daily
- Use lactic acid–containing moisturizers (e.g., AmLactin, Lac-Hydrin) on scaly patches without open breaks in the skin
- Use a humidifier during the winter months
- Drink plenty of water, and ensure appropriate intake of essential fatty acids
- Avoid irritating fabrics such as wool; use cotton clothing and cotton bedding
- Topical steroid ointments may be necessary to control pruritus in severe cases; systemic retinoids are sometimes used as adjuvant therapy for patients with certain genetic ichthyoses

DIFFERENTIAL DIAGNOSIS

Environmental etiologies
- Prolonged bathing in hot water
- Use of harsh soaps
- Infrequent use of emollients
- Use of degreasing agents (cleansers)
- Low humidity
- Cold temperatures ("winter itch")
- Excessive winds

Physiologic etiologies
- Decreased sebaceous or sweat gland activity
- Low keratin synthesis
- Increasing age (results in decreased rate of skin repair)

Nutritional etiologies
- Zinc deficiency
- Essential fatty acid deficiency

Severe xerosis in the elderly causing eczema craquelé
- Patient's legs often have a scale that resembles cracked porcelain
- Secondary erythema and excoriations occur because of the persistent itch

Ichthyoses vulgaris
- Very common cause of dry skin caused by a genetic defect in skin barrier function
- Patients often have hyperlinearity of the palmar skin and snake-like scale on the legs

Systemic disease
- Hypothyroidism and hyperthyroidism can also cause marked xerosis and/or itch
- Anemia
- HIV infection
- Sarcoidosis
- Liver/biliary disease and renal insufficiency are commonly associated with xerosis and marked pruritis
- Diabetes mellitus
- Malignancies
  - There is an uncommon association between lymphoma and marked xerosis

Other
- Many genetic conditions, such as the large family of ichthyoses (e.g., X-linked ichthyoses, Netherton's disease), lead to severely dry skin in association with other systemic manifestations
- Medications (e.g., niacinamide, diuretics, antispasmotics, antihistamines)
- Atopic dermatitis
- Allergic contact dermatitis
- Irritant contact dermatitis
- Nummular eczema
- Asteatotic eczema
- Mycosis fungoides
- Parapsoriasis
- Psoriasis

Dysarthria

INTRODUCTION

Dysarthria implies poor speech articulation due to impaired speech mechanics, such as motor weakness of the tongue or lips. It must be distinguished from aphasia and impoverished intelligence resulting from mental retardation or dementia. Pain is not a feature of dysarthria, nor is poor education. Speech, reading comprehension, and writing are completely unaffected in pure dysarthria. Speech therapy is an essential part of treatment to prevent aspiration and optimize communication.

DIAGNOSTIC WORKUP & INITIAL MANAGEMENT

History and physical examination
- Include complete neurologic and head and neck exams

Initial diagnostic workup
- Upper motor neuron lesions (voluntary motor pathways to cranial nerve nuclei 9, 10, and 12 are affected): Cerebral imaging (especially MRI) is indicated to distinguish ischemic from hemorrhagic infarction and an abscess from a tumor
- Lower motor neuron lesions: MRI is vastly superior to CT; labs may include TSH, glucose tolerance testing, and toxicology screening in patients with suspected metabolic causes or sedative drug intoxication
- Neuromuscular junction lesions often present with fluctuations of dysarthria as well as oropharyngeal or glossal weakness; myasthenia gravis antibody testing may be indicated; ECG and telemetry are indicated in various poisonings
- Muscle lesions: Genetic testing for heritable causes; creatine phosphokinase level and EMG for acquired causes
- Structural causes: Proper head and neck examination with indirect laryngoscopy and MRI of the oropharynx if suspect a mass
- EMG with nerve conduction tests in suspected cases of amyotrophic lateral sclerosis

Initial patient management
- Speech therapy is often necessary to relearn oral movements and communication skills, prevent aspiration, and motivate the patient
- Treat underlying etiologies as necessary
- Dysarthria may improve with treatment of diabetes and/or hypothyroidism
- Myasthenia gravis improves with pyridostigmine and immunosuppression
- Pralidoxime and atropine for nerve gas poisoning
- Antitoxin and close, intensive care observation for botulism
- Steroids for polymyositis and dermatomyositis
- Surgical intervention may be necessary for structural causes

DIFFERENTIAL DIAGNOSIS

Neurological causes
Lesions of upper motor neurons
- Stroke
- Tumor
- Abscess
- Degeneration (e.g., Parkinson's disease)

Lesions of lower motor neuron
- Brainstem stroke
- Amyotrophic lateral sclerosis
- Hypothyroidism
- Diabetic nerve infarction

Lesions of the neuromuscular junction
- Myasthenia gravis
- Prolonged effects of anesthesia
- Botulism
- Nerve gas
- Organophosphate poisoning

Lesions of muscle
- Polymyositis
- Dermatomyositis
- Inherited muscle diseases (e.g., myotonic muscular dystrophy)
- Mitochondrial diseases

Structural causes
- Tumors of the lips, tongue, and squamous cell epithelium of the vocal cords and oropharynx
- Polyps or salivary gland dysfunction resulting in xerostomia (dry mouth)
- Hypoglossal nerve damage from surgical traction (e.g., carotid endarterectomy)
- Glossitis (e.g., amyloidosis, hypothyroidism, anaerobic infection)
- Poor dentition or ill-fitting dentures
- Cleft palate

Other
- Acute dystonic reaction
- Unrecognized foreign accent
- Sedative or anticonvulsant intoxication
- Mild cerebral palsy

Dysmenorrhea

INTRODUCTION

Dysmenorrhea, or painful menstruation, is one of the most common gynecologic complaints. It is characterized into primary versus secondary disorders. Primary dysmenorrhea refers to severe uterine cramping during ovulatory menses and in the absence of demonstrable pelvic disease. Secondary dysmenorrhea is defined as painful menstruation caused by underlying pelvic disease, such as endometriosis or fibroids.

DIAGNOSTIC WORKUP & INITIAL MANAGEMENT

History and physical examination

- Obtain a complete menstrual and gynecologic history, history of symptoms, medical history, psychosocial history, and medication and dietary history
- Abdominal exam should assess for surgical scars, hernias, masses, tenderness, rigidity, rebound tenderness, and guarding
- Pelvic exam should evaluate for signs of infection (including vaginal wet mount and testing for chlamydia and gonorrhea, if warranted); uterosacral ligament abnormalities; cervical stenosis, motion tenderness, or lateral displacement of the cervix; and uterine or adnexal tenderness
- Rectal exam to rule out masses and assess for point tenderness

Initial workup and management

- An initial trial of lifestyle changes, NSAIDs, and oral contraceptives may be effective in patients with primary dysmenorrhea
  - Lifestyle changes include regular exercise, smoking cessation, decrease in alcohol and caffeine consumption, and weight reduction
  - Dietary interventions that may reduce pain severity include a low-fat vegetarian diet, fish oil supplementation, vitamin E, thiamine (vitamin B_1), and pyridoxine (vitamin B_6)
  - High-dose ibuprofen may be administered beginning the day before onset of menses
  - Oral contraceptives with or without NSAIDs may be effective when NSAIDs alone are inadequate
  - Use of heating pad on the lower abdomen or back
- Patients unresponsive to the above interventions or with symptoms suggesting pelvic pathology (secondary dysmenorrhea) require a complete workup for diagnosis
- Initial laboratory testing includes CBC, urinalysis, Pap smear, pregnancy testing (β-hCG), and testing for gonorrhea and chlamydia
- Pelvic and vaginal ultrasound may be used to assess for lower abdominal and pelvic pathology (e.g., ovarian/adnexal masses, nephrolithiasis, appendicitis, ovarian cysts, fibroids)
- Abdominal and/or pelvic CT may be indicated to evaluate for gynecologic and abdominal pathology
- If the diagnosis is still uncertain, further testing may include hysterosonography, hysteroscopy, or laparoscopy

DIFFERENTIAL DIAGNOSIS

Primary dysmenorrhea
- Accounts for nearly 75% of cases
- Symptoms develop before age 25 years (usually during adolescence)
- May present with cramping and lower abdominal discomfort, nausea, vomiting, diarrhea, and headache
- Pain is most severe at onset of menses and lasts 12–72 hours, then gradually diminishes
- Associated with high prostaglandin levels

Secondary dysmenorrhea
- Endometriosis (ectopic endometrial tissue)
- Adenomyosis (endometrial tissue in the myometrium)
- Acute pelvic inflammatory disease
- Chronic pelvic inflammatory disease
- Pelvic adhesions
- Uterine leiomyoma (fibroids)
- Ovarian cysts
- Ovarian or adnexal torsion
- Cervical stenosis
- Uterosacral ligament abnormalities
- Malignancy (e.g., uterine, ovarian)
- Intrauterine device (IUD) use
  - Most IUDs can cause dysmenorrhea, but the levonorgestrel-eluting IUD (Mirena) may be used as therapy for dysmenorrhea

Mental health issues
- Somatization
- Substance abuse
- Depression
- Sexual abuse

Extrapelvic disorders
- Irritable bowel syndrome (IBS)
- Appendicitis
- UTI
- Inflammatory bowel disease (IBD)
- Diverticulitis
- Cholecystitis
- Abdominal hernia
- Nephrolithiasis
- Constipation
- Malignancy

Other
- Fibromyalgia
- Malformations of the Mullerian ducts
- Interstitial cystitis
- Intestinal or uteropelvic junction obstruction
- Ectopic pregnancy

Dyspareunia

Dyspareunia is defined as painful and/or difficult sexual intercourse. The large differential diagnosis requires detailed history and physical examination and appropriate workup. Distinguish primary dyspareunia (occurring at the onset of sexual intercourse) from secondary dyspareunia (preceded by painless intercourse).

DIAGNOSTIC WORKUP & INITIAL MANAGEMENT

History and physical examination

- Note timing, onset (e.g., on entry, with deep penetration, postcoital), duration, location, persistence after intercourse, and previous occurrences
- Note associations of the pain; symptoms may occur with all vaginal or vulvar contact, with intercourse only, with exams only, with masturbation, or with memories or recollections of previous occurrences or traumatic experiences
  - Superficial dyspareunia: Pain or dysfunction is felt on initial penetration
  - Deep dyspareunia: Pain or dysfunction is felt deep within the pelvis during intercourse
- Note alleviating and aggravating factors during intercourse
- Note the quality of the pain (e.g., burning, sharp, dull, aching, throbbing, stabbing)
- Old medical records may be of crucial importance
- Include complete psychiatric history and exam
- Include pelvic and rectal exams

Initial workup and management

- Cervical and/or vulvar cultures, testing for gonorrhea and chlamydia, and microscopic evaluation of normal saline and potassium hydroxide wet mounts should be done
- Imaging studies may be indicated, including pelvic and/or abdominal ultrasound and/or CT
- Management of psychiatric causes is particularly challenging and requires specific and specialized therapy
- Consider gynecology and/or psychiatry consultation

DIFFERENTIAL DIAGNOSIS

- Sexual pain disorder: Persistent or recurrent genital pain of nonorganic cause associated with sexual stimulation
- Vaginismus: Painful, involuntary spasm of the vagina, preventing intercourse
- Vulvar vestibulitis: A chronic and persistent clinical syndrome characterized by severe pain with vestibular touch or attempted vaginal entry, tenderness in response to pressure within the vulvar vestibule, and physical findings confined to various degrees of vestibular erythema
- Vulvodynia: Chronic vulvar discomfort (e.g., burning, stinging, irritation, rawness)
- Female sexual dysfunction (disorders of desire, arousal, or orgasm)

Neurologic etiologies
- Genital nerve damage or infection
- Dysesthetic (essential) vulvodynia

Gynecologic etiologies
- Fibroids
- Gynecologic malignancy (e.g., vulvar, cervical, uterine, ovarian)
- Bartholin's gland inflammation
- Vaginal atrophy
- Vaginal trauma (e.g., laceration, ecchymoses)
- Severely retroverted uterus
- Imperforate hymen

Gastrointestinal etiologies
- Constipation
- Irritable bowel syndrome (IBS)
- Colitis
- Diverticulitis
- GI tumors (e.g., rectal cancer)

Urinary etiologies
- Interstitial cystitis
- Urethritis
- Urethral diverticulum

Infectious etiologies
- Endometritis
- Pelvic inflammatory disease
- Vulvovaginitis
- Postherpetic neuralgia
- Vaginitis
- Salpingitis
- Herpes genitalis
- Bartholin's abscess

Dermatologic etiologies
- Lichen sclerosis
- Behçet's syndrome
- Contact dermatitis

Musculoskeletal etiologies
- Pelvic floor myopathy
- Fibromyalgia
- Levator ani myalgia
- Dysfunctional vaginismus

Iatrogenic
- Surgical (e.g., pelvic adhesions, episiotomy, strictures)
- Pharmacologic (e.g., drying soaps or agents, topical medications, oral contraceptives)

Endocrine etiologies
- Estrogen deficiency
- Endometriosis

Dysphagia

INTRODUCTION

Dysphagia refers to difficulty swallowing (distinguish from odynophagia, which refers to painful swallowing). Difficulty swallowing results from difficulty transferring a food bolus from the oropharynx to the upper esophagus (oropharyngeal or transfer dysphagia) or from impaired transport of a food bolus through the body of the esophagus (esophageal or transport dysphagia). Pathologies that affect voluntary skeletal muscle generally present as difficulty initiating swallowing; if involuntary smooth muscle of the esophagus is affected, a sensation of incomplete swallowing tends to occur. Dysphagia may occur independently or with odynophagia, a sharp, substernal pain on swallowing that reflects severe erosive disease and is most commonly seen with infectious esophagitis or corrosive injury.

DIAGNOSTIC WORKUP & INITIAL MANAGEMENT

History and physical examination

- History should include onset, duration, and severity; dysphagia with liquid versus solids; medical history, including anxiety and other psychiatric illnesses; previous dysphagia or caustic substance exposure; and other head and neck problems
  - Mild weight loss may result from voluntary decrease in food intake; marked weight loss with anorexia suggests carcinoma or achalasia
  - Difficulty with solids suggests anatomic obstruction
  - Difficulty with both solids and liquids suggests motility problem
- Exam should include a thorough head, nose, mouth, neck/thyroid, and abdominal evaluation, and observation of the patient swallowing
- Oropharyngeal (transfer) dysphagia is difficulty initiating swallowing
  - May present with regurgitation of liquid through the nose, aspiration with swallowing, and inability to propel food out of mouth
- Esophageal (transport) dysphagia produces a sensation of food "sticking" in the throat
  - May present with retrosternal fullness after swallowing and relief upon regurgitation

Initial diagnostic workup

- If suspect esophageal dysphagia, barium swallow is often the first test indicated; it is less invasive than endoscopy and frequently sufficient for diagnosis
  - Identifies the area of the swallowing lesion
  - Differentiates motility disturbance from anatomic problems
- Endoscopy may be indicated as a complement to barium study; it can better detect mucosal lesions and allows biopsy and concomitant therapy (e.g., dilatation)
- Consider a video swallowing evaluation if suspect oropharyngeal dysphagia
- Esophageal manometry may be indicated in persistent dysphagia without a structural etiology
  - Evaluates motor function, measuring the strength, function, and coordination of the upper and lower esophageal sphincters and the body of the esophagus in response to a swallow
- Esophageal 24-hour pH study may be indicated if suspect GERD; provides temporal correlation between symptoms and reflux
- EMG and nerve conduction studies may be indicated to rule out neurologic causes (e.g., myasthenia gravis, amyotrophic lateral sclerosis)

Initial patient management

- Speech therapy evaluation may be indicated for cases without an apparent etiology
- Treat the underlying causes as necessary
- Acute mechanical obstructions require urgent endoscopy to relieve the obstruction and prevent potential perforation
- Chronic mechanical obstruction from webs, rings, and strictures requires endoscopic treatment or thoracic surgery; balloon dilation may be considered

DIFFERENTIAL DIAGNOSIS

Oropharyngeal (transfer) dysphagia

Neurologic
- Stroke
- Multiple sclerosis
- Dementia
- Pseudobulbar palsy
- Parkinson disease
- Brain mass
- Amyotrophic lateral sclerosis
- Tardive dyskinesia
- Postpoliomyelitis syndrome
- Huntington's disease
- Neuromuscular junction disorders (e.g., myasthenia gravis, botulism)
- Polyneuropathies (e.g., diabetic neuropathy, Guillain-Barré syndrome, toxin-related)

Rheumatologic
- Myopathy
- Oculopharyngeal dystrophy
- Polymyositis
- Sjogren's syndrome

Metabolic
- Thyrotoxicosis
- Cushing's disease
- Amyloidosis
- Wilson's disease
- Medication side effect (e.g., anticholinergics, phenothiazine)

Infectious
- Poliomyelitis
- Botulism
- Syphilis
- Diphtheria
- Lyme disease
- Viral mucositis

Structural lesions
- Zenker's diverticulum
- Cricopharyngeal bar
- Oropharyngeal tumor
- Cervical osteophytes
- Esophageal webs and rings
- Pill-induced injury
- Postsurgical or radiation changes (e.g., inflammation, stricture formation)

Motility disorders
- Upper esophageal sphincter dysfunction

Esophageal (transport) dysphagia

Mechanical obstruction
- Schatzki's ring
- Esophageal cancer
- Trauma
- Esophageal perforation
- Malignancy
- Anterior cervical osteophyte
- Enlarged thyroid
- Thyroglossal duct cyst
- Left atrial enlargement
- Peptic stricture
- Intrinsic esophageal lesions
- Foreign body retention
- Diverticula
- Mediastinal mass (e.g., thymoma, teratoma, lymphoma, carotid/aortic aneurysm)
- Postthoracic surgery or anterior cervical discectomy

Motility disorders
- Achalasia
- Diffuse esophageal spasm
- Scleroderma
- Gastric acid reflux
- Aberrant motility
- Nutcracker esophagus
- Chagas' disease
- Hypertensive lower esophageal sphincter

Other
- Globus hystericus (psychogenic dysphagia)

Dyspnea

INTRODUCTION

Dyspnea is defined as an abnormally uncomfortable awareness of breathing. Its mechanism is poorly understood. There is no single neural pathway or brain center for dyspnea; it is believed to arise from multiple sites (e.g., muscle and joint receptors, chemoreceptors, vagal afferents). A cardinal symptom of cardiac and pulmonary disease, dyspnea may also result from chest wall abnormalities, neurologic disorders, or anxiety. Complete evaluation focused on the cardiovascular, pulmonary, and GI systems is generally sufficient to narrow the differential, which can be further refined with appropriate diagnostic and laboratory evaluation. A marked, acute change in severity of dyspnea should be taken seriously; this may be a manifestation of a life-threatening underlying condition.

DIAGNOSTIC WORKUP & INITIAL MANAGEMENT

History and physical examination

- Determine the duration of dyspnea (acute or chronic) and rapidity of onset
- Note whether symptoms occur regularly (e.g., COPD, interstitial lung disease, pulmonary hypertension) or intermittently (e.g., asthma, congestive heart failure)
- Assess the rate of progression over the past months or years
- Note associated symptoms of left heart failure (e.g., paroxysmal nocturnal dyspnea, orthopnea, S_3, S_4), right heart failure (e.g., loud P_2, peripheral edema, jugular venous distension, hepatomegaly), bronchiectasis (e.g., purulent sputum, weight loss), obstructive airway disease (e.g., wheezing, chest tightness, recurrent bronchitis), pulmonary thromboembolism (e.g., acute dyspnea, pleuritic chest pain, hemoptysis, deep venous thrombosis), neuromuscular weakness, and rheumatologic symptoms (e.g., arthritis, skin rash)

Initial workup and management

- Evaluate airway, breathing, and circulation, including vital signs and pulse oximetry
- Administer supplemental oxygen to any patient in acute respiratory distress
  - Usually begin at higher oxygen flow rates (e.g., 6 L/min) and titrate down as appropriate
  - Oxygen can be administered via nasal cannula at 2–6 L/min (6 L provides 40% FiO_2), face mask (begin at > 40% FiO_2 for patients who are hypoxic despite nasal cannula oxygen), 100% nonrebreather (provides 100% FiO_2), CPAP, BiPAP, or intubation
  - In severe dyspnea, CPAP or BiPAP can be used to open the airway and alveoli and provide 100% FiO_2
  - Intubation and mechanical ventilation may be necessary to create a definitive airway or ventilate adequately
- After thorough history and physical, chest radiography is indicated in most patients
- If suspect lung disease, consider pulmonary function tests to differentiate between obstructive and restrictive physiology
  - Asthma is a common diagnosis; >12% improvement in FEV_1 on acute administration of bronchodilators is suggestive of asthma (also may be seen in COPD)
- Other laboratory studies may include CBC, BUN/creatinine, calcium, electrolytes, and thyroid function tests
- ABG will identify barriers to oxygen diffusion (increased A-a gradient), hypoxemia, and chronic hypercapnia
- If suspect cardiac ischemia, consider ECG, stress test, or coronary angiography
- In patients with normal pulmonary function, normal chest radiograph, and no heart disease:
  - Consider echocardiogram to evaluate for pulmonary vascular disease (e.g., pulmonary hypertension, chronic pulmonary thromboembolism); further testing may include right heart catheterization, V/Q scan, or pulmonary angiography
  - Consider neurologic evaluation if suspect neuromuscular disease
- Sputum culture and blood cultures may be necessary in cases of pneumonia
- Consider referral to specialists as necessary

DIFFERENTIAL DIAGNOSIS

Obstructive pulmonary disease
- Acute bronchospasm from asthma or COPD
- Bronchiectasis
- Pneumonia

Restrictive pulmonary disease
- Pleural effusion
- Interstitial lung diseases
- Neuromuscular disease
- Myopathies
- Obesity
- Kyphoscoliosis
- Chest wall abnormalities

Cardiac disease
- Congestive heart failure or "cardiac asthma"
- Valvular disease
- Pericardial effusion with cardiac tamponade
- Acute myocardial ischemia or infarction

Pulmonary edema (acute or chronic)
- Cardiogenic pulmonary edema
  - Left ventricular failure (e.g., MI, cardiomyopathy)
  - Valve disease
  - High-output states (e.g., thyrotoxicosis)
  - Volume overload
  - Hypertensive emergency
- Noncardiogenic pulmonary edema
  - Sepsis
  - Inhalation injury
  - Drugs (e.g., narcotics)
  - Renal failure
  - High altitude
  - Aspiration
  - Pancreatitis
  - Seizure
  - Trauma or CNS injury
  - Emboli (fat, air, amniotic fluid)
  - Airway obstruction (e.g., croup, foreign body)

Pulmonary vascular disease
- Acute or chronic pulmonary embolism
- Pulmonary hypertension

Pneumothorax
- Suspect in patients with history of COPD, *P. carinii* pneumonia, or recent placement of a subclavian or internal jugular central line
- Dyspnea and decreased breath sounds on the affected side are hallmarks
- Tension pneumothorax is a rare form that must be considered in patients with dyspnea, hypotension, jugular venous distension, and rapid deterioration

Psychogenic/anxiety attack
- A diagnosis of exclusion; most patients are anxious because they are short of breath, rather than short of breath because they are anxious

Other etiologies
- GERD
- Tracheal obstruction
- Deconditioning

Dysuria

INTRODUCTION

Dysuria is a painful or burning sensation during or immediately after urination caused by irritation of the urothelium and its innervation. This is a common symptom in primary care: Nearly 20% of women aged 20–55 will have at least one episode of dysuria per year, resulting in more than 8 million physician office visits annually. Women have episodes of acute dysuria much more frequently than men. The most common cause of dysuria in adult women is lower UTI.

DIAGNOSTIC WORKUP & INITIAL MANAGEMENT

History and physical examination

- Differentiate dysuria at initiation of, throughout, or at termination of urination
  - Pain at the start of urination usually indicates urethral involvement
  - Pain at the end of urination (strangury) suggests a bladder etiology
- History should assess for risk factors, including previous UTIs, STDs, urethral instrumentation, renal calculi, urothelial carcinoma, pelvic radiation, and atrophic vaginitis
- Female genital exam may include KOH prep, wet mount, Gram's stain, and DNA tests/culture
  - Thin, papery vaginal tissue suggests atrophic vaginitis
  - *Candida* discharge is thick, cheesy, and white; pruritic
  - Chlamydia discharge is scant, watery and has a gradual onset
  - Gonorrhea discharge is profuse, yellow-green with abrupt onset, intracellular gram-negative diplococci
  - Bacterial vaginosis discharge usually demonstrates clue cells on wet mount and a fishy odor on KOH whiff test
  - *Trichomonas* discharge is frothy and gray-green; associated with pruritis and mobile organisms on wet mount
- Male genital exam may include gonorrhea and chlamydia test, culture, and Gram's stain
  - A tender, boggy, swollen prostate suggests prostatitis (avoid prostatic massage because of risk of bacteremia)
  - Tender epididymitis and testicles suggest infection
  - A generally enlarged prostate associated with nocturia and increasing frequency suggests benign prostatic hyperplasia

Initial workup and management

- Urinalysis is indicated in all patients
  - Hematuria suggests urolithiasis, pyelonephritis, or cystitis
  - Painless hematuria may suggest bladder cancer
  - Positive nitrites, leukocyte esterase (highly sensitive and specific for infection), or white blood cells with suprapubic tenderness suggest uncomplicated cystitis
- Urine culture is indicated with positive urinalysis and in pregnant women, diabetic or immunocompromised patients, or males with urethral discharge
- Urine cytology to evaluate for uroepithelial carcinoma is indicated with persistent microscopic hematuria, dysuria, urinary urgency, or frequency without infection
- Cystoscopy may be indicated to visualize the bladder and perform biopsies
- Imaging of the genitourinary tract may be warranted in some cases: pelvic radiography (kidney, ureter, bladder) if suspect renal calculi or foreign body; pelvic CT is more definitive for calculi, urologic tumors, and to assess the upper urinary tract
- Symptomatic therapy with phenazopyridine can be given to alleviate dysuria (contraindicated in renal insufficiency and hepatic dysfunction); it will turn urine and body fluids orange (patients should be warned that contact lenses can be stained)

DIFFERENTIAL DIAGNOSIS

Lower urinary tract etiologies
Cystitis
- Infectious (e.g., *E. coli, Staphylococcus saprophyticus, Proteus, Klebsiella, Enterococcus*)
- Interstitial cystitis
- Noninfectious cystitis (e.g., drugs, radiation, granulomatous, allergic)
- Instrumentation

Urethritis
- Urethral infection (e.g., *Chlamydia, N. gonorrhea, E. coli, Staphylococcus aureus*)
- Urethral diverticulum
- Urethral strictures
- Caruncle (outgrowth of distal urethral tissue)
- Prolapse
- Radiation
- Instrumentation

Male-specific etiologies
- Acute prostatitis
- Benign prostatic hypertrophy
- Epididymitis (e.g., *Chlamydia, N. gonorrhea, E. coli, S. aureus*)

Female-specific etiologies
- Vaginitis (e.g., *Candida, Trichomonas*, bacterial vaginosis)
- Atrophic vaginitis

Upper urinary tract etiologies
- Pyelonephritis
- Nephrolithiasis/urolithiasis

Anatomic abnormalities
Outflow obstruction
- Nephrolithiasis/urolithiasis
- Bladder neck contracture
- Posterior urethral valves
- Prostatic hyperplasia
- Urethral stricture
- Meatal stenosis

Malignancy
- Uroepithelial cancer
- Prostate cancer
- Bladder cancer
- Tumors adjacent to or invading the lower urinary tract (e.g., colorectal)

Other etiologies
- Foreign bodies (e.g., urethral catheter, recent instrumentation)
- Intravesicle chemotherapy
- Systemic medications
- Inflammation of adjacent organs
- External infections (e.g., herpes)
- Allergic reaction to contraceptives, soaps, or lotions
- Reiter's syndrome
- Behçet's syndrome
- Rectal fissure
- Psychogenic (e.g., conversion disorder)
- Trauma

Ear Pain

INTRODUCTION

Ear pain is an extremely common presenting complaint in both primary care and otolaryngology practices. Otitis media (infection and inflammation of the inner ear) and otitis externa (infection and inflammation of the ear canal) cause most cases of ear pain. The vast majority of otitis media cases are caused by viruses; thus, deciding when to use antibiotics is a common clinical issue. Not all ear pain, however, is otologic. The ears have rich sensory innervation from multiple nerves, and secondary pain is common. Most cases of otologic ear pain have some associated physical findings; if not, a complete head and neck examination, including imaging, may be required to search for a source of referred pain.

DIAGNOSTIC WORKUP & INITIAL MANAGEMENT

History and physical examination

- Include an otoscopic exam with pneumatic otoscopy and complete head and neck exam
- Note ability to localize the pain, which may distinguish otologic from nonotologic disease
- Pain upon traction of the pinna suggests otitis externa (hyperemic external canal)
- Bulging, red, immobile tympanic membrane is consistent with acute otitis media (with or without otorrhea secondary to perforation)
- A retracted, immobile tympanic membrane may be seen in serous otitis media
- A mass lesion behind the tympanic membrane suggests cholesteatoma or tumor
- Tonsillar asymmetry or uvular deviation suggests peritonsillar abscess or mass

Initial diagnostic workup

- Tympanometry may reveal otitis media with effusion, eustachian tube dysfunction, or tympanostomy tube obstruction
- Audiometry to evaluate for hearing loss
- Consider culture of otorrhea for bacterial and fungal etiologies if suspect perforation or complicated disease (e.g., recurrent infection, spread of infection as occurs in meningitis or mastoiditis)
- Lateral neck radiography will diagnose retropharyngeal mass or abscess
- Head CT is indicated if suspect an intracranial lesion, abscess, or basilar skull fracture or to delineate the extent of cholesteatoma, mastoiditis, or tumor
- Consider CBC and ESR if suspect malignant necrotizing otitis media
- Check glucose in cases of recurrent severe otitis externa

Initial patient management

- If the patient is in distress, immediately stabilize airway, breathing, and circulation
- Pain control with acetaminophen, NSAIDs, warm compress, and topical benzocaine solution
- Remove cerumen and foreign bodies with a curette, if appropriate
- Otitis media guidelines suggest that most cases can be initially observed without antibiotic treatment; antibiotics may be necessary in some patients, especially those with risk factors for bacterial infection (e.g., persistent fever, immunocompromise)
- Serous otitis media that persists for >3 months may require a course of corticosteroids or myringotomy
- Otitis externa is treated with aluminum acetate and 2% acetic acid, antibiotics, and/or steroid drops
- Malignant otitis externa is treated with IV antipseudomonal or antistaphylococcal antibiotics

DIFFERENTIAL DIAGNOSIS

External ear

Otitis externa
- Pain occurs on movement of the tragus or pinna

Malignant (necrotizing) otitis externa
- Mostly occurs in diabetics, usually from *Pseudomonas aeruginosa* infection

Impacted cerumen
- May result in hearing loss and aural fullness

Foreign bodies
- Items include beads, toys, and extruded tympanostomy tubes

Trauma
- Any object inserted into the ear canal may cause trauma, including Q-tips

Perichondritis
- Inflammation or infection of the cartilage of the pinna and ear canal

Myringitis

Middle ear and mastoid

Otitis media
- Most cases are of viral origin and occur in children 6–18 months of age
- Exam reveals a red tympanic membrane with decreased mobility
- Risk factors include day care, supine bottle feeding, smoking in household, siblings with otitis media, anatomic abnormalities (e.g., Down's syndrome)

Barotrauma
- Deep-sea diving, airplane travel
- Pretreatment with topical nasal decongestants may be effective

Mastoiditis
- Associated with postauricular pain and normal typmanic membrane

Eustachian tube dysfunction

Nonotologic

Cranial nerve referred pain
- Cranial nerve 3: Dental infection, TMJ, dental trauma, orthodontic intervention (e.g., tightening of braces)
- Cranial nerve 7: Herpes zoster oticus (Ramsay-Hunt syndrome)
- Cranial nerve 9: Tonsillitis, pharyngitis
- Cranial nerve 10: Laryngitis, GERD, thyroiditis

Cervical nerve referred pain
- Neck infection
- Inflamed lymph nodes, cervical adenitis
- Cyst
- Cervical spine disorders

Other causes of referred pain
- Posttonsillectomy or adenoidectomy
- Retropharyngeal abscess and other deep-space infections
- Paranasal sinusitis, rhinitis, laryngitis, or esophagitis
- Migraine
- Trigeminal neuralgia
- Parotiditis or sialoadenitis (including mumps)
- Angina or acute coronary syndrome
- Cholesteatoma

Edema, Periorbital

INTRODUCTION

Periorbital, or eyelid, edema has many possible causes, including mechanical, hemodynamic, infectious, inflammatory, and neoplastic causes. A careful history and physical examination are necessary to determine whether the problem is localized or generalized and to uncover the underlying etiology.

DIAGNOSTIC WORKUP & INITIAL MANAGEMENT

History and physical examination

- History should include symptom onset and course, exposure history (allergens, irritants, chemicals, ultraviolet, or thermal injury), associated symptoms, medical and family history, and medication history
- Physical exam, including a full ophthalmologic exam for erythema, tenderness, cutaneous vesicles, discharge, proptosis, vision changes, and conjunctival injection or chemosis
- Preseptal cellulitis is not associated with conjunctival hyperemia, proptosis, extraocular motility restriction, or vision loss; orbital cellulitis may have some or all of these

Initial diagnostic workup

- Initial laboratory evaluation may include CBC with differential, electrolytes, BUN and creatinine, TSH, ESR, ANA, albumin, and urinalysis
- Culture and Gram's stain of eye discharge if suspect infection
- Consider CT or MRI of the orbits, neck, and/or chest
- Consider biopsy of suspicious or persistent lesions
- Consider echocardiogram if suspect congestive heart failure

Initial patient management

- Consider ophthalmology consultation
  - Orbital cellulitis is an ophthalmic emergency with a risk of cavernous sinus thrombosis or orbital apex syndrome; it requires immediate imaging studies to look for the cause (e.g., extension from adjacent infectious sinusitis), possible drainage, and IV antibiotics
- Treat the underlying cause as appropriate
- Treat blepharitis with lid hygiene and bland antibiotic ointment (e.g., erythromycin) or antibiotic-steroid ointment (e.g., tobramycin-dexamethasone)
- Treat infectious etiologies with topical and/or systemic antibiotics
- For allergic causes, remove the inciting allergen or medication and treat with oral antihistamines and cool compresses; consider topical steroids for local processes or systemic steroids for systemic disorders
- Allergic conditions can generally be treated with cold compresses and chilled, preservative-free artificial tears
- Blepharoplasty may be indicated in cases of herniated orbital fat if it interferes with vision or is cosmetically unappealing

DIFFERENTIAL DIAGNOSIS

Conjunctivitis

- Bacterial etiologies include *S. aureus, S. pneumoniae, H. influenzae, N. gonorrhoeae, C. trachomatis,* and *N. meningitidis*
- Viral etiologies include adenovirus, enterovirus, coxsackievirus, vaccinia virus, molluscum contagiosum, HSV-1 and -2, varicella-zoster virus, EBV, human papillomavirus, congenital rubella, influenza viruses, and measles
- Toxic conjunctivitis may result from neomycin, aminoglycosides, atropine, and other topical medications, as well as cosmetics and preservatives
- Seasonal allergic conjunctivitis (hay fever) usually results from exposure to airborne allergens; allergic conjunctivitis may also result from rubbing the eyes with allergen (e.g., cat dander)
- Immunogenic conjunctivitis is associated with systemic immune disorders (e.g., Graves disease, rheumatoid arthritis, Sjogren's syndrome, SLE, Wegener's granulomatosis, relapsing polychondritis, polyarteritis nodosa)

Allergy

- Systemic (e.g., reaction to medication, urticaria, angioedema)
- Local (e.g., insect bite)

Dermatitis

- Contact dermatitis
- Dermatitis medicamentosa

Chalazion

- Zeis or meibomian gland obstruction of eyelid

Orbital disease

- Thyroid-associated orbitopathy
- Orbital cellulitis
- Orbital tumors
- Orbital vasculitis
- Trauma

Autoimmune disease

- Dermatomyositis/polymyositis
  - Associated with a heliotropic (violet-colored) rash on the upper eyelids
- Hypothyroidism
  - Associated with fatigue, pretibial edema, and delayed relaxation of reflexes
- Discoid lupus

Systemic disease

- Congestive heart failure
- Renal failure
- Nephrotic syndrome
- Superior vena cava syndrome

Other

- Preseptal/periorbital cellulitis
- Acute dacryocystitis (infection of the lacrimal ducts)
- Ocular cicatricial pemphigoid (symblepharon)
- Orbital fat herniation through attenuated or dehiscent orbital septum and/or orbicularis oculi muscle (associated with aging)
- Herpes simplex or herpes zoster blepharitis/dermatitis
- Trauma/postsurgical
- Chemical, ultraviolet, or thermal burn
- Blepharitis/rosacea
- Dacryoadenitis
- Sebaceous gland carcinoma
- Squamous or basal cell carcinoma

Edema, Peripheral

INTRODUCTION

Peripheral edema can be pitting or nonpitting. Pitting edema suggests fluid in the surrounding tissue caused by an imbalance in the forces holding fluid within the vascular space. Remember Starling's equation and the forces involved in fluid movement across a capillary membrane. Nonpitting edema suggests swelling of the cells themselves, as in myxedema. It is also helpful to assess whether the edema is unilateral or bilateral. Unilateral swelling suggests a lesion to the vein or lymphatic drainage on the affected side or an inflammatory process, such as infection or gout. Bilateral swelling suggests a systemic cause.

DIAGNOSTIC WORKUP & INITIAL MANAGEMENT

History and physical examination

- In most cases, the cause will be suggested by the history and physical exam; focus on the time course, associated symptoms (e.g., dyspnea, urinary changes, fever), unilateral versus bilateral involvement, pitting versus nonpitting edema, and risk factors for deep venous thrombosis (e.g., stasis, hypercoagulability, vessel trauma)

Initial diagnostic workup

- Initial labs may include CBC, electrolytes, BUN and creatinine, urinalysis, coagulation studies, liver function tests, serum albumin, and thyroid function tests
- Chest radiography may reveal signs of pulmonary edema or cardiomegaly
- Duplex ultrasound of the legs is useful in diagnosing deep venous thrombosis
- Echocardiography may reveal depressed ejection fraction in congestive heart failure
- Blood cultures are often indicated in immunocompromised or systemically ill patients
- Renal or liver biopsy may be necessary to diagnose cirrhosis or renal pathology leading to nephrotic syndrome

Initial patient management

- Venous insufficiency: Mild cases should respond to leg elevation, avoidance of standing for prolonged periods, and compression stockings; surgical stripping of varicosities may relieve pain in severe cases
- Congestive heart failure: Use dietary salt restriction, diuretics, digoxin, ACE inhibitors, and β-blockers to improve cardiac function and control fluid overload
- Cellulitis: Elevate extremity; use antibiotics to cover skin flora (e.g., streptococci, staphylococci)
- Deep venous thrombosis: Use anticoagulation with unfractionated heparin or low-molecular-weight heparin; duration of therapy (often 3–6 months) varies with the clinical situation
- Cirrhosis: Liver disease is typically progressive; symptoms may respond to diuretics and low salt diet; hepatic bypass procedures (e.g., TIPS) or transplantation may be necessary
- Nephrotic syndrome: 80% of cases in children are caused by minimal change disease and can be treated effectively with steroids; adults tend to have progressive illness; dialysis or renal transplant may be necessary

DIFFERENTIAL DIAGNOSIS

Venous insufficiency
- Usually bilateral swelling, but may be unilateral if caused by vessel injury (e.g., previous leg vein harvesting in cardiac bypass surgery)
- Incompetent venous valves may manifest as varicose veins
- Swelling is typically worse after the legs are held in a dependent position and is least noticeable after a night's sleep
- With long-standing disease, the overlying skin may have superficial varicose veins associated with a reddish-brown pretibial discoloration ("venous stasis skin changes")

Congestive heart failure
- Usually bilateral swelling
- Associated with pitting peripheral edema
- Other signs of heart failure include S_3, cardiomegaly, and hepatomegaly

Cirrhosis
- Usually bilateral swelling
- Advanced liver disease results in hypoalbuminemia and poor venous return through cirrhotic liver tissue
- Other stigmata of chronic liver disease include caput medusae, ascites, and spider angiomata

Nephrotic syndrome
- Usually bilateral swelling
- Glomerular damage results in protein loss and decreased oncotic pressure

Cellulitis
- Usually unilateral swelling
- The edematous leg is typically red, warm, and inflamed
- The patient may exhibit signs of systemic toxicity with fever and leukocytosis

Gout
- Usually unilateral swelling
- Mimics cellulitis with redness, warmth, and inflammation; the patient is not toxic as in cellulitis, although pain can be severe

Deep venous thrombosis
- Usually unilateral swelling
- May exhibit a palpable cord representing a thrombosed vein
- Homan's sign may be elicited: Pain in the calf occurs on passive dorsiflexion of the foot
- Hypercoagulable states, venous stasis, and vessel injury (Virchow's triad) are risk factors

Less common etiologies
- Filariasis (lymphatic infection by *Wuchereria bancrofti* worm)
- Myxedema (seen in patients with severe hypothyroidism)
- Milroy's disease (congenital lymphedema)

Epistaxis (Nosebleed)

INTRODUCTION

Bleeding from the nose may be anterior (through the nares) or posterior (through the nasopharynx or oropharynx). Anterior epistaxis (90% of cases) is generally a benign process that quickly resolves with therapy; it usually originates in Kiesselbach's plexus of vessels in the anterior nasal septum. Posterior epistaxis is a much more serious bleed that originates in the large posterior nasal vessels and is more difficult to control; it may result in significant blood loss, hypotension, or airway compromise. Bilateral or posterior nasal epistaxis suggests a medical etiology; unilateral epistaxis suggests a physical cause or local structural lesion. Because the nose protrudes from the face, trauma is common. The thin mucosal surface also often becomes dry and cracked, exposing the rich blood supply beneath.

DIAGNOSTIC WORKUP & INITIAL MANAGEMENT

- Assess vital signs and evaluate airway, breathing, and circulation
  - Ensure that patients are tolerating the bleeding and secretions; suction or intubation may be indicated in those unable to tolerate secretions or with altered mental status
  - Place 2 large-bore IVs (18 gauge) if hemodynamic compromise is a concern
- Unstable patients (hypotension, tachycardia, or hypoxia) require immediate treatment with IV fluids; if vital signs remain unstable after 2 L of fluid, blood transfusion may be indicated

History and physical examination

- History should include onset and duration of bleeding, location, quantity of blood, previous occurrences, and precipitating events (e.g., trauma, nose picking, recent nasogastric tube insertion, use of nasal cannula oxygen)
- Medical history, including previous episodes of epistaxis, previous nasal surgery, personal or family history of bleeding diathesis (e.g., hemophilia, von Willebrand's), current anticoagulant therapy, or history of hypertension (unclear whether hypertension precipitates epistaxis)
- Physical exam should evaluate for respiratory distress and accessory muscle use, identification of bleeding site, bleeding from posterior oropharynx, and signs of a bleeding diathesis (e.g., petechiae, bruising, telangiectasias)
  - Inspect for evidence of septal perforation or deviation and for the source of bleeding
  - Washing the area with normal saline or 1:1,000 epinephrine may increase visibility
  - Blood seen in the mouth without evident nasal bleeding suggests a posterior bleed

Initial workup and management

- In stable patients with active bleeding, have the patient sit upright in the "sniffing" position, compress the nares, and hold pressure for ≥10 minutes
- Following direct pressure, examine both nares and nasal passages using a nasal speculum
- If an anterior bleeding site is identified (90% of cases), consider cautery with silver nitrate
- For patients who continue to bleed but are not hypertensive and do not have a cardiac history, vasoconstrictive agents (e.g., Neo-Synephrine) can be used
- Patients who continue to bleed despite the above interventions require nasal packing or balloon catheter tamponade, preferably by an ENT specialist
  - Patients who receive nasal packing require prophylactic antibiotic therapy (e.g., amoxicillin, amoxicillin/clavulanate, clindamycin) to prevent toxic shock syndrome
- Laboratory testing may include CBC and coagulation studies, especially for patients taking anticoagulant medications, with significant bleeding, or cardiac history
  - Hematocrit may not reflect current bleeding; serial hematocrits may be indicated
  - Consider blood transfusion in patients with cardiovascular disease and a low hematocrit
  - Patients who are anticoagulated and have severe epistaxis should be rapidly reversed with a transfusion of fresh-frozen plasma
- CT of the sinuses and nasal area may be indicated to search for neoplasms
- Consider biopsy of suspicious areas and/or nasolaryngoscopy, especially in smokers

DIFFERENTIAL DIAGNOSIS

Bilateral or posterior epistaxis usually indicates a medical etiology

- Bleeding disorder (e.g., leukemias, aplastic anemia, thrombocytopenia, von Willebrand's disease, hemophilia, liver failure)
- Coagulopathy (e.g., liver failure, snake bite, infection, idiopathic thrombocytopenic purpura, TTP, uremia, disseminated intravascular coagulation, anticoagulant or antiplatelet medications)
- Trauma (e.g., nasal or facial fracture)
- Hypertension (usually severe)
  - Probably does not cause epistaxis but may inhibit the cessation of bleeding

Unilateral or anterior epistaxis usually indicates a physical cause or local structural lesion

- Irritation of the nose resulting from the common cold
- Dryness of nasal mucosa (e.g., low humidity, chronic nasal oxygen canula use without supplemental humidification)
- Allergic rhinitis
- External trauma (e.g., fistfight)
- Internal trauma (e.g., nose picking)
- Iatrogenic (e.g., nasogastric tube insertion, nasotracheal intubation)
- Foreign body
- Nasal polyps (often secondary to allergy, aspirin, or cystic fibrosis)
- Acute sinusitis
- Postsinus surgery
- Bleeding from a sinus is an uncommon presentation of bony fracture from trauma or infection
- Neoplasm (especially squamous cell carcinoma)
- Telangiectasias
- Arteriovenous malformation

Infection

- Sinusitis
- Rhinitis
- Scarlet fever
- Malaria
- Typhoid fever

Septal deviation or perforation

- Can alter nasal airflow, resulting in mucosal crusting and bleeding
- Consider the diagnosis in patients with a history of nasal fracture
- Risk factors for perforation include septal surgery, cocaine use, rheumatologic diseases, vasculitis (e.g., Wegener's granulomatosis), and sarcoidosis

Hereditary hemorrhagic telangiectasias (Osler-Weber-Rendu syndrome)

- An autosomal dominant condition that leads to small arteriovenous malformations on mucosal surfaces, including the nasal mucosa and GI tract

Nasal mass

- Juvenile nasopharyngeal angiofibroma is a rare, benign mass that most commonly presents in teenage males with recurrent epistaxis

Fatigue

INTRODUCTION

Fatigue is a very common, although nonspecific, presenting symptom that refers to the sensation of exhaustion during or after usual activities or a feeling of inadequate energy to begin such activities. Fatigue is a difficult clinical complaint, because many explanations are possible. This difficulty is compounded by the subjective nature of the complaint and the potential seriousness of some of the etiologies. A thorough history and physical examination are crucial in narrowing down the differential diagnosis and identifying serious causes.

DIAGNOSTIC WORKUP & INITIAL MANAGEMENT

History and physical examination

- Complete history and physical exam are essential, including screening for malignancy, chronic infection, chronic cardiopulmonary disease, sleep disorders, and psychiatric disease

Initial diagnostic workup

- Initial laboratory testing may include CBC, chemistries, glucose, calcium, urinalysis, liver function studies, TSH, vitamin D level, pregnancy test in women, and stool guaiac testing
- Consider age-appropriate cancer screening, possibly including Pap smear, mammography, flexible sigmoidoscopy, and PSA levels
- Further testing based on history and physical findings may include chest radiography (for dyspnea, cough, abnormal lung exam), ECG (for chest pain, dyspnea), echocardiography (for heart murmur, signs of infection, or signs of congestive heart failure), appropriate cultures and/or serologies if infection is suspected (e.g., PPD, HIV, hepatitis), ANA, ESR, RF, and Lyme disease titers
- Further testing based on abnormal initial labs may include anemia workup (reticulocyte count, iron studies, vitamin B_{12} and folate levels, hemoglobin electrophoresis), hepatitis workup (γ-glutamyl transferase, viral hepatitis serologies, liver ultrasound), renal ultrasound, bone marrow biopsy, colonoscopy, and/or thyroid function tests
- Appropriate imaging studies based on initial workup may include head CT or MRI, abdominal ultrasound or CT, cardiac stress testing, bone radiography, and/or bone scan

Initial patient management

- Treatment is targeted at the specific underlying medical problems, if determined
- Discontinue or change offending medications
- Consider regularly scheduled physical activity
- Improve sleep hygiene (e.g., regular sleep/wake times; avoidance of caffeine, alcohol, and food consumption in the late evenings; use the bedroom for sleep and sexual activity only—not television watching)
- Referral to support groups
- Chronic fatigue syndrome and fibromyalgia are often treated with supportive care, healthy diet, moderate exercise, and low-dose antidepressants
- Weight loss is advised in overweight patients
- If screening is positive for depression, consider a trial of antidepressants or referral to counseling or psychiatry

DIFFERENTIAL DIAGNOSIS

Infectious
- Acute viral or bacterial infection
- Chronic infection (e.g., subacute bacterial endocarditis, osteomyelitis, tuberculosis, HIV, viral hepatitis, mononucleosis)

Hematologic
- Anemia
- Thrombotic thrombocytopenia purpura (TTP)
- Polycythemia vera

Cardiac
- Congestive heart failure
- Congenital heart disease
- Valvular heart disease
- Coronary artery disease

Pulmonary
- COPD
- Obstructive sleep apnea
- Poorly controlled asthma

Endocrine
- Hypothyroidism or hyperthyroidism
- Diabetes mellitus, type 1 or 2
- Pregnancy
- Perimenopause
- Addison's disease

Rheumatologic
- Rheumatoid arthritis
- Systemic lupus erythematosus (SLE)
- Sjogren's syndrome
- Polymyalgia rheumatica

Gastrointestinal
- Inflammatory bowel disease (IBD)
- Portal hypertension (e.g., cirrhosis)
- Irritable bowel syndrome (IBS)

Neurologic
- Parkinson's disease
- Multiple sclerosis

Medications or drug withdrawal
- Medication side effects: β-blockers, phenytoin, digitalis, antidepressants, muscle relaxants, hypnotics
- Drug intoxication or withdrawal: alcohol, opioids, benzodiazepines, barbiturates, cocaine

Other
- Poor sleep hygiene or interrupted sleep
- Chronic fatigue syndrome
- Fibromyalgia
- Malignancy
- Acute or chronic renal failure
- Psychiatric (e.g., depression, anxiety or panic disorder, anorexia nervosa or bulimia, somatization disorder)
- Headache syndromes (e.g., tension headache)
- Primary obesity

Fever

INTRODUCTION

Fever is a nonspecific response to a variety of environmental and internal factors and is among the most frequent emergency room and outpatient presentations. Most fevers are of short duration, resolve without specific therapy, and are induced by polypeptide molecules called endogenous pyrogens, which are produced in response to infection, injury, inflammation, or antigenic challenge. True fever occurs when the body adopts a new thermoregulatory "set point" secondary to the release of pyrogenic cytokines in response to bacteria, viruses, or other sources (e.g., malignancy). In contrast, hyperthermia is an elevation of temperature without resetting of thermoregulation that occurs when heat production outstrips the body's ability to disperse excess heat (e.g., heat stroke).

DIAGNOSTIC WORKUP & INITIAL MANAGEMENT

History and physical examination

- In most cases, the cause of fever will be suggested during the history and physical exam
- Normal temperature is 36–37.8°C, with circadian rhythmicity (daily variation of 1°C); body temperature is lowest in early morning and highest in late afternoon
- Temperature is measured either orally, rectally, axillary, or tympanic (oral temperatures measured after intake of hot/cold beverages, smoking, hyperventilation may be inaccurate)
- Note characteristics of fever, maximum temperature, and presence of diurnal variation
- Evaluate current illness, symptom chronology, details of fever (e.g., duration, remitting/relapsing), and medical history, with attention to immune status
- Careful epidemiological and risk factor history is important in raising suspicion for specific diagnoses, including immunosuppression, sick contacts, employment history, exposures (e.g., animal, water, soil), sexual history, recent travel (including pretravel vaccinations and precautions, and known endemic areas), and new medications
- Physical exam should include careful search to identify clues to diagnosis (e.g., skin rash, lymphadenopathy, hepatosplenomegaly, embolic phenomena, clinical signs of meningitis or focal neurological signs, joint effusion or tenderness over spine, signs of pneumonia, costovertebral angle tenderness)

Initial diagnostic workup

- Initial tests may include CBC with differential, electrolytes, glucose, urinalysis and urine culture, blood cultures, and CRP or ESR measurement
  - Blood cultures may include a thick smear to evaluate for parasites (e.g., malaria)
- Chest radiography in patients with respiratory symptoms may reveal a focus of infection (e.g., pneumonia, tuberculosis, malignancy)
- Further investigations may include CT of the chest, abdomen, and pelvis (may reveal occult infection, abscess, or malignancy); tagged white blood cell scans (may localize an abscess); and rheumatologic tests (e.g., ANA)
- If deep venous thrombosis is suspected clinically or based on high risk, perform Doppler studies of the lower extremities without delay
- Lumbar puncture for CSF analysis may be indicated
- Echocardiography is indicated if suspect infective endocarditis or aortitis (syphilis)
- Further workup for malignancy may be warranted in certain patients (e.g., bone marrow biopsy may be indicated if suspect leukemia or a myelodysplastic syndrome)

Initial patient management

- Treat the etiology rather than the fever: Only extreme fevers (>106°F) are in themselves potentially harmful
- Young children are at risk for febrile seizures when rectal temperature exceeds 38.9°C
- Empiric therapy with antibiotics is not necessary unless the patient is hemodynamically unstable, immunocompromised, or is suspected of having bacterial meningitis

DIFFERENTIAL DIAGNOSIS

Infectious
- Respiratory, urinary, GI, and skin/soft tissue infections are the most common causes

Viral
- Influenza, acute HIV, hepatitis, herpes simplex encephalitis, mononucleosis, adenovirus, upper respiratory infection, cytomegalovirus, Epstein-Barr virus, and many others

Bacterial
- Pneumonia, endocarditis, tuberculosis, osteomyelitis, head/neck infection (e.g., meningitis, pharyngitis, dental abscess, sinusitis, otitis media), UTI (especially pyelonephritis), appendicitis, cholecystitis, cellulitis, Lyme disease, erhlichiosis, syphilis, tularemia, leptospirosis, and many others

Parasitic
- Malaria and many others

Fungal
- Candidiasis, aspergillosis, and many others

Abscess
- Intra-abdominal, brain, liver, paraspinal, occult abscess, and others

Noninfectious

Malignancy
- Lymphoma (Hodgkin's and non-Hodgkin's)
- Lymphoproliferative disorders
- Renal cell carcinoma
- Leukemia
- Hepatocellular carcinoma

Rheumatologic disorders
- Temporal arteritis/giant cell arteritis
- Adult-onset Still's disease
- SLE or rheumatoid arthritis
- Sarcoidosis

Allergy and inflammation
- Drugs (e.g., antibiotics, antineoplastic agents, anticonvulsants)
- Autoimmune disorders
- Gout or pseudogout
- Malignancy
- Fecal impaction
- Dressler's syndrome

Tissue ischemia or infarction
- Venous thromboembolism, MI, stroke, hematoma, subarachnoid hemorrhage, intramuscular injections, intestinal infarction, renal infarction, splenic infarction, pancreatitis, atheroembolic syndrome, heterotopic ossification

Postoperative or postprocedure
- Major surgery, endoscopy, transfusion reaction, infusion-related phlebitis or chemical injury, atelectasis

Autonomic and endocrine dysfunction
- CNS or spinal cord dysfunction, delirium tremens, neuroleptic malignant syndrome, thyrotoxicosis, Addison's disease

Malignant hyperthermia
- An inherited, life-threatening disorder often triggered by anesthetics (e.g., inhalational agents, succinylcholine) can cause hypermetabolism, skeletal muscle damage, and death

Fever with Rash

INTRODUCTION

Patients with fever and rash require immediate attention because some cases are life-threatening. The etiologies of rash with fever are vast, but a systematic approach will help to narrow the differential quickly. Patients who appear "toxic" with fever and prostration must be rapidly and thoroughly evaluated to rule out life-threatening infections and illnesses. Patients with fever and skin rash are categorized according to the character of the rash (e.g., petechial eruption, maculopapular, vesicobullous, erythematous), and associated symptoms and signs (e.g., cough, upper respiratory symptoms, pharyngitis, myalgias) may give clues to the diagnosis. Empiric treatment may be necessary before the results of cultures or biopsies are available.

DIAGNOSTIC WORKUP & INITIAL MANAGEMENT

History and physical examination

- History should include medication and drug history, site of rash onset, rate and direction of spread, presence or absence of pruritus, whether any topical or oral therapies have been attempted, recent travel or animal exposure and seasonality, contact with ill persons, and specific associated conditions (e.g., valvular heart disease, STDs, immune status)
- Skin lesions should be examined for character (blanching vs. nonblanching; macular, papular, or petechial), distribution and spread (truncal vs. peripheral, centripetal vs. centrifugal), configuration, excoriations, and tenderness
  - Petechial eruption: Small, red or brown lesions that do not blanch with pressure
  - Morbilliform rash: Diffuse erythematous macules or papules that may be confluent
  - Vesicobullous rash: Small vesicles, large blisters, and bullae
- Assess vital signs, general appearance, and signs of toxicity
- Note adenopathy, hepatosplenomegaly, and oral, genital, or conjunctival lesions
- Note nuchal rigidity or neurologic dysfunction

Initial workup and management

- Initial laboratory studies include CBC with differential, chemistry panel, liver function tests, and blood and urine cultures
- Aspirates, scrapings, and pustular fluid may be obtained for Gram's stain and culture
- Biopsy nonhealing or persistent purpuric lesions and inflammatory dermal nodules/ulcers
- Send urethral secretions for Gram's stain and culture if suspect STD; test for HIV and syphilis
- Evaluate ANA, RF, and ESR if suspect vasculitis
- Obtain bacterial cultures from any wounds, culture the pharynx if indicated, and consider skin biopsy and culture; blood cultures are indicated in toxic patients; consider immediate lumbar puncture for CSF culture and Gram's stain if suspect meningococcemia
- Acute and convalescent antibody titers can confirm Rocky Mountain spotted fever (RMSF); skin biopsy with immunofluorescence may demonstrate vasculitis with visible rickettsial organisms
- Toxic shock syndrome is often diagnosed by history and exam alone; recent cutaneous injury and nonspecific morbilliform rash in a hypotensive patient suggests the diagnosis
- Infectious disease and dermatology consultations are often required
- Stop all unnecessary drugs
- Typical empiric antibiotic regimens do not cover most microbial causes of fever and rash
- Think first about life-threatening causes: Fever and rash that are associated with shock (e.g., meningococcemia, gonococcemia, toxic shock syndrome) or multi-organ failure (e.g., RMSF) require emergent therapy
- Unusual antibiotics may be indicated (e.g., tetracyclines, antivirals, antifungals, macrolides, fluoroquinolones), though many causes do not benefit from antibiotics
- Corticosteroids are rarely indicated empirically and may increase morbidity and mortality

DIFFERENTIAL DIAGNOSIS

Petechial eruption with fever
- Infectious etiologies include endocarditis, meningococcemia, gonococcemia, bacteremia of any origin, hepatitis B, hepatitis C, EBV, rubella, enteroviral infection, and RMSF
- Noninfectious etiologies include allergy, thrombocytopenia, Henoch-Schönlein purpura, hypersensitivity vasculitis, acute rheumatic fever, hyperglobulinemia, amyloidosis, and SLE

Morbilliform rash with fever
- Infectious etiologies include secondary syphilis, Lyme disease, mycoplasma, meningococcemia, psittacosis, typhoid fever, rickettsiosis, RMSF, ehrlichiosis, epidemic typhus, primary HIV, and parvovirus B19
- Noninfectious etiologies include allergy, SLE, erythema multiforme, erythema marginatum, and serum sickness

Vesicobullous rash with fever
- Infectious etiologies include herpes, varicella, vaccinia virus, *Candida*, coxsackievirus, parvovirus, *Staphylococcus*, gonococcemia, *Pseudomonas*, HIV, folliculitis, erythema multiforme
- Noninfectious etiologies include allergy, eczema vaccinatum, Stevens-Johnson syndrome, toxic epidermal necrolysis

Erythematous rash with fever
- Infectious etiologies include group A *Streptococcus*, staphylococcal infection, *Streptococcus viridans*, scarlet fever, ehrlichiosis, and enteroviral infection
- Noninfectious include allergy, eczema, vasodilatation, psoriasis, pityriasis rubra

Urticarial rash with fever
- Infectious include Lyme disease, HIV, viral hepatitis, EBV, mycoplasma, adenovirus, enterovirus
- Noninfectious include allergy, malignancy, vasculitis

Important etiologies to rule out
Viral exanthems
- Leading cause of fever and rash in childhood; most children present with low-grade fevers, viral prodromal symptoms, and secondary, diffuse, morbilliform exanthem
Drug reactions
- Immune complex disease or serum sickness with many medications
Meningococcemia
- Most common in patients < 1 year, military recruits, and college students
- Abrupt onset with spiking fevers, diffuse purpuric lesions, delirium, and possibly, death
- DIC and purpura fulminans with secondary necrosis of digits and limbs can occur
Rocky Mountain spotted fever
- A fulminant and deadly rickettsial disease transmitted by a tick bite
- Characteristic rash starts acrally on wrists and ankles, spreads toward the trunk
- Initially, pink macules evolve over 10–24 hours into red papules, then purpuric macules and violaceous patches involving most of the body surface area
- Necrosis and DIC may occur
Toxic shock syndrome
- Results from *Staphylococcus aureus* or streptococci
- Rapid onset of fever, hypotension, and skin/mucosa (especially palms and soles) erythema, and subsequent multi-organ failure
- Palmar and solar desquamation occurs in 1–3 weeks
- A morbilliform rash and skin "pain" or hyperesthesia is common
- Nonsurgical and surgical wounds are often the source of infection

Flank Pain/CVA Tenderness

INTRODUCTION

Pain and/or tenderness on the side of the trunk from the ribs to the ilium is often associated with kidney or urologic disease; however, nonrenal etiologies are very common. Renal disease should be strongly suspected when costovertebral angle tenderness (CVA) occurs with concurrent urinary signs and symptoms. The absence of urinary findings should direct attention toward musculoskeletal, neurologic, vascular, and retroperitoneal etiologies.

DIAGNOSTIC WORKUP & INITIAL MANAGEMENT

History and physical examination

- Assess onset, duration, quality, intensity, aggravating or mitigating factors, location, and radiation of pain
  - Patients with urolithiasis typically have colicky pain, cannot get comfortable, and are often fidgety because of the intense discomfort
- Note associated symptoms (e.g., nausea, vomiting, fever, dysuria, hematuria, rash)
- Note history of recent trauma or illness
- Note history of spine disease
- Note family history of renal disease or cancer
- Exam should include complete cardiovascular, pulmonary, abdominal, and genitourinary exams as well as a pelvic exam if suspect ectopic pregnancy
  - Turner's sign (bluish discoloration at the flank) and/or Cullen's sign (bluish discoloration at the umbilicus) indicate retroperitoneal hemorrhage and may occur in pancreatitis or ruptured AAA
  - Pain on rib palpation may suggest fracture or metastatic disease

Initial diagnostic workup

- Workup should be guided by findings of the history and physical examination
- Initial laboratory testing may include CBC, ESR, electrolytes, BUN and creatinine, amylase and lipase, liver function tests, pregnancy test, blood cultures, urinalysis, and urine culture
- Renal ultrasound or abdominal CT may be warranted
  - Noncontrast CT is the gold standard to diagnose urolithiasis
  - Contrast CT may reveal pancreatitis, renal or splenic infarction, renal carcinoma, and renal obstruction
  - Renal ultrasound may demonstrate renal obstruction without contrast exposure
- Lumbosacral imaging may be useful if the history and exam suggest musculoskeletal or neurological etiology
  - Thoracolumbar radiography can quickly show vertebral compression fracture or degenerative joint disease
  - Thoracolumbar MRI may reveal spinal radiculopathy
- Urine cytology or cystoscopy may be indicated if suspect bladder cancer; however, bladder cancer does not usually present with flank pain (unless associated with renal obstruction)
- IV pyelography is almost never used today

DIFFERENTIAL DIAGNOSIS

Infectious etiologies
- Bacterial cystitis
- Pyelonephritis (acute or chronic)
  - *E. coli* is the most common cause of upper and lower UTIs, followed by *Staphylococcus saprophyticus*
  - Acute pyelonephritis is usually a complication of a lower UTI
  - Chronic pyelonephritis may be associated with obstruction or abnormal vesicoureteral anatomy
- Perirenal (kidney) abscess
- Herpes zoster

Nephro-urologic etiologies
- Urolithiasis is the most common urinary tract etiology
- Obstructive nephropathy
- Polycystic kidney disease
- Renal infarction or trauma
- Renal cancer
- Papillary necrosis

Musculoskeletal etiologies
- Degenerative disk disease and/or disk herniation with or without nerve root compression is the most frequent cause overall
- Muscle spasm or cramping
- Rib fracture
- Trauma

GI etiologies
- Acute pancreatitis
- Cholecystitis or biliary colic
- Appendicitis

Other
- Pneumonia
- Ectopic pregnancy
- Vasculitis (e.g., polyarteritis nodosa)

GI Bleeding, Hematemesis

INTRODUCTION

Hematemesis is defined as vomiting of blood or coffee ground–like material and suggests upper GI tract bleeding (i.e., proximal to the ligament of Treitz). The clinical presentation of upper GI bleeding varies, depending on the location, volume, briskness, and duration of the bleeding, and may include hematemesis, melena (black, tarry stools), life-threatening hemorrhage that results in hypotension and shock, occult blood loss, iron deficiency anemia, or abdominal pain. Be sure to distinguish hematemesis from hemoptysis (coughing up blood) and epistaxis (oropharyngeal bleeding).

DIAGNOSTIC WORKUP & INITIAL MANAGEMENT

- Assess severity of bleeding by measuring vital signs and orthostasis
- Administer supplemental oxygen in most patients, and ensure adequate IV access by placing 2 large-bore peripheral IVs ($\geq$18 gauge) or a central venous catheter
- Anticoagulation should be withheld, if possible
- Consider intubation for airway protection if massive bleeding or altered mental status

History and physical examination

- Note duration and amount of bleeding, presence of abdominal pain (ulcer disease, esophageal perforation, mesenteric ischemia), retching (Mallory-Weiss tear), change in bowel habits, anorexia, weight loss, medication use that may predispose to ulcers (e.g., aspirin, NSAIDs, steroids), and alcohol use
- Note previous GI disease, endoscopic procedures, and bleeding episodes
- Evaluate for alcohol abuse and liver disease (suggests bleeding esophageal varices)
- Physical exam may reveal stigmata of chronic liver disease, abdominal tenderness (ulcer disease, ischemic colitis), or evidence of non-GI bleeding (epistaxis, dental bleeding)

Initial workup and management

- First priority: Ensure patient is adequately resuscitated with IV fluids and blood
- Evaluate hematocrit, platelet count, coagulation studies, and liver function tests
  - Blood transfusion may be necessary to maintain appropriate hematocrit based on age, rate of bleeding, and comorbidities (e.g., heart disease, heart failure, renal failure)
  - Hematocrit of 30% is recommended for patients with hemodynamic instability (shock, orthostatic hypotension), serious comorbid conditions, persistent bleeding, or need for multiple blood transfusions; do not transfuse patients with documented portal hypertension to a hematocrit > 28%, because overtransfusion can elevate portal pressure
  - INR should be corrected with fresh frozen plasma if > 1.5
  - Transfuse platelets if count < 50,000/mm^3
- Diagnostic nasogastric lavage is essential in all patients with upper GI bleeding
  - Nasogastric lavage revealing bright-red blood that does not clear is an emergency requiring immediate gastroenterology consultation for emergent endoscopy
  - Nasogastric lavage revealing coffee-ground material or blood that clears confirms upper GI tract bleeding but suggests the bleeding has ceased
  - A positive lavage is confirmatory; a negative lavage does not necessarily exclude upper GI bleeding if it originates beyond the pylorus
- Upper GI endoscopy (esophagogastroduodenoscopy) is diagnostic in most cases (identifies the source of bleeding in 90% of patients) and may be therapeutic
- Angiography is indicated for severe bleeds or if endoscopy is not available or inconclusive
- EKG may be indicated to rule out cardiac ischemia secondary to severe anemia
- Upper GI bleeding generally requires monitoring in an intensive care unit
- Consider gastroenterology or general surgery consultation

DIFFERENTIAL DIAGNOSIS

Peptic ulcer disease

- The most common cause of acute upper GI hemorrhage
- Risk factors include NSAIDs (including aspirin), *H. pylori* infection, and excess acid production (e.g., Zollinger-Ellison syndrome)
- High-dose, IV proton pump inhibitor therapy reduces incidence of ulcer rebleeding and should be considered in all patients with significant upper GI bleeding; H_2-receptor antagonists do not significantly reduce the risk of ulcer rebleeding

Portal hypertension

- Can cause bleeding from many sources, including esophageal varices, gastric varices, ectopic varices, and gastropathy
- Bleeding from esophageal varices is usually massive, and patients are usually hemodynamically unstable; suspected variceal bleeding is not a contraindication to nasogastric tube placement
- Patients suspected of having portal hypertension and possible variceal bleeding should be treated with octreotide infusion
- A Sengstaken-Blakemore tube may be necessary to stabilize the patient while preparing for emergent endoscopy; if unable to control bleeding endoscopically, an emergent TIPS procedure may be indicated

Gastric erosions (erosive gastritis)

- Common cause of mild bleeding; rarely causes hemodynamically significant bleeding
- Risk factors include NSAIDs, alcohol, stress-related medical illnesses (e.g., severe trauma, extensive burns, respiratory failure, sepsis, renal failure, intracranial disease), coagulopathy, and respiratory failure

Mallory-Weiss tear

- A mucosal tear at the gastroesophageal junction; may occur during vomiting or retching
- Bleeding is usually self-limited and recurrent bleeding is uncommon

Upper GI tract malignancies

- Can rarely present with hematemesis
- Gastric carcinoma is the most common upper GI tumor associated with significant bleeding

Dieulafoy's lesion

- Uncommon, but usually results in massive bleeding
- Occurs when a mucosal blood vessel erodes through the surface epithelium
- Usually occurs within 6 cm of the gastroesophageal junction

Erosive esophagitis

- Infectious (e.g., *Candida*, HSV, cytomegalovirus)
- Corrosive ingestion
- Pill-induced (e.g., NSAIDs, aspirin, corticosteroids)

Arteriovenous malformations

- Osler-Weber-Rendu syndrome, idiopathic angiomas, radiation-induced telangiectasias, hereditary hemorrhagic telangiectasia, blue-rubber bleb nevus syndrome

Other etiologies

- Nasopharyngeal or oropharyngeal sources (e.g., epistaxis)
- Esophageal or gastric polyps
- Gastric varices secondary to splenic vein thrombosis
- Erosion of pancreatic tumor into the duodenum
- Aortoenteric fistula [suspect in any patient with known aortic graft (e.g., previous AAA repair) or occlusive aortic disease]
- Coagulopathies (e.g., hemophilia, excessive anticoagulation therapy)
- Thrombocytopenia
- Leukemia
- Connective tissue disease

GI Bleeding, Melena & Hematochezia

INTRODUCTION

Lower GI tract bleeding occurs distal to the ligament of Treitz, which separates the duodenum from the jejunum, and refers to the passage of either bright-red blood per rectum (hematochezia), maroon stools, or black, tarry stools (melena). Hematochezia suggests either bleeding from the lower intestinal tract or very brisk bleeding from higher in the intestinal tract; melena suggests the blood has had time to be processed, implying slower bleeding that usually originates higher in the intestinal tract. Most cases are isolated and self-limited. Gastroenterology consultation is often indicated to assist with patient management and timing of interventions. General surgery consultation is indicated with severe or recurrent bleeding or if the patient is hemodynamically unstable.

DIAGNOSTIC WORKUP & INITIAL MANAGEMENT

- Assess the severity of bleeding by measuring vital signs and orthostasis
- Administer supplemental oxygen in most patients, and ensure adequate IV access by placing 2 large-bore, peripheral IVs ($\geq$18 gauge) or a central venous catheter
- Anticoagulation should be withheld, if possible

History and physical examination

- Age is an important component of the history because the differential diagnosis varies based on age: Elderly patients are more likely to bleed from diverticula, angiodysplasia, ischemia, and cancer; younger patients are more likely to bleed from ulcers, IBD, infectious colitis, varices, or Meckel's diverticula
- Note duration and amount of bleeding, presence of abdominal pain (IBD, ischemic colitis), change in bowel habits, anorexia, weight loss (malignancy, IBD), medication use that increases risk of ulcers (e.g., aspirin, NSAIDs, steroids), previous aortic surgery (aortoenteric fistula, ischemic colitis), previous radiation therapy (radiation colitis), alcohol use
- Note previous GI disease, endoscopic procedures, and bleeding episodes
- Perform rectal and pelvic exams, which may reveal evidence of non-GI bleeding (e.g., vaginal bleeding, hemorrhoids)

Initial workup and management

- First priority: Ensure patient is adequately resuscitated with IV fluids and blood transfusions
- Laboratory testing may include CBC, coagulation workup (PT/PTT/INR, bleeding time, platelet count), glucose, electrolytes, BUN/creatinine, liver function tests, albumin, toxicology screen (e.g., for alcohol), and stool ova/parasites culture
  - Blood transfusion may be necessary to maintain appropriate hematocrit based on age, rate of bleeding, and comorbidities (e.g., heart disease, heart failure, renal failure)
  - Hematocrit of 30% is recommended for hemodynamic instability (shock or orthostatic hypotension), serious comorbidities, persistent bleeding
  - INR should be corrected with fresh-frozen plasma if > 1.5
  - Transfuse platelets if count $< 50,000/mm^3$
- Determine source of bleeding:
  - Rule out upper GI bleeding by nasogastric tube aspiration or upper GI endoscopy
  - Perform abdominal radiography before colonoscopy to rule out perforation or obstruction
  - Colonoscopy is the test of choice; it allows direct visualization of the mucosa and provides a means of treatment; flexible sigmoidoscopy if a lesion is in the distal colon
  - Angiography may be indicated in active bleeding or if colonoscopy is inconclusive; it is highly specific and permits therapeutic intervention to stop bleeding
- EKG may be indicated to rule out cardiac ischemia secondary to severe anemia
- Nasogastric lavage is necessary in cases of massive bleeding or hemodynamic instability
- Red blood cell scintigraphy is a highly sensitive, non-invasive test (but poorly specific)
- Consider capsule endoscopy or enteroscopy if the source of bleeding is not identified

DIFFERENTIAL DIAGNOSIS

Anatomic lesions
- Diverticular bleeding: Most common cause of massive hematochezia in the elderly
  - Often associated with mild, crampy pain, but may be painless
  - Most episodes ($\sim$ 75%) are isolated and self-limited
  - Patients with recurrent bleeding may require surgery
- Meckel's diverticulum: Common cause of acute bleeding in patients <30 years
  - The diverticulum contains acid-secreting gastric cells, which can cause ulceration of the GI mucosa
  - Bleeding is usually brisk and painless
  - A radiolabeled technetium scan (Meckel's scan) is diagnostic

Vascular lesions
- Angiodysplasia (arteriovenous malformation) accounts for 20%–30% of cases
  - More common in the elderly and in patients with renal failure
  - Most patients present with occult bleeding, but some have acute, painless hematochezia or episodic, self-limited bleeding

Neoplastic lesions
- Colon cancer accounts for 10% of cases in patients > 50 years but is rare in younger patients
  - Generally presents as low-grade, recurrent bleeding
  - Bright-red blood suggests left-sided lesions; right-sided lesions may present with maroon blood or melena
- Polyps and masses of the small bowel and colon usually present with occult blood loss but may present as hematochezia
  - Postpolypectomy hemorrhage complicates < 1% of polypectomies but can occur from 24 hours to 3 weeks following the procedure
- Rectal cancer
- Small bowel tumors

Inflammatory lesions
- Inflammatory bowel disease often presents in a young patient with abdominal pain, weight loss, and bloody diarrhea
  - Mild to moderate hematochezia is a common feature of ulcerative colitis; bleeding usually occurs from the rectum
- Colitis (e.g., infectious colitis, ischemic colitis, radiation colitis)
  - Ischemic colitis generally presents with abdominal pain, distension, and bloody diarrhea in patients > 50 years; most cases mild and self-limited, and treatment is supportive
  - Radiation colitis and radiation proctitis generally present 2–3 weeks after a course of radiation but can occur as early as 24 hours or as late as years afterward
  - Infectious colitis is most commonly caused by *Salmonella*, *Shigella*, and *Campylobacter*

Anorectal lesions
- Hemorrhoids are the most common cause of rectal bleeding (usually painless) in patients < 50 years
- Fissures
- Polyps
- Idiopathic rectal ulcers

Other diagnoses
- Aortoenteric fistula is a surgical emergency
  - Suspect diagnosis in any patient with aortic graft (e.g., previous aortic aneurysm repair, occlusive aortic disease) or known AAA
- Idiopathic in up to 15% of cases
- Brisk upper GI tract bleeding
- Systemic bleeding disorders (e.g., hemophilia, excessive anticoagulation, thrombocytopenia)

Gynecomastia

INTRODUCTION

Gynecomastia, or breast swelling, refers to a noninflammatory enlargement of the male breast. It typically results from an excess of estrogen relative to androgens/testosterone. It is defined histologically as a benign proliferation of the glandular tissue of the male breast and clinically by the presence of a mass extending concentrically from the nipple. Gynecomastia is common in infant, adolescent, and middle-aged or older males. Differentiate from lipomastia, which is swelling of the breast caused by fatty tissue proliferation. Diagnosis is usually clinical, but further laboratory or radiologic evaluation may be necessary to determine the etiology.

DIAGNOSTIC WORKUP & INITIAL MANAGEMENT

History and physical examination
- Assess medical history, family history, developmental and growth history, and medication history
- Note decreased libido or erectile dysfunction
- Signs of breast cancer may include a rubbery or firm mass, asymmetric growth, skin dimpling or other rash, nipple retraction, discharge, and axillary lymphadenopathy
- Assess for jaundice, ascites, and edema
- Assess for goiter, thyroid nodule, tremor, and tachycardia
- Include a testicular exam for masses or pain

Initial diagnostic workup
- If gynecomastia is of recent onset, painful, or tender, initial laboratory testing may include β-hCG level, LH, testosterone, TSH, estradiol, liver function tests, BUN and creatinine, prolactin, and DHEA-S
- Mammography may be indicated to evaluate for cancer
- Ultrasound may distinguish normal glandular tissue from worrisome solid lesions
- Karyotype analysis may be indicated to diagnose Klinefelter's syndrome (XXY)

Initial patient management and follow-up
- Many cases regress spontaneously without treatment
- In adolescents with a normal physical exam, the diagnosis is likely pubertal gynecomastia; gradual improvement with age supports this diagnosis
- Discontinue offending medications (listed below), if possible
- Three types of medical therapy are available for elderly patients with severe pain, tenderness, or embarrassment:
  - Androgens (e.g., testosterone, dihydrotestosterone, danazol)
  - Antiestrogens (e.g., clomiphene, tamoxifen)
  - Aromatase inhibitors (e.g., testolactone)
- Surgical therapy (liposuction, direct surgical excision) may be indicated if there is no response to medical therapy, especially if the condition is present for >1 year
- Treat underlying medical conditions as necessary

DIFFERENTIAL DIAGNOSIS

- Physiologic gynecomastia of puberty
- Persistent postpubertal or elderly gynecomastia
- Lipomastia (e.g., obesity)
- Idiopathic
- Medications (e.g., estrogens, antiandrogens, spironolactone, nifedipine, digitalis, isoniazid, phenytoin, griseofulvin, cimetidine, omeprazole, tricyclic antidepressants, metoclopramide)
- Illicit drugs (especially marijuana, also heroin)
- Anabolic steroids
- Liver disease
  - Cirrhosis
  - Hepatitis
  - Hemochromatosis
- Chronic renal insufficiency
  - 50% of men on dialysis have gynecomastia
- Hypogonadism
  - Klinefelter's syndrome
  - Enzymatic defects in androgen synthesis or action (e.g., 3β-and 17β-hydroxysteroid dehydrogenase)
  - Testicular trauma
  - Infection
- Thyroid disease (especially hyperthyroidism)
- Pituitary disease
  - Acromegaly (excess growth hormone)
  - Chromophobe adenoma
- Androgen insensitivity or resistance (e.g., testicular feminization syndrome)
- Neoplasms
  - Breast cancer
  - Testicular cancer
  - Adrenal cancer
  - Hepatocellular carcinoma
  - Lung cancer
  - Carcinoid
- Ulcerative colitis
- Refeeding after starvation
- Local irradiation

Halitosis

INTRODUCTION

Halitosis, or bad breath, may be acute or chronic, depending on the underlying cause. It may indicate the need for improved dental hygiene or be a symptom of an underlying infection or chronic disease. Acute halitosis is usually caused by an upper respiratory infection, such as stomatitis, tonsillitis, sinusitis, or postnasal drip. Chronic halitosis is more likely to be caused by dental problems, such as dental caries, faulty dentistry, or periodontal disease. Oral disease constitutes ~90% of the etiologies of halitosis, whereas upper respiratory and stomach disease causes much of the remainder of cases. Other etiologies are relatively uncommon.

DIAGNOSTIC WORKUP & INITIAL MANAGEMENT

History and physical examination

- Careful dental and medical history, including dental hygiene habits and dietary history
  - Note onset, duration, and severity of symptoms, including associated symptoms that may suggest a systemic etiology (e.g., cough, nasal congestion, fever, sore throat, tachypnea)
  - Note medical history, including history of recurrent pneumonia, GI upset, or digestive problems
  - Odor after sleeping, dieting, or exercising suggests xerostomia
  - Odor on talking suggests postnasal drip
  - Bleeding gums suggests periodontal disease
- Dental examination to rule out treatable dental causes (e.g., periodontal disease, dental decay, uncemented prostheses)
- Physical exam should include oral, nasal, sinus, neck, pulmonary, and abdominal exams
  - Examine the oral cavity for dental hygiene, dental caries, gingival swelling, and orthodontic devices or dentures that are poorly fitting or poorly maintained
  - Assess odor from the mouth and nose separately
  - Small, malodorous, whitish stones on the tongue suggest tonsilloliths
  - Place dentures into plastic bag for several minutes, then smell to evaluate for denture odor
  - Spoon test involves scooping mucus/saliva from back of tongue and evaluating for malodor; if present, suggests postnasal drip

Initial diagnostic workup

- Consider throat culture if suspect streptococcal pharyngitis
- Radiography or CT of the sinuses may be indicated to assess for mucosal thickening or air-fluid levels
- Lateral radiography may be indicated to assess for adenoid hypertrophy
- Nasolaryngoscopy may be indicated if suspect nasal cause
- Chest radiography if suspect a pulmonary lesion
- Endoscopy may be necessary if suspect GERD or bezoar
- Zenker's diverticulum is diagnosed by contrast barium swallow

Initial patient management

- Improve oral hygiene (e.g., brush teeth at least twice per day, floss daily, treat underlying periodontal disease)
- Avoid exacerbating medications or foods
- Brush the tongue during toothbrushing
- Gargle with chlorhexidine mouthwash twice a day for a week and assess improvement
- Treat postnasal drip (e.g., saline rinse, antihistamines, nasal steroids, polyp removal)
- Decrease or eliminate alcohol and tobacco use
- Treat sinusitis and other nonviral infections with appropriate antibiotics
- Treat other underlying medical diseases (e.g., diabetic ketoacidosis, uremia, GERD)

DIFFERENTIAL DIAGNOSIS

Head and neck etiologies
Consumption of odor-producing foods
- Such as onion or garlic

Dental conditions
- Dry mouth (xerostomia)
  - Results in alteration of the oral mucosa
  - May be caused by chronic mouth breathing (e.g., nasal polyps, adenoid hypertrophy, allergic rhinitis, chronic sinusitis), side effect of medications, salivary gland disease, or dehydration
- Periodontal disease/gingivitis
- Bacterial accumulation on the teeth or tongue
- Denture odor
- Orthodontic devices
- Dental abscess (may result from untreated dental caries, dental fracture, or poor hygiene)
- Food concretions within the tonsillar crypts
- Food particles not cleaned from teeth

Upper respiratory disorders
- Stomatitis
- Sinusitis (most commonly the maxillary sinuses)
- Pharyngitis
- Tonsillitis
- Tonsillar abscess
- Allergic rhinitis
- Postnasal drip
- Nasal foreign body

Systemic etiologies
Pulmonary disorders
- Pulmonary abscess
- Bronchiectasis
- Pneumonia
- Neoplasms
- Tuberculosis

Gastric and esophageal disorders
- GERD
- Zenker's (pharyngoesophageal) diverticulum
- Bezoar

Other
- Tobacco or alcohol use
- Diabetes mellitus, especially with ketoacidosis
- Uremia
- Trimethylaminuria (fishy breath odor)
- Liver failure (fetor hepaticus)
- Menstruation may exacerbate halitosis

Hallucinations

INTRODUCTION

Hallucinations are psychotic symptoms in which patients perceive stimuli that do not exist. Any of the five senses (auditory, visual, tactile, gustatory, or olfactory) may be involved, with auditory hallucinations being the most common. Patients may believe the hallucinations to be true, or they may identify them as false. Distinguish all hallucinations from illusions (i.e., the misinterpretation of real but ambiguous stimuli). The patient's medical and psychiatric condition as well as the type and duration of hallucinations are important in reaching the correct diagnosis.

DIAGNOSTIC WORKUP & INITIAL MANAGEMENT

History and physical examination

- In caring for patients with major psychiatric illness, follow three important principles:
  - Know the patient's drug regimen
  - Work with a psychiatrist if changes are needed
  - Remember that chronic psychiatric patients have difficulty communicating medical history and needs
- A diagnosis of schizophrenia requires two positive or negative symptoms present for a month and signs continuing for at least 6 months (DSM-IV criteria)
- Assess for suicidal and homicidal ideations
- Note the timing of hallucinations (e.g., following alcohol or drug use, at random, under stress)

Initial diagnostic workup

- Initial testing may include electrolytes, glucose, calcium, BUN and creatinine, albumin, liver function tests, alkaline phosphatase, magnesium, phosphate, CBC, ECG, pulse oximetry, urinalysis, toxicology screen, and drug levels
- Chest radiography may be indicated for infectious etiologies of delirium
- Lumbar puncture may be indicated
- If suspect delirium, further tests include vitamin B_{12} and folate levels, ANA, ammonia, and heavy metal screen
- EEG may reveal slowing activity in delirium, low-voltage fast activity in alcohol withdrawal
- Consider psychiatric consult after medical causes of psychosis are ruled out

Initial patient management

- Treat hallucinations symptomatically with antipsychotic drugs (e.g., haloperidol, risperidone, olanzepine)
- In cases of delirium, treat the underlying cause (e.g., hydration, proper nutrition, oxygen, thiamine, glucose)
- In cases of alcohol or sedative withdrawal, monitor closely and treat for seizures with benzodiazepines
- Treat schizophrenia with traditional antipsychotics (e.g., haloperidol, chlorpromazine)
  - Extrapyramidal side effects (parkinsonism, akathesia, dystonia) are common
  - Neuroleptic malignant syndrome (hyperthermia, rigidity, hypertension, tachycardia) may rarely occur during the first week of treatment and can be fatal
  - Clozapine has a 1% chance of fatal agranulocytosis

DIFFERENTIAL DIAGNOSIS

Delirium
- Develops over hours to days
- Fluctuates throughout the day
- Causes include dehydration, drug-induced, electrolyte imbalance, UTI, hypoglycemia, and alcohol or drug withdrawal
- Occurs in 10%–30% of hospitalized patients
- Drug-induced delirium (e.g., cocaine, β-blockers, alcohol, corticosteroids, pseudoephedrine, dopaminergic drugs)

Alcohol withdrawal (delirium tremens)
- Often presents in hospitalized patients ~3 days after admission
- Commonly presents with tactile hallucinations (e.g., formication, which is the sense of insects crawling over the body)
- May be accompanied by seizure activity

Hallucinogenic syndromes
- LSD
- Marijuana
- Mescaline
- Phencyclidine
- Mushrooms
- Amphetamines

Schizophrenia
- Auditory hallucinations are most frequent; visual hallucinations occur in ~50% of patients, tactile in ~20%, olfactory in ~6%
- Progresses to positive psychotic symptoms (e.g., hallucinations, delusions, thought disorder) and/or negative symptoms (e.g., anhedonia, poor concentration, flattened affect, poor social/personal function)
- 1% incidence in the general population

Charles Bonnet syndrome
- Also referred to as "release hallucinations"
- Formed and unformed hallucinations can occur with visual loss caused by ocular problems or damage to the occipital lobe
- Reassure patients they are not having mental problems when they experience release hallucinations

Other
- Schizophreniform disorder
- Schizoaffective disorder
- Posttraumatic stress disorder
- Dementia
- SLE (auditory hallucinations may be caused by corticosteroids; visual and tactile hallucinations may be caused by lupus psychosis)
- Bipolar disorder
- Psychotic depression
- Postpartum major depression
- Mass lesions
- CNS infections/encephalitis
- Seizures
- Occipital lobe injury
- Heavy metal ingestion
- Lewy body dementia

Headache

INTRODUCTION

Headache is one of the most common primary care complaints. It may be an isolated or a recurrent event, idiopathic or secondary to an underlying structural lesion, and simply require an analgesic for pain relief or a complete and detailed workup for its source. One must distinguish benign from malignant and life-threatening causes and treat appropriately. The pathophysiology of primary headaches is poorly understood. Proposed mechanisms include vascular (vascular spasm, dilatation, constriction), neuronal (release of inflammatory cytokines), and serotonin imbalance. Other causes include increased intracranial pressure, compression of cranial or spinal nerves, muscle spasms, and inflammation of cranial or cervical musculature.

DIAGNOSTIC WORKUP & INITIAL MANAGEMENT

History and physical examination

- History should focus on onset, duration, frequency, location, possible triggers, severity, quality (e.g., throbbing, band-like), accompanying symptoms (e.g., aura, photophobia, visual changes, nausea/vomiting, lacrimation, nasal congestion), constitutional symptoms (e.g., weight loss, fever), medications, and dietary history
- Assess whether this is "the first or worst headache of your life"
- Note signs of increased intracranial pressure (papilledema) and focal neurologic symptoms
- Include neurologic, visual/retinal, head and neck, and gait exams
- Search for "red flags" that increase the likelihood of a more serious diagnosis
  - "Red flag" symptoms include sudden onset; new onset of severe headache in a patient >50 years; presence of systemic illness, malaise, nausea, vomiting (especially early morning vomiting), or stiff neck; accompanying seizure or history of chronic disease with frequent neurologic complications (e.g., HIV, cancer)
  - "Red flag" signs include abnormal vital signs (e.g., fever, hypertension, tachycardia), altered level of consciousness, meningeal irritation (e.g., Brudzinski's and Kernig's signs), papilledema and retinal hemorrhages, or neurological signs (e.g., weakness, numbness, gait problems, aphasia, changes in personality)

Initial workup and management

- Order head CT without contrast emergently if suspect head trauma, subarachnoid hemorrhage, cerebral infarct, pseudotumor cerebri, or subdural or epidural hematomas; CT with contrast may be indicated if suspect brain abscess or neoplasm and in patients with AIDS or cancer
- Initial blood tests may include CBC and blood cultures if suspect infection, ESR if suspect temporal arteritis, electrolytes to evaluate for metabolic abnormalities, and coagulation studies if suspect hemorrhage or bleeding abnormalities
- Lumbar puncture may be indicated to evaluate for infection, meningitis, pseudotumor, or hemorrhage (CT may be indicated before lumbar puncture to rule out increased intracranial pressure); measure opening pressure and send for CSF analysis
- Serologies for bacterial, viral, and other causes of meningitis or encephalitis
- ESR suggests temporal arteritis or infection
- Carboxyhemoglobin measurement if history suggests carbon monoxide poisoning

Initial patient management

- Assess for serious underlying conditions, and treat accordingly
- Eliminate potentially causative medications, including over-the-counter and alternative/complementary medications
- Educate the patient to identify triggers; a log of headache frequency and timing may help

DIFFERENTIAL DIAGNOSIS

Primary headache syndromes

- Migraine headache: Results from inflammation and hyperreactivity of the cerebral vasculature; may present with throbbing headache, photophobia or phonophobia, and nausea or vomiting that generally lasts several hours; usually has identifiable triggers (e.g., bright light, stress, chocolate, cheese, alcohol, oral contraceptives)
- Cluster headache: Results in abrupt onset of steady, unilateral, retro-orbital pain that generally lasts 45 minutes to 2 hours; patients are often restless (i.e., won't lie down)
- Tension-type headache: a bilateral, "bandlike" headache caused by muscle spasm

Meningitis

- A serious etiology of headache that requires emergent head CT, lumbar puncture, and empiric antibiotics (administer antibiotics immediately on suspicion of meningitis)
- Characteristic symptoms include headache, fever, neck stiffness, and altered mental status
- Pneumococcal meningitis has a mortality rate that approaches 30%
- Brudzinski's sign: Neck pain on passive flexion of neck *hip*
- Kernig's sign: Neck pain and flexion on passive extension of knee with hips flexed

Subarachnoid hemorrhage

- Sudden onset of severe headache (often termed "the worst headache of my life")
- Most commonly results from rupture of a cerebral aneurysm or head trauma
- Head CT may reveal blood in the cisterns but is only 95% sensitive (during the first 12 hours); if strongly suspect, lumbar puncture is necessary to rule out the diagnosis
- On lumbar puncture, evidence of hemoglobin breakdown products (xanthochromia) may indicate recent subarachnoid hemorrhage (within past 2 weeks)
- Immediate neurosurgery consult if subarachnoid hemorrhage is discovered

Intracranial hemorrhage secondary to stroke

- 25% of cases of sudden onset of severe headache result from intracranial hemorrhage
- Presents as a sudden, severe headache with neurologic deficits (e.g., aphasia, paralysis)
- Head CT is the best test to reveal the hemorrhage
- Immediate blood pressure control is necessary to the minimize size of hemorrhage
- Neurosurgery should be consulted immediately

Pseudotumor cerebri

- Occurs primarily in young, obese females
- Headache is caused by increased intracranial pressure
- In contrast to stroke, focal neurologic findings are absent
- Headache may be associated with blurred vision, nausea, tinnitus, and papilledema
- CT may reveal slitlike ventricles; lumbar puncture reveals high opening pressure

Temporal arteritis

- A common cause of headache in patients >60 years
- Often presents with unilateral temporal headache, myalgias, jaw claudication, elevated ESR (>100), and visual changes (may include blindness)
- Temporal artery biopsy is indicated for definitive diagnosis
- Steroids should be administered immediately

Other etiologies

- Allergic rhinitis and chronic sinusitis
- Head trauma
- Medications
- Carbon monoxide exposure
- TMJ syndrome or dental pain
- Withdrawal from alcohol, barbiturates, caffeine, or other substance
- Mass lesions (e.g., tumor, hematoma)
- Glaucoma
- Chronic daily headache or rebound headache (i.e., secondary to chronic analgesic use)
- Benign intracranial hypertension

Hearing Loss

INTRODUCTION

Hearing loss affects ~10% of the U.S. population. Two broad categories of hearing loss exist: conductive and sensorineural. Conductive hearing loss results from any process that prevents sound from reaching the inner ear. Sensorineural hearing loss refers to nerve-type hearing loss in either the inner ear or the auditory nerve. Early diagnosis allows early intervention, which has important implications for speech and language development in children. Acute or chronic exposure to excessive loud noises is a common cause.

DIAGNOSTIC WORKUP & INITIAL MANAGEMENT

History and physical examination

- Otologic history should include duration of hearing loss, laterality, associated symptoms (e.g., otorrhea, tinnitus, dizziness), risk factors for sensorineural hearing loss, family history, and a focused medical history (e.g., exposure to gentamicin, history of infections)
- Physical exam should assess the external auditory canal for patency and evaluate the tympanic membrane for perforation or cholesteatoma
- Weber's and Rhinne's tuning fork testing may be used to determine conductive versus sensorineural hearing loss; however, audiography is the definitive test

Initial diagnostic testing

- Audiometric testing provides an objective test of nerve function
  - Classifies hearing loss as conductive, sensorineural, or mixed
  - Quantifies the extent of hearing loss for the full spectrum of sound frequencies
  - If too young for ear-specific behavioral testing, obtain otoacoustic emission and auditory brainstem response testing; this is increasingly used to screen for hearing loss in newborns
- CT of the temporal bones may be helpful in evaluating conductive hearing loss
- MRI with gadolinium is indicated for all patients with unilateral sensorineural hearing loss or tinnitus to evaluate for acoustic neuroma

Initial patient management

- In many cases, the physical exam is therapeutic, because it involves cleaning the ear canal
- For middle ear effusions, a course of antibiotics and observation is usually sufficient; if symptoms persist, myringotomy and tube placement may be indicated
- Hearing aids are helpful in most cases of conductive or sensorineural hearing loss
- Acute, profound hearing loss is sometimes treated with steroids, which may prevent permanent hearing loss
- Middle-ear implantable devices may be indicated for moderate to severe sensorineural hearing loss
- Cochlear implants may be indicated for severe to profound sensorineural hearing loss if hearing aids are of minimal to no benefit
- Reconstructive middle ear surgery may be necessary and includes tympanoplasty and stapedectomy
- Prevent additional hearing loss with ear protection
- In the case of cholesteatoma, immediate attention by an otolaryngologist is necessary for resection and possible mastoidectomy to preserve hearing

DIFFERENTIAL DIAGNOSIS

Conductive hearing loss
Obstruction of the ear canal
- Usually caused by cerumen impaction or foreign body in external auditory canal
Otitis media with middle ear effusion
- Most common in children, but also occurs in adults
Chronic otitis media
- Results in permanent insult to the ear, such as tympanic membrane perforation, ossicular chain discontinuity and fixation, cholesteatoma, or external auditory canal stenosis
Middle ear tumor
- Paraganglioma (glomus tympanicum)
- Facial neuroma
- Histiocytosis X
Ossicular erosion or fixation
- Results from middle ear disease
Cholesteatoma
- May be congenital or acquired
Tympanic membrane perforation
- Usually occurs secondary to trauma or chronic otitis media
Congenital atresia of the external auditory canal

Sensorineural hearing loss
Presbycusis (age-related hearing loss)
- The most common form of sensorineural hearing loss
Acoustic trauma (noise-induced hearing loss)
- Often results from occupational exposure
Hereditary sensorineural hearing loss
- Usually autosomal recessive heritance
Ototoxic medications
- Aminoglycosides, cytotoxic chemotherapeutic agents (e.g., cisplatin), diuretics (especially loop diuretics), and salicylates have been implicated
Meniere's disease
- Usually presents with hearing loss, tinnitus, vertigo, and aural fullness
Cerebellopontine angle tumor (unilateral hearing loss)
- Vestibular schwannoma (acoustic neuroma)
- Meningioma
Alport's syndrome
- Presents as hereditary nephritis, sensorineural deafness, and ocular abnormalities
Autoimmune disease
- Such as vasculitis, scleroderma, or Kawasaki's disease
Congenital long QT syndrome

Mixed hearing loss (both conductive and sensorineural hearing loss)
- Wardenberg's syndrome and other hereditary congenital deafness syndromes
- Other causes of congenital hearing loss (infection, kernicterus, temporal bone anomaly)
- Meningitis
- Vascular (e.g., embolism, thrombosis, hemorrhage)
- Viral (e.g., mumps, measles, influenza, varicella, adenovirus, Epstein-Barr virus)

Heart Murmurs

INTRODUCTION

Systolic heart murmurs may be either benign or pathologic. Diastolic, continuous, or very loud murmurs are never normal and should always be further evaluated. The part of the cardiac cycle that the murmur falls into (early, middle, or late) and the specific characteristics of the murmur will help in determining the etiology.

DIAGNOSTIC WORKUP & INITIAL MANAGEMENT

History and physical examination
- Complete history and physical exam, emphasizing the cardiac and pulse exams
  - Careful cardiac auscultation should be done from the patient's right side with the patient's clothing or gown removed
  - Note the timing, tempo, quality, shape, location, and radiation of the murmur
  - Note the effect of cardiac maneuvers (e.g., Valsalva, squatting, amyl nitrate, and deep inspiration) on the murmur
- Assess associated symptoms, if any
- Assess medical history of heart disease, murmurs, or rheumatic fever
- Note family history of sudden cardiac death

Initial diagnostic workup
- Initial tests may include ECG, chest radiography, and/or echocardiography
- Laboratory studies may include CBC, electrolytes, glucose, BUN and creatinine, TSH, liver function tests, pulse oximetry, and ABG analysis
- Consider cardiac enzymes and blood cultures, if indicated

Initial patient management
- Consider cardiology consultation
- Pay close attention to symptoms and hemodynamic status
- Treat the underlying cause (e.g., anemia, infection, hyperthyroidism, MI)
- Perform serial examinations to track progression of the underlying cause
- Valve repair or replacement may be indicated for severe valvular disease
- Antibiotic prophylaxis may be indicated for dental work or invasive procedures

DIFFERENTIAL DIAGNOSIS

Systolic murmurs

- Mitral valve prolapse
  - Late systolic murmur with midsystolic click; murmur shifts with cardiac maneuvers
- Aortic stenosis
  - A harsh, crescendo-decrescendo ejection murmur heard best at right second intercostal space with radiation to neck; if severe, may be associated with a diminished carotid pulse with classic "pulsus parvus et tardus" upstroke and associated systolic thrill
- Aortic sclerosis
  - Heard best at the right second intercostal space at midsystole; carotid pulse is normal (in contrast to aortic stenosis)
- Cervical venous hum
  - Disappears upon pressing of the jugular vein
- Hepatic venous hum
  - Disappears with epigastric pressure
- Mammary souffle
  - Occurs in pregnancy; disappears upon compression of the breast
- Bicuspid (or unicuspid) aortic valve
  - Systolic ejection click heard best at right second intercostal space during early systole
- Mitral insufficiency
  - A holosystolic murmur that radiates to the axilla and is heard best in the left lateral decubitus position; S_1 is usually diminished in intensity
- Tricuspid insufficiency
  - A holosystolic murmur at the second or third intercostal space
- Hypertrophic cardiomyopathy
  - Prominent S_4 and loud, late-peaking, crescendo-decrescendo murmur; may have a holosystolic murmur at the apex that radiates to the axilla if mitral regurgitation coexists
- Innocent systolic murmur
  - Also known as a flow, vibratory, or Still's murmur
  - May be caused by increased flow states (e.g., anemia, hypovolemia, fever)

Diastolic murmurs

- Aortic insufficiency
  - Decrescendo or "blowing" murmur heard best at the right second intercostal space associated with bifid or bisferiens carotid upstroke; Austin Flint murmur is a late diastolic rumble from severe aortic regurgitation that causes mitral regurgitation
- Mitral stenosis
  - Opening snap with middiastolic rumble, especially in left lateral decubitus position
- Pulmonic valve insufficiency
  - Accentuated P_2 and decrescendo murmur at the left second or third intercostal space
- Tricuspid stenosis
  - Mid-diastolic rumble at the left sternal border that increases with inspiration
- Carey-Coombs murmur
  - Mid-diastolic murmur associated with acute rheumatic fever

Other etiologies of systolic or diastolic murmurs

- Endocarditis
- Coarctation of the aorta
- Prosthetic valve noises
- Papillary muscle dysfunction
- Patent ductus arteriosus
- Pulmonary artery stenosis
- Atrial myxoma ("tumor plop")
- Pericardial friction rub
- Hyperthyroidism
- Pericardial knock (constrictive pericarditis)
- Atrial or ventricular septal defect
- Left ventricular outflow tract obstruction
- Pulmonic valve stenosis or outflow obstruction
- Coronary or pulmonary arteriovenous fistula
- Bronchial collaterals (congenital heart disease)
- Anomalous pulmonary venous drainage with left-to-right shunt

Heart Rate, Bradycardia

INTRODUCTION

Bradycardia is defined as heart rate of < 60 beats per minute (bpm). It may be caused by primary cardiac dysfunction or be secondary to the influence of extrinsic, noncardiac factors. It is often benign and generally does not require treatment in the absence of symptoms. In fact, bradycardia is a normal finding in well-trained athletes with good vagal tone. Rarely, syncope may occur. The classical syncopal episode caused by a bradyarrhythmia is a Stokes-Adams attack, characterized by a sudden, immediate collapse with loss of consciousness. Patients appear pale and still, as if dead, for up to 1–2 minutes and then recover rapidly. More commonly, patients with bradyarrhythmia may simply feel fatigued or dizzy. Some are completely asymptomatic despite a heart rate as low as 30 bpm and complete heart block.

DIAGNOSTIC WORKUP & INITIAL MANAGEMENT

History and physical examination

- Thorough review of systems to identify associated symptoms (e.g., palpitations, dyspnea, dizziness, presyncope or syncope, chest pain, mental status changes) and precipitants of increased vagal tone (e.g., nausea, pain, headache)
- Thorough medication history, including over-the-counter medicines; consider the possibility of inadvertent administration of an incorrect medication or overdose
- Exam may reveal irregular heartbeat, jugular venous distension (cannon A waves suggest AV dissociation), S_4 gallop, variable intensity of carotid upstrokes, or heart failure

Initial diagnostic workup

- ECG is often diagnostic
  - Sinus bradycadia: P waves have normal contour and occur before each QRS complex; P-R interval is constant
  - 1st-degree AV block: Prolonged P-R (>200 ms), each P wave is followed by a QRS
  - 2nd-degree AV block, Mobitz I: Progressive prolongation of P-R interval and shortening of R-R interval until a p wave is not conducted; usually has a narrow QRS complex
  - 2nd-degree AV block, Mobitz II: Regular sinus or atrial rhythm with intermittent, nonconducted p waves; QRS complex may be wide; P-R interval is fixed and may be prolonged
  - 3rd-degree AV block: Atrial impulses consistently fail to reach ventricles; atrial and ventricular rhythms are independent; P-R interval varies; P-P and R-R intervals are constant; atrial rate exceeds ventricular rate (maintained by junctional or escape rhythm)
- Consider thyroid tests, electrolytes, calcium, magnesium, glucose, and toxicology screen
- Consider 24–48 hour ambulatory ECG monitoring (e.g., Holter monitor)
- Electrophysiology testing may be indicated if bradycardia mechanism is uncertain
- Exercise stress testing may be useful to evaluate for sinus node dysfunction

Initial patient management

- Asymptomatic cases (sinus bradycardia 1st-degree block, Mobitz I) do not require therapy
- Emergent treatment is indicated for symptomatic bradycardia: Atropine and epinephrine are indicated for asystole, symptomatic bradycardia, or symptomatic AV block
  - Dopamine may also be used if hypotension and bradycardia
  - Repeated coughing may also help in some cases
  - Emergency transcutaneous and/or transvenous cardiac pacing is indicated for asystole, symptomatic bradycardia, and patients at high risk of progression to asystole (e.g., Mobitz II or 3rd-degree heart block)
- Bradycardia induced by β-blockers or calcium channel blockers is treated by discontinuing the offending medications and administration of IV glucagon and calcium
- Bradycardia due to digoxin toxicity may be treated with Digibind if life-threatening
- Permanent pacemaker implantation may be indicated for symptomatic, irreversible cases

DIFFERENTIAL DIAGNOSIS

Etiologies intrinsic to the heart
- Idiopathic degeneration (occurs in elderly due to fibrosis of the conduction system)
- Acute myocardial ischemia or infarction (especially of inferior or anterior walls)
- Congenital heart disease (disruption between the atrium and AV node occurs in a significant proportion of congenital heart diseases)
- Paravalvular abscess caused by endocarditis
- Surgical trauma, including valve replacement (due to the conduction system edema)
- Infiltrative diseases (e.g., sarcoidosis, amyloidosis, hemochromatosis)
- Infectious diseases (e.g., Chagas' disease, Lyme disease, endocarditis, myocarditis)

Etiologies extrinsic to the heart
- Autonomically mediated syndromes (e.g., neurocardiogenic syncope, carotid artery hypersensitivity, coughing, micturition, defecation)
- Medications and antiarrhythmic agents (e.g., β-blockers, calcium channel blockers, digoxin, amiodarone, clonidine, lithium)
  - Atrial fibrillation with complete heart block is pathognomonic for digitalis toxicity
- Hypothyroidism
- Myxedema
- Hypothermia
- Electrolyte disturbances (e.g., hypo- or hyperkalemia)
- Collagen vascular disease (e.g., SLE, rheumatoid arthritis, scleroderma)
- Neuromuscular disease (e.g., muscular dystrophy)
- Tumors (intracranial, cervical, mediastinal)
- Trauma (e.g., myocardial contusion)

Sinus bradycardia
- Most often results from increased vagal tone or medications (e.g., β-blockers)
- Normally seen in healthy young adults and well-trained athletes
- May occur with hypothermia, advanced liver disease, hypothyroidism, sinoatrial node disease, anorexia nervosa, sleep disorders, and increased intracranial pressure

Sinus node dysfunction
- Sinus node dysfunction may present with marked sinus bradycardia, sinus arrest, tachycardia-bradycardia syndrome, or various degrees of sinus exit block
- May result from sinus node fibrosis (e.g., aging) or infiltrative diseases (e.g., amyloidosis)
- Sick sinus syndrome: symptomatic bradycardia with sinus node dysfunction
- Tachycardia-bradycardia syndrome: sick sinus syndrome manifested by tachyarrhythmias alternating with bradyarrhythmias

Heart block
- AV block is a failure of appropriate conduction of atrial impulse to the ventricles; the atrial impulse is either delayed or not conducted to the ventricles
- 1st-degree AV block results from slowed conduction through the AV node and is benign
- 2nd-degree AV block, Mobitz I (Wenckebach) results from delayed conduction through the AV node and is often benign
- 2nd-degree AV block, Mobitz II results from disease in the bundle of His (may be life-threatening because of risk of complete heart block or ventricular asystole)
- Complete heart block results from complete dissociation between the atria and ventricles

Other
- Atrial fibrillation
- Atrial flutter with variable conduction
- Normal athletic heart
- Symptomatic bradycardia can manifest with a variety of nonspecific complaints (e.g., dizziness, syncope, fatigue), which may mimic numerous conditions
- Aortic stenosis
- Obstructive sleep apnea could lead to severe nocturnal bradycardia

Heart Rate, Tachycardia

INTRODUCTION

Tachycardia is defined by a heart rate exceeding 100 bpm. Most tachyarrhythmias result from triggered activity, increased automaticity, or re-entry circuits. A 12-lead ECG is essential to determine the type of tachyarrhythmia. Wide-complex tachycardia must be worked up and treated as ventricular tachycardia until proven otherwise. Patients should generally be transferred to a monitored setting or an ICU if unstable. Many tachyarrhythmias result from underlying electrolyte imbalances (e.g., hyperkalemia, hypomagnesemia), hypoxia, acidosis, infection, thyroid disease, or hypovolemia and therefore respond well to treatment of the underlying cause. Other etiologies may require antiarrhythmic therapy or cardioversion.

DIAGNOSTIC WORKUP & INITIAL MANAGEMENT

- Assess general appearance, level of consciousness, airway, vital signs, and pulse oximetry
- Administer supplemental oxygen and ensure IV access, if appropriate
- If unstable, begin rescue maneuvers (IV fluids, vasopressors, cardioversion)

History and physical examination

- If the patient is hemodynamically stable, perform a focused history and physical exam with emphasis on the cardiovascular, neurologic, and pulmonary systems
- Confirm the onset and duration of the tachycardia
- Assess associated symptoms (e.g., chest pain, fever, dyspnea, orthopnea, palpitations)
- Obtain medical history and review current medications

Initial workup and management

- All patients require a 12-lead ECG; it should be compared to previous ECGs
  - Cardioversion is indicated for ventricular fibrillation, ventricular tachycardia, or SVT with hypotension
  - Determine if p waves are present before each QRS complex and if the P-R interval is regular
  - Assess the QRS complex; determine if it is wide (>120 ms, or 3 small squares)
- Order routine labs, including CBC, electrolytes, cardiac markers, TSH, toxicology screen, and pregnancy test, if indicated
- If the QRS complex is narrow and regular, consider vasovagal maneuvers (e.g., carotid massage, Valsalva) or IV adenosine (6–12 mg) to possibly restore sinus rhythm or slow down the ventricular response to allow easier identification of arrhythmias (e.g., atrial flutter)
- IV drips of other AV-blocking agents may be indicated to control ventricular response
  - Diltiazem may be effective in SVT; use caution in left ventricular dysfunction
  - β-Blockers (e.g., esmolol, metoprolol) are effective for SVT; use with caution in COPD
  - Digoxin can be used for atrial fibrillation if hypotension; cardioversion may be necessary, and toxicity can occur in the elderly or those with renal dysfunction
  - Amiodarone is useful for both ventricular and supraventricular arrhythmias
  - AV nodal blockers should not be used in patients with WPW and atrial fibrillation, because ventricular fibrillation may result from rapid preferential conduction down the accessory pathway; instead, use procainamide or cardioversion
- Assess and treat underlying causes (e.g., pain, hypovolemia, ischemia, acidosis, hypoxia, electrolyte imbalances)
- Echocardiography may be needed to rule out structural heart disease
- Electrophysiology testing and/or implantable defibrillator or pacemaker may be necessary in some cases

DIFFERENTIAL DIAGNOSIS

Sinus tachycardia

- A very common cardiac response to a systemic injury or illness
- Nearly always results from a primary underlying physiologic stimulus (e.g., infection, pain, thyrotoxicosis, fever, volume depletion, pulmonary embolism, anxiety)
- Determined by a p wave with normal vector (positive in lead II) preceding every QRS
- Heart rate is usually 100–160 bpm

Atrial fibrillation

- Other than sinus tachycardia, atrial fibrillation is the most common arrhythmia
- Distinguish new-onset (<72 hours) versus chronic (unknown onset, or >72 hours): Restoration to sinus rhythm **should not** be attempted in patients with atrial fibrillation of unknown duration, unless a 4–6 week cycle of anticoagulation had been completed or a transesophageal echocardiogram demonstrates absence of left atrial thrombus or stasis (often described as "smoke" on an echocardiogram)
- Workup should rule out ischemic or structural heart disease and metabolic causes (e.g., thyroid disease)

Atrial flutter

- Usually presents in younger patients
- Atrial activity is organized and fast (p wave rate of 200–400 per minute in a "sawtooth" pattern), with regular or irregular ventricular response; be very suspicious of a regular tachycardia at 150 bpm as being atrial flutter with 2:1 conduction
- Etiology and management are similar to atrial fibrillation; it may respond to lower energy levels with cardioversion (25–50 Joules)
- Rule out structural heart disease via echocardiogram
- Catheter ablation therapy may be an option in younger patients

Multifocal atrial tachycardia

- Common in patients with severe, chronic pulmonary disease
- Usually occurs in the elderly with underlying hypoxia or cardiopulmonary disease
- ECG is characterized by ≥3 different p wave morphologies and an irregularly irregular ventricular response
- Treatment is guided toward resolution of the respiratory or metabolic trigger; rate control with AV nodal blocking agents (e.g., calcium channel blockers, β-blockers) can be used

AV nodal re-entry tachycardia

- The most common regular paroxysmal SVT
- ECG shows a narrow QRS tachycardia without discernible p waves, or an additional p wave immediately after the QRS with opposite vector to normal p wave
- Usually self-limited and responsive to vagal maneuvers or adenosine

Ventricular tachycardia

- A medical emergency that may result in sudden cardiac death
- Patients can be hemodynamically stable and asymptomatic
- Patients who are hemodynamically unstable require immediate electrical cardioversion
- ECG usually demonstrates a regular, wide QRS complex tachycardia; if irregular, consider atrial fibrillation with aberrant conduction
- Usually a sign of severe electrolyte disturbance, acidosis, myocardial ischemia or scarring, QT prolongation, drug toxicity, left ventricular dysfunction, or structural heart disease
- Torsade de pointes may be associated with electrolyte abnormalities, drug toxicity
- Electrophysiology testing, catheter ablation, or implantable defibrillator may be necessary

Ectopic atrial tachycardia

- A regular rhythm, narrow QRS complex tachycardia that results from an atrial focus other than the sinus node; p waves are often inverted in the inferior leads

Orthodromic AV reentrant tachycardia

- A regular, narrow QRS arrhythmia with abrupt onset; due to a reentrant circuit at AV node

Heart Sounds (Abnormal)

INTRODUCTION

Abnormal heart sounds are fairly common, particularly in children, and are usually benign. Distinguishing benign from pathologic heart tones is extremely important. Cardiac auscultation should be performed in a systematic manner while standing on the patient's right side with the patient's gown or shirt removed. Normal heart sounds (S_1, S_2) should be identified, and the precordium should be examined for gallops (S_3, S_4) and additional heart sounds. It may be prudent to focus on only one part of the cardiac cycle at a time during auscultation so that little will be missed. Refer also to the *Heart Murmurs* entry.

DIAGNOSTIC WORKUP & INITIAL MANAGEMENT

History and physical examination
- Assess associated symptoms, if any
- Assess medical history (e.g., previous MI, rheumatic fever), surgical history (e.g., previous valve replacement, congenital heart disease surgery), medications (e.g., ergotamines, anthracyclines for chemotherapy), social history (e.g., IV drug use), and family history of cardiovascular diseases (e.g., familial cardiomyopathies, valve diseases)
- Perform a complete cardiovascular and pulse exams
- Muffled or absent heart tones are also important to note, because they may signify a potentially life-threatening condition (e.g., cardiac tamponade)

Initial diagnostic workup
- ECG is indicated in all patients
  - Atrial fibrillation is often seen in mitral stenosis (particularly advanced cases) and may be the presenting cardiac rhythm or the initial manifestation
  - Left atrial enlargement is seen in mitral stenosis or mitral regurgitation
  - Left ventricular hypertrophy is seen in hypertensive heart disease and aortic stenosis
- Chest radiography may reveal valvular calcification, pulmonary edema, or left ventricular enlargement
- Transthoracic echocardiography is used to assess chamber size, wall thickness, ventricular function, valvular abnormalities, and pericardium
  - Transesophageal echocardiography may be used when transthoracic echocardiograms are unclear

Initial patient management
- Consider cardiology consultation, if appropriate
- Treat underlying causes as appropriate
- Endocarditis prophylaxis according to published guidelines for valve disease

DIFFERENTIAL DIAGNOSIS

S$_3$ gallop
- A low-frequency diastolic sound following S$_2$, best heard with the stethoscope bell
- May be heard normally in healthy young adults
- An S$_3$ in a patient > 40 years suggests ventricular enlargement, often secondary to chronic mitral regurgitation, decreased left ventricular ejection fraction, elevated left atrial pressure, acute pulmonary edema, or high-output states (e.g., thyrotoxicosis, pregnancy)
- Other etiologies include right ventricular infarction and hypertrophic cardiomyopathy

S$_4$ gallop
- A low-frequency diastolic sound preceding S$_1$, best heard with the stethoscope bell
- May be normally heard in healthy older adults
- May occur with hypertensive heart disease, aortic stenosis, hypertrophic cardiomyopathy, pulmonary hypertension, acute mitral regurgitation, and coronary artery disease

Midsystolic click
- Most commonly results from mitral valve prolapse

Summation gallop
- Fusion of S$_3$ and S$_4$ with tachycardia that results in a loud diastolic filling sound

Pericardial knock
- An early, loud, high-pitched diastolic sound that is common in patients with constrictive pericarditis

Opening snap
- A high-frequency, early diastolic sound most commonly resulting from mitral stenosis
- Can also be seen in patients with tricuspid stenosis, ventricular septal defect, or thyrotoxicosis

Early systolic ejection sound (ejection click)
- Associated with a bicuspid aortic valve, mitral or tricuspid prolapse, aortic stenosis, or prosthetic valves
- Tumor "plop" may occur secondary to atrial myxoma

Abnormal S$_2$ (single or loud) in children
- May indicate a large left-to-right shunt, pulmonary hypertension (loud P$_2$ component of S$_2$), or pulmonary atresia
- A fixed split S$_2$ is common in patients with atrial septal defects
- Delayed S$_2$ splitting is common in patients with pulmonic stenosis or right bundle branch block
- A paradoxically split S$_2$ is common in patients with left bundle branch block

Loud S$_1$
- Short P-R interval
- Stiff left ventricle
- Mitral stenosis

Soft S$_1$
- Long P-R interval
- Acute aortic regurgitation
- Left bundle branch block
- Obesity

Heartburn

INTRODUCTION

Heartburn is a term commonly used by patients and must be carefully evaluated to ensure accurate understanding of the symptoms. Typically, patients use the term to describe a substernal or epigastric, burning pain associated with a "sour stomach" sensation and/or a sour, acidic taste in the back of the mouth or throat. Esophageal pathologies are most common, but clinicians must immediately assess for life-threatening conditions, such as myocardial ischemia, ruptured aortic aneurysm, aortic dissection, esophageal rupture, pulmonary embolism, and perforating peptic ulcer disease.

DIAGNOSTIC WORKUP & INITIAL MANAGEMENT

History and physical examination

- Immediately obtain vital signs, including pulse oximetry
- Assess the onset, duration, and characteristics of the pain; aggravating and alleviating factors; associated symptoms; medical history; and current medications
- Distinguish between esophageal pain (reflux) and cardiac pain (angina)
  - Coronary artery disease typically presents as chest discomfort (often a "crushing" pain, as if someone is sitting on the patient's chest) exacerbated by physical or emotional stress and relieved by rest; lasts up to 20 minutes and may radiate to the shoulder, neck, jaw, or arm; may occur with diaphoresis, palpitations, dyspnea, nausea/vomiting
  - GERD typically presents as squeezing or burning chest discomfort lasting minutes to hours, often after eating; may be associated with burning in the throat and dyspepsia
- Perform complete cardiovascular, pulmonary, and abdominal exams

Initial diagnostic workup

- If acute ischemia cannot be ruled out in the office, transport the patient to the emergency department for further evaluation and management
- Initial testing for cardiac ischemia may include ECG and cardiac enzymes
- ECG may reveal ischemia (e.g., new bundle branch block, ST segment or T wave changes) or arrhythmias; widespread ST elevations suggest pericarditis
- If suspect CAD, consider stress testing, echocardiography, and catheterization
- Initial diagnostic test for esophageal etiologies may be a therapeutic challenge with H_2-blockers or proton pump inhibitors; further evaluation only for patients who fail initial therapy or have signs or symptoms suggesting serious pathology
- Upper GI endoscopy (with biopsy and *H. pylori* testing) will verify reflux esophagitis and other pathology (e.g., stricture) and rule out Barrett's esophagus and esophageal carcinoma; endoscopy if the patient has dysphagia, odynophagia, weight loss, hematemesis, black or bloody stools, chest pain, choking, persistent vomiting, or anemia
- Ambulatory esophageal pH monitoring may be used to evaluate patients with atypical reflux symptoms and normal endoscopy
- Double-contrast barium swallow may identify early stages of reflux esophagitis, ulcers, strictures, folds, and hiatal hernia
- Esophageal manometry diagnoses motility disorders, decreased peristalsis, and spasm
- Biopsy is diagnostic for Barrett's esophagus, carcinoma, sclerosis, and infection
- Consider chest radiography to rule out chest masses, pneumothorax, and pneumonia

Initial patient management

- Lifestyle modifications for most cases of esophageal pathology: elevate the head of bed (for nocturnal symptoms); avoid reflux-inducing foods (e.g., chocolate, fats, caffeine, alcohol, acidic food, licorice); decrease caloric intake, smoking, and stress
- Acid suppression medications for significant reflux and/or failed lifestyle modifications

Chapter 69

DIFFERENTIAL DIAGNOSIS

Cardiovascular disease
- Angina/ischemia
- MI
- Pericardial disease
- Aortic dissection
- Valvular disease
- Myocarditis

Esophageal pathology
- GERD
- Hiatal hernia
- Esophageal motility disorders with decreased peristaltic clearance (e.g., achalasia)
- Esophageal spasm
- Infectious esophagitis (e.g., *Candida*, HIV, cytomegalovirus, HSV)
- Barrett's esophagus
- Esophageal carcinoma (commonly squamous cell)
- Strictures, webs, or rings
- Esophageal diverticulum
- Scleroderma
- Esophageal varices
- Mallory-Weiss tear
- Esophageal atresia or fistula
- Caustic agent ingestion with resultant mucosal injury

Other gastrointestinal etiologies
- Peptic ulcer disease
- Gastritis
- Pancreatitis
- Cholecystitis

Musculoskeletal etiologies
- Muscle strain
- Rib fracture
- Costochondritis
- Arthropathy
- Fibromyalgia
- Tietze's syndrome

Other
- Pulmonary embolism
- Pneumonia
- Sarcoidosis
- Pleuritis
- Asthma
- Pregnancy
- Herpes zoster
- Panic attack or anxiety disorder
- Factitious disorder
- Myasthenia gravis
- Chagas' disease

Hematuria

INTRODUCTION

Hematuria is the presence of red blood cells in the urine. It is relatively common, can arise from nearly any site in the urinary tract, and has a variety of etiologies, ranging from benign and self-limited to malignant and lethal. The amount of blood can be grossly evident or microscopic. Significant microscopic hematuria may lend the urine a cola- or tea-like color. About 2.5% of the general population has asymptomatic hematuria. A single urinalysis showing hematuria may result from exercise, fever, menstruation, mild trauma, sexual activity, or viral illness; persistent hematuria warrants further investigation. Gross, painless hematuria in older adults is considered a urinary tract cancer until proven otherwise.

DIAGNOSTIC WORKUP & INITIAL MANAGEMENT

History and physical examination

- Distinguish between gross and microscopic hematuria
  - Gross hematuria suggests urologic disease, IgA nephropathy, Alport's disease, or anti-GBM disease
  - Microscopic hematuria is more likely of renal origin and carries a worse prognosis
- Note the timing of hematuria during urination:
  - Hematuria throughout urination suggests renal or ureteral disease
  - Hematuria at the onset of urination suggests urethral disease
  - Hematuria at the culmination of urination suggests bladder or prostate disease
- Note irritative voiding symptoms (e.g., dysuria, increased frequency, nocturia, urgency), which may suggest infection or uroepithelial malignancy
- Note previous history of hematuria, renal or urologic disease, proteinuria, and infection
- Perform a complete review of systems, with attention to arthralgias, fatigue, fever, pain, pulmonary symptoms, rash, weakness, and weight loss
- Review medications and duration of use; commonly implicated medications include analgesics, cyclophosphamide, and extended-spectrum penicillins
- Physical exam includes evaluation for hypertension, abdominal and back pain or masses, rash, arthritis, and pulmonary, prostatic, urethral, and vaginal disease

Initial diagnostic workup

- Nearly all patients require urinalysis with microscopic evaluation of urinary sediment; consider catheterization to distinguish vaginal bleeding from other sources
  - Blood clots can occur with significant bleeding, typically from urologic etiologies
  - Glomerular sources of bleeding result in RBC casts, dysmorphic RBCs, and proteinuria
  - UTI results in pyuria, leukocyte esterase, and often nitrites
  - Pyuria suggests infection; verify by urine Gram's stain or culture
- Labs include urinalysis with microscopic analysis of a freshly voided, midstream, clean-catch urine specimen; urine protein/creatinine ratio; coagulation studies; BUN and creatinine
- Urine cytology and cystoscopy may be necessary for patients at risk of bladder cancer (e.g., smoking, cyclophosphamide use)
- Microscopic hematuria is classified by associated findings in the urine sediment:
  - Glomerular origin is suggested by RBC casts or >20% dysmorphic RBCs and is often accompanied by proteinuria on dipstick; however, most laboratories are not equipped to identify dysmorphic RBCs
- If clinically indicated, glomerular hematuria can be further evaluated with ESR, ANA, ANCA, complement levels (C3, C4), ASO titers, anti-DNAse B antibodies, anti-GBM antibodies, SPEP, UPEP, and viral serologies
- Renal biopsy is often necessary to fully evaluate glomerular bleeding
- Consider urology or nephrology referral

DIFFERENTIAL DIAGNOSIS

Transient hematuria
- UTI/pyelonephritis
- Urolithiasis
- Exercise
- Trauma, instrumentation, catheterization, or foreign bodies
- Endometriosis
- Hemolytic uremic syndrome
- Coagulopathy or excess anticoagulation
- Prostatitis or epididymitis

Persistent hematuria
- Sickle cell trait (papillary necrosis)
- Cancer (e.g., prostate, bladder, kidney)
- Benign prostatic hyperplasia
- Polycystic kidney disease
- Intrinsic glomerular disease

Glomerular bleeding
- Thin basement membrane disease (benign familial hematuria)
- Alport's syndrome
- Diabetic nephropathy
- Glomerulonephritis
  - IgA nephropathy (Berger's disease) and Henoch-Schönlein purpura
  - Focal sclerosis
  - Postinfectious glomerulonephritis
  - SLE
  - ANCA-associated (Wegener's granulomatosis and microscopic polyangiitis)
  - Viral-associated (e.g., hepatitis B and C, HIV)
  - Anti-GBM disease

Nonglomerular bleeding
- Infection (urethritis, cystitis, pyelonephritis)
- Urolithiasis
- Uroepithelial malignancy
- Benign prostatic hyperplasia
- Prostate cancer
- Renal cell cancer
- Stricture
- Polycystic kidney disease
- Arteriovenous malformation
- Renal infarction
- Renal trauma
- Sickle cell trait or disease

Other causes of red or brown urine (pseudohematuria)
- Beeturia (from excretion of betalaine, a reddish pigment contained in beets)
- Myoglobinuria (usually secondary to rhabdomyolysis)
- Hemoglobinuria
- Medications (e.g., rifampin, phenazopyridine, phenytoin, metronidazole)
- Food dye
- Porphyria

Hemiparesis & Hemiplegia

INTRODUCTION

Hemiplegia (complete lack of motor function on one side of the body) and hemiparesis (decreased motor function on one side of the body) are almost always the result of a problem with the central nervous system. The tempo of onset, history, and associated findings on examination are usually helpful in localizing the problem and suggesting an etiology. Emergent stabilization and treatment are essential to save lives and decrease disability, but correct diagnosis is necessary to limit untoward risks of treatment, such as hemorrhagic stroke in a patient who receives thrombolytic therapy.

DIAGNOSTIC WORKUP & INITIAL MANAGEMENT

History and physical examination

- Acute onset of hemiparesis or hemiplegia suggests a vascular cause until proven otherwise (although exacerbation of multiple sclerosis may present relatively acutely)
- More gradual onset of hemiparesis suggests a more slowly evolving process (e.g., tumor)
- The pattern of weakness noted on exam and the associated deficits help to localize the lesion:
  - Right hemiparesis with greater weakness of the face and arm than the leg and associated aphasia suggest a cerebral infarction in the territory of the left middle cerebral artery
  - Equal weakness of the face, arm, and leg without associated cortical deficits suggests a subcortical lesion (e.g., internal capsule)
  - Cranial nerve abnormalities and weakness of the contralateral limbs suggest a brainstem lesion
  - Bilateral hemiparesis without cognitive or cranial nerve findings suggests a spinal cord disorder

Initial diagnostic workup

- Initial laboratory studies may include CBC, electrolytes, calcium, glucose, BUN and creatinine, and coagulation studies
- Head MRI and/or CT are the imaging modalities of choice
- CSF exam is useful in suspected cases of multiple sclerosis (reveals oligoclonal bands and elevated IgG index)

Initial patient management

- Identify and treat the underlying cause
- General measures (e.g., physical and occupational therapy, assistive devices, orthotics) may all be beneficial in improving the functional abilities of patients with hemiplegia or paresis
- Cerebral infarction is best managed medically
  - Thrombolytics within 3 hours of symptom onset in carefully selected patients improves the outcome of ischemic stroke patients
  - General measures include careful management of blood pressure, blood sugar, and avoiding infectious complications (e.g., pneumonia caused by bed rest)
  - Identify the underlying cause to direct long-term therapy (usually antiplatelet or anticoagulant therapy with risk factor management) to prevent recurrence
- Mass lesions affecting the brain, including tumors and hematomas, may require surgical management
- Multiple sclerosis is treated with steroids during acute exacerbations and other medical therapies chronically

DIFFERENTIAL DIAGNOSIS

Cerebrovascular disease

- Infarction (thromboembolic)
- Intracerebral hemorrhage
- TIAs may produce a transient hemiplegia or paresis (although they are defined as cerebrovascular deficits that resolve within 24 hours, most cases last only minutes)

Other etiologies

- Chronic subdural hematoma
- Demyelinating disease (e.g., multiple sclerosis, Guillain-Barré syndrome)
- Trauma
- Congenital (e.g., cerebral palsy, congenital structural anomalies)
- Brain tumors (primary or metastatic)
- Cerebral abscess
- Complicated migraine
- Inflammatory conditions (e.g., cerebral vasculitis)
- Postictal (Todd's) paralysis
- Psychogenic or hysterical weakness
  - These patients usually lack associated physical findings (e.g., hyperreflexia, Babinski's sign) and may exhibit inconsistent or nonphysiologic patterns of weakness
- Amyotrophic lateral sclerosis
  - May present initially with asymmetric weakness, but more diffuse involvement develops over time
- Brown-Sequard syndrome (spinal cord hemisection)
  - Leads to weakness, upper motor neuron signs, and impaired proprioception and vibratory sensation ipsilateral to the lesion
  - Impaired pain and temperature sensation contralateral to the lesion
- Meningitis
- Syphilis
- Transverse myelitis
- Periodic paralysis

Hemoptysis

INTRODUCTION

Hemoptysis is the expectoration of blood or blood-tinged sputum from the lower respiratory tract (i.e., below the vocal cords). It is important to distinguish hemoptysis from other sites of bleeding (nose, mouth, throat, GI tract). It can be particularly difficult to discern hemoptysis from hematemesis. Massive hemoptysis (expectoration of >600 mL within 24 hours), although uncommon, is a medical emergency that may be fatal because of asphyxiation or respiratory failure. Although the mortality rate of patients who present with acute hemoptysis is low, the amount of blood expectorated is a major determinant of morbidity, while the underlying etiology remains an important determinant of long-term survival.

DIAGNOSTIC WORKUP & INITIAL MANAGEMENT

Emergent management of massive hemoptysis
- Patients with massive hemoptysis are at high risk of asphyxiation and require emergent management, which may include intubation to protect the airway and facilitate treatment
- Evaluate the patient and assess the severity of the situation; assess vital signs, especially respiratory rate and pulse oximetry; and estimate the amount of hemoptysis
- Set up a bedside suction apparatus
- Ensure that 2 large-bore IVs (≥18 gauge) are available for access
- Hemodynamic monitoring is critical, given the potential for hypotension and shock
- Administer supplemental oxygen via nasal cannula; have a nonrebreather mask and Ambu-bag ready if the patient continues to oxygenate poorly
- With major hemoptysis with active bleeding, consider urgent bronchoscopy
  ○ Stable patients may undergo initial chest CT to identify the area of bleeding

History and physical examination
- Assess mental status, ability to clear secretions, and use of accessory muscles for breathing; auscultate heart and chest; assess nares and oral cavity to evaluate for signs of a bleeding source; evaluate skin for signs of coagulopathy (petechiae, purpura)
- Distinguish hemoptysis (bleeding from below the vocal cords) from nasopharyngeal or upper GI bleeding; note whether the hemoptysis is sudden or progressive and whether it occurs in the context of recent illness or fever
- Review medications (e.g., warfarin, NSAIDs); note whether the patient smokes
- Evaluate for recent trauma (e.g., intubation, inhalation injury, Swan-Ganz manipulation)

Initial workup and management
- Ensure the patient is receiving supplemental oxygen and IV fluids, suction is available to maintain the airway, hemodynamics are monitored, and the bleeding lung is in the dependent position to prevent blood drainage into the opposite lung
- Initial testing may include chest radiography (may reveal a parenchymal etiology, such as lung mass, cavitary lesion, or infiltrate, and may localize the area of bleeding), blood type and cross for ≥2 units of packed RBCs, and ABG analysis
- Further testing in massive hemoptysis includes CBC, chemistries, urinalysis, sputum analysis (cytology, Gram's stain, culture, acid-fast stain), and coagulation studies
  ○ Compare current hematocrit to previous results; note hematocrit may fall slowly despite significant volume depletion and fall precipitously after volume repletion
- In cases of active bleeding, immediate bronchoscopy must be considered
- Bronchoscopy and/or chest CT may be indicated, particularly if the chest X-ray is abnormal, hemoptysis persists longer than 1–2 weeks, the volume of hemoptysis increases, or in smokers older than 40 (bronchoscopy allows direct visualization of the airways, lateralization of bleed, and collection of samples for pathology and microbiology)

DIFFERENTIAL DIAGNOSIS

- The most common causes of massive hemoptysis are tuberculosis, bronchitis, bronchiectasis, necrotizing pneumonia, lung abscess, lung cancer, bronchovascular fistula, fungal infection, and coagulopathy
  - Pulmonary infarction and CHF are common causes of ordinary hemoptysis ($<$ 200 mL/day)
- Other (nonhemoptysis) sources of bleeding (e.g., hematemesis, epistaxis, other causes of upper airway bleeding) must be ruled out
  - ABG of expectorated blood may distinguish hemoptysis (alkaline pH) from hematemesis (acidic pH)

Pulmonary etiologies

- Bronchitis (acute or chronic) is thought to be the most common etiology of massive hemoptysis and causes $>$25% of cases
- Bronchiectasis causes up to 10% of cases
- Pulmonary embolism
- Cystic fibrosis
- Bullous emphysema
- Foreign body
- Diffuse alveolar hemorrhage syndromes: (e.g., crack cocaine, SLE, cytotoxic drug use)

Infectious etiologies

- Tuberculosis
- Lung abscess
- Necrotizing pneumonia
- Fungal pneumonia (e.g., aspergillosis)
- Parasitic infection

Trauma

- Penetrating chest injury
- Fat embolism
- Ruptured bronchus
- Iatrogenic trauma (e.g., postbronchoscopy, Swan-Ganz catheter infarction, pulmonary artery rupture, and transtracheal aspiration)

Malignancy

- Lung cancer (most often squamous cell carcinoma) frequently causes hemoptysis but usually not massive hemoptysis
- Metastatic and other primary lung cancers may also cause hemoptysis
- Kaposi's sarcoma in HIV-positive patients

Toxins

- Anticoagulants, crack cocaine, thrombolytics, solvents, penicillamine

Cardiovascular etiologies

- Mitral stenosis, tricuspid endocarditis, congenital anomalies, CHF, aortic aneurysm, fistula between the vasculature and the airway

Congenital etiologies

- Hereditary telangiectasias (e.g., Osler-Weber-Rendu), AV malformation

Systemic and inflammatory etiologies

- Wegener's granulomatosis, SLE, Goodpasture's syndrome, vasculitis, Behçet's disease, sarcoidosis, Henoch-Schönlein purpura, idiopathic pulmonary hemosiderosis, antiphospholipid antibody syndrome

Hematologic etiologies

- Thrombocytopenia, von Willebrand's disease, anticoagulant use, DIC

Other

- Catamenial hemoptysis (intrathoracic endometriosis)
- Idiopathic (20% of cases)

Hemorrhoids

INTRODUCTION

Hemorrhoids are common, affecting up to 50% of the population. They are *not* protruding "varicose veins" and are distinct from the rectal varices of portal hypertension. Rather, hemorrhoids are downwardly displaced anal cushions, which are normal vascular tissue (sinusoids) that protects the anal canal during defecation. The supporting tissue deteriorates over time and, with increased anal pressure (straining), leads to sliding, engorgement, bleeding, and prolapse of the cushions. Hemorrhoids become symptomatic when venous pressure is increased. Over time, redundancy and enlargement of venous cushions occur, leading to hemorrhoidal bleeding or protrusion.

DIAGNOSTIC WORKUP & INITIAL MANAGEMENT

History and physical examination

- Assess onset and duration, associated symptoms (e.g., anal mass, bleeding, itching), medical and surgical histories, and medications
- The most common presenting complaints are painless, bright-red bleeding after defecation (in toilet or on paper), itching, and prolapse of a hemorrhoid
  - Hemorrhoids are usually not painful unless thrombosed, ulcerated, or gangrenous
  - Sudden onset of excruciating perirectal pain with palpable mass usually suggests acute thrombosis of a hemorrhoid
- Perianal exam will directly reveal external hemorrhoids; nonprolapsed, internal hemorrhoids are not visible but may protrude through the anus with gentle straining; prolapsed hemorrhoids appear as protuberant, purple nodules covered by mucosa
  - The perianal region should also be inspected for fistulas, fissures, skin tags, and dermatitis
- On digital exam, uncomplicated internal hemorrhoids will not be palpable or painful; pain on rectal exam implies proctitis and/or complicated hemorrhoidal disease
- Evaluate for prolapse by having patient strain (may place patient on a toilet to facilitate)
  - 1st-degree Hemorrhoid: No prolapse
  - 2nd-degree: Prolapse during defecation, followed by spontaneous return to anal canal
  - 3rd-degree: Prolapsed but manually reducible
  - 4th-degree: Constant, irreducible prolapse

Initial diagnostic workup

- Anoscopy, proctoscopy, or sigmoidoscopy are used to evaluate symptoms and bleeding and will provide optimal visualization of hemorrhoids
  - Colon mucosa should be well-evaluated to rule out colitis and other mucosal diseases
- Full colonoscopy is indicated in all patients > 50 years or if diagnosis is unclear
- Rectal manometry is indicated if the patient complains of incontinence
- Biopsy is indicated for any rectal polyp or palpable lesion

Initial patient management

- Treatment is initially conservative: High-fiber diet ($\geq$25 g/day), stool softeners, appropriate anal hygiene, warm sitz baths, and topical steroids
- Surgical options for internal hemorrhoids or large external hemorrhoids:
  - Asymptomatic internal hemorrhoids should be left alone
  - Symptomatic hemorrhoids not responding to conservative therapy may be treated in an outpatient setting by infrared coagulation or bipolar cautery, which causes fixation of the hemorrhoidal tissue to the underlying connective tissue and reduces the blood supply
  - 3rd-degree hemorrhoids can be treated surgically with rubber band ligation
  - 4th-degree hemorrhoids are treated with surgical excision
- Acute thrombosis of a hemorrhoid may require surgical drainage

DIFFERENTIAL DIAGNOSIS

External hemorrhoids
- Located below the dentate line, which defines the junction of the rectum (columnar epithelium) with the anus (squamous epithelium)
- Typically painful
- External hemorrhoids, when enlarged, can easily thrombose; the thrombus is usually at the level of sphincteric muscles, which often results in anal spasm

Internal hemorrhoids
- Located above the dentate line
- Typically not painful, unless thrombosis occurs

Pregnancy
- Up to 35% of pregnant females will develop hemorrhoids around the time of delivery, with most cases occurring after vaginal delivery and/or prolonged labor

Rectal prolapse
- Complete prolapse
- Partial full-thickness prolapse
- Prolapse of the mucosa only

Papilloma (warts)
- Condylomata acuminatum are genital warts caused by syphilis

Other
- Rectal polyp
- Rectal or anal cancer
- Hypertrophied anal papilla (polypoid structure at pectinate line)
- External skin tag (a redundant fold of tissue along the external anal margin)
- Perirectal abscess
- Anal fissure or fistula
- Inflammatory bowel disease (IBD)
- Diverticular disease
- Infectious proctitis
- Rectal varices secondary to portal hypertension
- Rectal cavernous hemangioma

Hepatomegaly

INTRODUCTION

The liver is the largest parenchymal organ in the body. It receives a dual blood supply via the portal venous system, which drains the GI tract, and the hepatic arterial system via the aorta. Hepatic blood flow is ~1,500 mL/min, representing ~25% of cardiac output. Hepatomegaly, or enlargement of the liver, usually refers to a liver span >12 cm at the right midclavicular line or a palpable left lobe extending into the epigastrium. However, liver size on physical exam is only an approximation and should be measured accurately with an abdominal ultrasound, CT, or MRI. The liver is the most common site for hematogenously spread metastatic cancer, particularly from colon cancer. Abnormalities such as a low-lying liver or other abdominal masses must be also considered.

DIAGNOSTIC WORKUP & INITIAL MANAGEMENT

History and physical examination

- History should include history of present illness, associated symptoms (e.g., vomiting, jaundice, fever, other constitutional symptoms), medical history, alcohol and drug use, medications (including herbal remedies), and family history of liver disease
  - Metastatic liver tumors are often asymptomatic and found on metastatic workup
  - The classic presentation of hepatocellular carcinoma is right upper quadrant or epigastric pain (caused by distention of the liver capsule by the tumor and/or hemorrhage), abdominal swelling, and weight loss in a patient with existing cirrhosis
  - Patients may present with jaundice caused by liver disease or compression of a large bile duct
- Physical exam should include palpation of the liver surface for tenderness (may suggest an inflammatory disorder), consistency, nodularity, pulsations, bruits, and rubs; skin exam (e.g., for jaundice, spider angiomata); cardiac exam; rectal exam; and evaluation for lymphadenopathy

Initial diagnostic workup

- Liver function tests (ALT, AST, GGTP, albumin, alkaline phosphatase, bilirubin) and coagulation tests (PT, PTT, INR) to assess liver function
- Hepatitis serologies may be indicated, including hepatitis (A, B, and C), cytomegalovirus, and Epstein-Barr virus
- Ultrasound will discriminate solid masses from cysts
- Abdominal CT to evaluate masses and fatty liver
- Doppler ultrasound to determine blood flow
- Abdominal MRI is useful to diagnose excess deposition of iron (hemochromatosis) or copper (Wilson's disease)
- Radionuclide scanning to characterize inflammatory and neoplastic lesions
- Angiography is the gold standard to differentiate hemangioma from solid tumor
- Consider iron panel (hemochromatosis) and ceruloplasmin (Wilson's disease)
- Workup for cancer may include serum α-fetoprotein and alkaline phosphatase, liver biopsy, PET scan, and CT of the abdomen, pelvis, and chest

Initial patient management

- Gastroenterology consultation may be warranted
- Treat underlying etiologies as appropriate (e.g., diuretics and afterload reduction for heart failure, antivirals and supportive care for viral hepatitis, antimicrobials for other infections, abstinence from alcohol, steroids for sarcoidosis, chelation therapy for hemochromatosis and Wilson's disease)
- Resection, chemotherapy, radiation therapy, and other modalities for cancers
- Advanced liver disease may require liver transplantation

DIFFERENTIAL DIAGNOSIS

Right heart failure
- May also be associated with congestion of the GI tract and limb edema

Inflammatory disorders
- Hepatitis (viral, drug-induced, or autoimmune)
- Other infections (e.g., HIV, malaria, amebiasis, schistosomiasis, tuberculosis, *B. burgdorferi*, toxocariasis)
- Alcoholic liver disease
- SLE
- Liver toxins (e.g., tyrosinemia, galactosemia, vitamin A)

Infiltrative disorders
- Fatty liver (nonalcoholic steatohepatitis)
- Sarcoidosis
- Hemochromatosis
- Wilson's disease
- Amyloidosis
- Chronic granulomatous disease
- Extramedullary hematopoiesis
- Histiocytosis
- Lipid storage diseases (e.g., Gaucher's disease, Wolman's disease, Niemann-Pick disease)
- Glycogen storage diseases
- Mucopolysaccharidoses
- α_1-Antitrypsin deficiency

Neoplasms
- Metastatic cancer (e.g., colon, lung, breast) is more common than primary liver cancers
- Hepatocellular carcinoma is the most common primary liver cancer (often caused by chronic hepatitis or cirrhosis)
- Hepatic adenoma or hepatic cysts
- Hemangioma
- Hepatoblastoma
- Leukemia or lymphoma
- Liver abscess

Portal hypertension
- Prehepatic causes: Narrowed portal vein, occlusive thrombosis
- Intrahepatic causes: Cirrhosis (most common cause in U.S.), schistosomiasis (most common cause worldwide), biliary cirrhosis, sarcoidosis, tuberculosis, and noncirrhotic hepatic fibrosis
- Posthepatic causes: Hepatic vein thrombosis (Budd-Chiari syndrome), inferior vena cava obstruction, right heart failure, constrictive pericarditis, restrictive cardiomyopathy
- Portal hypertension secondary to extrahepatic causes: Adjacent inflammation (e.g., pancreatitis), obstructing mass, splenic vein thrombosis

Ascites secondary to extrahepatic causes
- Nephrotic syndrome
- Congestive heart failure
- Carcinomatosis

Medications
- Acetaminophen, NSAIDs, isoniazid, sodium valproate, propylthiouracil, halothane

Less common causes
- Tricuspid regurgitation
- Kala-azar (visceral leishmaniasis)
- Amyloidosis
- HIV/AIDS

Hirsutism

INTRODUCTION

Hirsutism is excessive growth of androgen-dependent terminal hairs (stiff, coarse, dark hair) along a male pattern of distribution in women. Some degree of hirsutism is estimated to affect 5–15% of all women. It usually results as a response to excess adrenal or ovarian androgens. The etiology and significance depend on whether the patient is hirsute only (excessive hair) or is also virilized (increased weight, clitoromegaly, acne, deep voice). Polycystic ovarian syndrome (PCOS) is the most common etiology and may affect up to 10% of women. Be sure to differentiate hirsutism from hypertrichosis, which refers to diffusely increased, non–androgen dependent total body hair and is reversible.

DIAGNOSTIC WORKUP & INITIAL MANAGEMENT

History and physical examination

- History should include time course of symptoms as well as menstrual, pregnancy, medical, family, and medication history
  - Progressive worsening, late age of onset, or abrupt onset suggest a tumor
- Physical exam should confirm and document the extent of hirsutism, rule out hypertrichosis, assess for virilization, and assess for abdominal or ovarian masses
  - Assess for male body hair distribution on face (mustache, beard, sideburns) and body (chest, areolae, linea alba, abdominal trigone, inner thighs)
  - Assess for other manifestations of excess androgens/virilization: breast atrophy, frontal balding, acne, deepening voice, clitoromegaly, or a change in normal female body habitus (increased musculature, absence of female contours)
  - Acanthosis nigricans (velvety, hyperpigmented skin) may occur in axillae and neck

Initial diagnostic workup

- Obtain labs when menses are irregular; hirsutism is abrupt, late in onset, or rapidly progressive; or signs of virilization are present
- Serum testosterone level of 50–150 ng/dL suggests an endocrine disorder; >200 ng/dL requires imaging studies to assess for an androgen-producing tumor
- LH:FSH ratio > 3 may suggest polycystic ovarian syndrome
- DHEA-S should be measured if progressive symptoms, irregular menstrual cycles, or signs of virilization (>700 μg/dL suggests adrenal hyperplasia or tumor)
- 17-OH progesterone level < 300 ng/dL or suppressible rules out adrenal hyperplasia
- Measure prolactin and TSH if menstrual cycles are irregular
- Imaging studies are indicated if suspect tumor (e.g., abdominal CT to rule out adrenal tumor, pelvic ultrasound or CT to rule out ovarian tumor or polycystic ovaries)
- Endometrial biopsy may be indicated to evaluate for endometrial hyperplasia if periods are irregular and polycystic ovarian syndrome is a concern

Initial patient management

- Combination low-dose estrogen and nonandrogenic progestin oral contraceptive pills are effective in >60% of women; they will inhibit adrenal and ovarian androgen production, stimulate production of sex hormone–binding globulin by the liver (which reduces free testosterone), and diminish terminal hair growth
- Spironolactone (antiandrogen therapy) blocks testosterone binding to its receptors
- Remove terminal hair via waxing, depilatories, electrolysis, or laser treatment
- GnRH agonists (e.g., luprolide) with oral contraceptives or estrogen may be tried
- Topical eflornithine hydrochloride cream (13.9%) is FDA approved for unwanted facial hair; acts by inhibiting hair growth; requires 8 weeks for peak effectiveness
- All currently available medications for hirsutism must be stopped if pregnancy is desired
- Dexamethasone will reduce virilization caused by adrenal hyperplasia

DIFFERENTIAL DIAGNOSIS

Polycystic ovarian syndrome
- A syndrome of androgen excess, possibly from excess LH stimulation of the ovaries
- Presents with classic clinical triad of hirsutism, anovulation, and obesity
- Polycystic ovaries each contain at least eight small (2–8 mm) follicles
- Approximately 4%–6% of women have PCOS; it may be the most common endocrinopathy in reproductive-aged women
- Patients have insulin resistance and compensatory hyperinsulinemia and hyperandrogenism; the abnormal insulin function causes the cascade of diverse syndrome presentations and the ultimate morbidity in these patients
- Associated with increased risk of cardiovascular disease, infertility, and endometrial hyperplasia

Tumors
- Pituitary tumors resulting in hyperprolactinemia
- Adrenal tumors
- Ovarian tumors

Congenital adrenal hyperplasia
- A family of diseases caused by an inherited deficiency of any enzyme needed in cortisol biosynthesis from cholesterol precursors; nearly all these enzymes are members of the cytochrome P450 family
- 90% of cases result from 21-hydroxylase deficiency, which is responsible for conversion of 17-hydroxyprogesterone to 11-deoxycortisol
- Cortisol deficiency causes ACTH hypersecretion, resulting in adrenal hyperplasia, overproduction of precursors, and increased steroids in alternative pathways
- Three types exist: classic salt-losing disease (complete enzyme deficiency), classic simple virilizing/non–salt losing disease (partial enzyme deficiency), and nonclassic form (mild disease, late onset)
- There is no cure for virilization caused by adrenal hyperplasia; however, it can usually be controlled with ongoing dexamethasone treatment

Hypertrichosis
- Often related to medications (e.g., steroids, phenytoin, diazoxide, cyclosporine, minoxidil)
- May be associated with hypothyroidism, anorexia, or malnutrition

Drug-induced
- Cyclosporine, steroids, oral contraceptives, phenytoin, some diuretics (e.g., acetazolamide, hydrochlorothiazide), minoxidil, penicillamines

Idiopathic hirsutism
- Usually not reversible; if untreated, however, terminal hair growth may gradually increase with age
- There is often a family history of hirsutism

Other
- Cushing's syndrome
- Normal hair growth for race and ethnicity
- Androgenized ovary syndrome
- Gonadal dysgenesis
- 5α-reductase deficiency
- HAIR-AN syndrome
- Porphyria
- Genetic syndromes (e.g., Cornelia de Lange's syndrome, trisomy 18, Hurler's syndrome, Bloom's syndrome, Seckel's syndrome, Marshall-Smith syndrome, Rubinstein-Taybi syndrome, Achard-Thiers syndrome, leprechaunism)

Hoarseness

INTRODUCTION

Hoarseness is any undesirable alteration of the voice. A rough sound of the voice, change in pitch, or increased effort of speaking can all be considered as hoarseness. "Acute" hoarseness refers to a sudden onset and/or duration of <2 weeks. "Chronic" hoarseness implies duration >2 weeks. Evaluation of possible airway obstruction and stridor should take precedence in the examination.

DIAGNOSTIC WORKUP & INITIAL MANAGEMENT

- Assess for airway compromise, and treat emergently if present
- In cases of trauma or airway obstruction, emergent cricothyrotomy or tracheostomy may be necessary to establish an airway

History and physical examination

- Assess previous history, onset, and duration
- Assess exposure to irritants, allergens, tobacco and/or alcohol, and medications
- Inquire about voice use or abuse
- Note recent trauma
- Evaluate associated symptoms (e.g., cold symptoms, heartburn, vomiting, weight loss, dysphagia)
- Assess medical and surgical history, including immunizations and prolonged or repeated intubations
- Physical exam should focus on head and neck, thyroid, lung, and cardiac exams, including evaluation of voice quality

Initial diagnostic workup

- Chest radiography may be useful to assess for a mediastinal lesion
- Lateral neck radiography may be indicated if history and physical exam suggest epiglottitis or a foreign body
- Direct or fiberoptic nasolaryngoscopy is best to assess the larynx and vocal cord mobility; flexible fiberoptic nasopharyngoscopy can often be done in an outpatient office setting, but if suspect epiglottitis, the exam must be done in an operating room
- Biopsy may be indicated for masses seen on direct laryngoscopy (usually refer to ENT specialist)
- If indicated by history or exam, consider thyroid function tests, upper GI endoscopy (esophagogastroduodenoscopy), upper GI radiographic series, CT of the sinuses, and/or CT of head and neck

Initial patient management

- Repeatedly assess airway, breathing, circulation if airway compromise is a concern
- Vocal abuse may be treated with voice rest (whispering is not voice rest); if speaking is absolutely necessary, oral steroids may be used; voice therapy may be necessary in chronic voice abuse to correct faulty vocal habits
- Avoid irritants, if necessary (e.g., smoking cessation, protective clothing or masks)
- Treat infections with symptomatic measures (e.g., hydration, decongestants, cough suppression), antibiotics if appropriate, and voice rest; surgery may be indicated for abscess
- Treat GERD, sinusitis, allergic rhinitis, endocrine, neurologic, rheumatologic, and other disorders as necessary
- Masses usually require surgical intervention

DIFFERENTIAL DIAGNOSIS

Acute (<2 weeks)

Infections
- Laryngitis
- Tracheitis
- Epiglottitis (accompanied by stridor and "thumb sign" on lateral neck radiograph)
- Croup
- Upper respiratory infections
- Deep-space face and neck infections (e.g., peritonsillar abscess, retropharyngeal abscess, parapharyngeal abscess)

Voice abuse
- May occur upon shouting, speaking, or singing loudly
- May cause chronic hoarseness if the abuse is recurrent

Trauma
- Laryngeal trauma secondary to motor vehicle collision
- Strangulation
- Assault
- Sporting injuries
- Arytenoid cartilage dislocation
- Iatrogenic (e.g., intubation, damage to recurrent laryngeal nerve during thyroid surgery)
- Foreign body

Irritants
- Vomiting
- Chemical inhalation

Anaphylaxis

Chronic (>2 weeks)

Allergic rhinitis, chronic sinusitis, or GERD

Irritants
- Tobacco smoke
- Occupational

Endocrine
- Puberty, menopause, hypothyroidism, normal aging

Vocal cord disease
- Polyps, nodules ("singer's nodules"), neoplasm (primary, metastatic), papilloma (infants, children), corditis (Reinke's edema, vocal cord edema), vocal cord paralysis

Malignancy
- Laryngeal, esophageal, lung, or head and neck (e.g., tonsillar, tongue) cancers

Iatrogenic
- Medication side effect (e.g., pioglitazone, aerosolized steroids), postsurgical recurrent laryngeal nerve damage with vocal cord paralysis, radiation therapy

Neurologic disease
- Multiple sclerosis, amyotrophic lateral sclerosis, Parkinson's disease, muscular dystrophy, brainstem stroke, injury to recurrent laryngeal nerve

Less common etiologies
- Hemorrhage into the vocal folds
- Psychogenic (laryngeal conversion disorders)
- Rheumatologic disease (e.g., rheumatoid arthritis, sarcoidosis, amyloidosis)

Hypercalcemia

INTRODUCTION

Calcium is the most abundant mineral in the body, with 99% stored in bone. Calcium in the plasma is either protein-bound (mostly to albumin; thus, hyperalbuminemia caused by dehydration or multiple myeloma can cause pseudohypercalcemia) or ionized and readily available for use. Serum calcium is regulated by parathyroid hormone (PTH) and vitamin D. The storage form of vitamin D, 25-hydroxyvitamin D, is converted to the active form, 1,25-dihydroxyvitamin D, in the kidney. Hypercalcemia, defined as serum calcium > 10.5 mg/dL, is relatively uncommon. Ninety percent of cases result from primary hyperparathyroidism or an underlying malignancy. Serum calcium levels up to 12.0 mg/dL rarely cause clinical symptoms. Higher levels can be tolerated if the rise in serum calcium occurs slowly.

DIAGNOSTIC WORKUP & INITIAL MANAGEMENT

History and physical examination

- Most cases are asymptomatic (fatigue and other nonspecific symptoms may occur)
- "Stones, bones, abdominal groans, and psychic overtones" are the classic symptoms of chronic hypercalcemia, but these are often not present initially
  - Stones: Renal stones occur in up to 20% of cases of primary hyperparathyroidism
  - Bones: Bone pain, weakness, osteoporosis
  - Groans: Abdominal pain, nausea/vomiting, constipation, PUD, pancreatitis
  - Psychic overtones: Psychosis, depression, anxiety, personality changes, mood disorders
- Other presentations: Cardiac (hypertension, arrhythmias), renal (nephrogenic diabetes insipidus, type 1 distal renal tubular acidosis, chronic renal insufficiency, acute renal failure), rheumatologic (gout or pseudogout, chondrocalcinosis), neurologic (hyporeflexia)

Initial diagnostic workup

- Initial testing includes repeat total calcium, ionized calcium, phosphorus, PTH, creatinine, albumin, total protein, chest radiography, and ECG
  - Calcium correction for albumin: [0.8 × (normal albumin − measured albumin) + calcium]
  - A cornerstone of diagnosis is PTH level: Elevated in primary hyperparathyroidism; decreased in nonparathyroid causes
  - Phosphorus is elevated or normal in vitamin D–mediated diseases and decreased in parathyroid-mediated diseases and malignancies
- PTH-related peptide (PTHrp) is secreted by certain cancers
- If PTH and PTHrp are normal, check 25-vitamin D and 1,25-vitamin D levels
  - 1,25-vitamin D (active form) is elevated in granulomatous diseases (converted to active form by granuloma-associated macrophages)
  - 25-vitamin D (storage form) may be elevated in exogenous vitamin D intoxication (rare)
- Alkaline phosphatase is elevated in etiologies associated with bone resorption (e.g., hyperparathyroidism, malignancy)
- ECG may show ST depression, wide T waves, short ST segments, or QT shortening, bradyarrhythmias, or heart block
- Other labs and imaging are directed toward specific etiologies or complaints (e.g., CT for nephrolithiasis, ACE for sarcoidosis); search for underlying malignancy may be indicated, including mammography, Pap smear, colonoscopy, chest radiography, and PSA

Initial patient management

- Severe hypercalcemia (>13.0 mg/dL or with symptoms) requires immediate intervention
- IV rehydration with large volumes of normal saline (3–4 L may be necessary)
- Once rehydrated, loop diuretics may be used to increase renal calcium excretion
- Bisphosphonates (IV pamidronate or zoledronate) may be used to inhibit bone resorption
- Calcitonin is sometimes used (decreases bone resorption via osteoclast inhibition)

DIFFERENTIAL DIAGNOSIS

Primary hyperparathyroidism

- Most commonly caused by a single parathyroid adenoma (85% of cases)
- Less commonly caused by parathyroid hyperplasia (may be associated with multiple endocrine neoplasia syndromes) or parathyroid carcinoma
- Symptoms may include weakness, confusion, polyuria, renal stones, nausea, and anorexia
- Symptoms are usually present only when calcium rises over 12.0 mg/dL

Malignancy

- Most common cause of hypercalcemia in hospitalized patients
- The higher the plasma calcium level, the more likely it is caused by a malignancy
- Hypercalcemia results from stimulation of bone resorption by PTHrp produced by the tumor or by locally acting cytokines released from tumor cells
- Symptoms are identical to primary hyperparathyroidism
- Causative malignancies include multiple myeloma, leukemia, lymphoma, breast cancer, lung cancer, renal cell cancer, and others

Drugs

- Thiazides
- Lithium

Other

- Pseudohypercalcemia (elevated albumin levels)
- Dehydration
- Vitamin A or D intoxication
- Renal failure
- Hyperthyroidism
- Pheochromocytoma
- Familial hypocalciuric hypercalcemia
- Granulomatous disease (e.g., sarcoidosis, tuberculosis)
- Adrenal insufficiency
- Paget's disease
- Immobilization
- Hypophosphatemia
- Acromegaly
- Excess calcium ingestion (e.g., milk-alkali syndrome caused by excessive ingestion of milk or calcium supplements)

Hypocalcemia

INTRODUCTION

Hypocalcemia is a common clinical finding, particularly with the increasing numbers of patients on chronic hemodialysis. Calcium is the most abundant mineral in the body, with 99% stored in bone. In plasma, calcium is either protein bound (most commonly to albumin) or ionized and readily available. Decreased plasma calcium stimulates parathyroid hormone (PTH) release, which counteracts decreased serum calcium by stimulating calcium reabsorption from bone and kidney and activation of vitamin D to promote calcium absorption from the gut. Hypocalcemia is defined as serum calcium < 8.5 mg/dL; however, "true" metabolic hypocalcemia requires a low level of ionized (active) calcium. Up to 10% of hospitalized, terminal cancer patients and 50% of ICU patients may be hypocalcemic.

DIAGNOSTIC WORKUP & INITIAL MANAGEMENT

History and physical examination

- Severity of symptoms depends on the rate of drop in the calcium level
- Symptoms may include weakness, fatigue, muscle cramping and spasm (difficulty speaking may indicate laryngeal spasm), paresthesias (perioral or digital), abdominal pain, nausea, vomiting, irritability, and depression
- Severe acute symptoms are rare but warrant prompt recognition and intervention
  - CNS changes may include psychosis, seizures, retardation (in children), dementia, dystonia, parkinsonism, ataxia, oculogyric crisis, or mood disorders
  - Cardiac arrhythmias (including torsades de pointes from prolonged QT interval)
  - CHF and hypotension caused by decreased cardiac contractility
- Skin exam may reveal patchy hair loss, dry and/or scaly skin, hyperpigmentation, brittle nails, and mucocutaneous candidiasis
- Chvostek's sign: Twitching of the corner of the mouth or eyelid upon tapping on the facial nerve in the preauricular area
- Trousseau's sign: Inflation of blood pressure cuff on upper arm for 3 minutes results in extension at IP joints, flexion at MCP joints, and flexion of the wrist

Initial diagnostic workup

- Initial labs include repeat total calcium, ionized calcium, phosphorus, magnesium, PTH, albumin, 25- and 1,25-vitamin D, creatinine, CBC, amylase, and lipase
  - Hypocalcemia is defined as calcium < 8.5 mg/dL
  - Correct calcium level for hypoalbuminemia: Calcium is decreased by 0.8 for each 1 g/dL drop in albumin (ionized calcium does not need correction)
  - Hypoparathyroidism is suggested by decreased PTH and increased phosphorus
  - Pseudohypoparathyroidism is suggested by increased PTH and increased phosphorus
  - Vitamin D deficiency is suggested by increased PTH and decreased phosphorus
- ECG may show prolonged QT interval (most common), heart block, or dysrhythmias
- Radiography may reveal cortical thinning, bone demineralization, or fractures

Initial patient management

- Asymptomatic hypocalcemia can be treated with oral calcium supplements (e.g., calcium carbonate, calcium citrate) plus vitamin D
- Symptomatic hypocalcemia (ionized calcium usually < 0.7 mmol/L) is generally treated with IV calcium gluconate via a central line (may cause cardiac arrest if infused too rapidly)
- Correct other electrolyte abnormalities (e.g., hypomagnesemia)
- Thiazides can be used in patients at risk for stones to decrease renal calcium excretion

DIFFERENTIAL DIAGNOSIS

Hypoparathyroidism

- May be caused by dysfunction of the parathyroid glands caused by autoimmune destruction, infiltrative disease (e.g., hemochromatosis, Wilson's disease, sarcoidosis, tuberculosis), hypomagnesemia, or devitalization of tissue during thyroid or parathyroid surgery
- PTH activity can be overwhelmed (i.e., calcium is deposited in bone despite high parathyroid and low serum calcium) in cases of shock, sepsis, burns, pancreatitis, acute renal failure, or osteoblastic metastases
- Ineffective PTH activity occurs in pseudohypoparathyroidism (end-organ PTH resistance)

Hypoalbuminemia ("pseudohypocalcemia")

- Hypoalbuminemia causes a decreased total calcium level but does not necessarily result in symptoms if the ionized (active) calcium level is normal

Vitamin D deficiency

- Poor oral intake and/or absent sun exposure
- Malabsorption
- Hepatic and/or renal failure
- Anticonvulsant use

Medications

- Diuretics
- Heparin
- Foscarnet
- Cimetidine
- Glucagon
- Phosphates
- Aminoglycosides
- Theophylline
- Cisplatin

Other

- Pancreatitis
- Alkalosis (especially respiratory alkalosis)
- Sepsis
- Shock
- Burns
- Magnesium deficiency (often seen in alcoholism)
- Hyperphosphatemia
- Alcoholism (may directly suppress PTH and/or deplete magnesium)
- Postoperative (usually transient)
- Postblood transfusion with citrated blood
- Malignancy (e.g., medullary carcinoma of the thyroid, osteoblastic metastases)
- Familial hypocalcemia
- DiGeorge's syndrome (congenital absence of the parathyroid glands)
- Polyglandular autoimmune syndrome type I (hypoparathyroidism, adrenal insufficiency, and mucocutaneous candidiasis)
- Rickets
- Pseudohypocalcemia caused by contrast agents

Hyperglycemia

INTRODUCTION

The American Diabetes Association criteria for diagnosis of diabetes mellitus requires a random plasma glucose of ≥200 mg/dL *or* a fasting plasma glucose of ≥126 mg/dL *or* a 2-hour plasma glucose of ≥200 mg/dL during an oral glucose tolerance test. Fasting plasma glucose (after at least 8 hours of fasting) is generally considered the best test: A plasma glucose of <100 mg/dL is normal; a plasma glucose of 100–125 mg/dL is classified as IFG; and a plasma glucose of ≥126 mg/dL is classified as diabetes. Diagnosis should usually be reconfirmed by repeat testing on a different day. Diabetes is usually diagnosed by these criteria as an outpatient case; inpatient management of hyperglycema is discussed below.

DIAGNOSTIC WORKUP & INITIAL MANAGEMENT

- Hyperglycemia is relatively common in hospitalized patients because of increased insulin demands and resistance during times of stress or illness, altered oral intake, and altered medication regimens
- The target glucose level is < 110 mg/dL pre-meal, with no values > 180 mg/dL; patients may require IV insulin to reach these goals
- Patients with hyperglycemia in the hospital setting can be classified into 3 groups: known diabetics, undiagnosed diabetics (i.e., patients who are true diabetics but have not yet been diagnosed), and nondiabetics with new-onset hyperglycemia

History and physical examination

- Assess vital signs and evaluate for symptoms of DKA, such as abdominal pain, nausea/vomiting, and diaphoresis; also evaluate for symptoms of nonketotic hyperosmolar hyperglycemia, including weakness, visual disturbances, and confusion
- Perform a focused history, review of systems, and physical exam including medication usage (e.g., note when last doses of insulin and oral hypoglycemic medications given), diet history and restrictions, and reason for hospitalization
  - In patients receiving IV medications, ensure they are not being administered with dextrose solution (versus saline solution)
- Initial labs include CBC with differential, chemistries, magnesium, phosphorus, urinalysis, serum ketones (e.g., acetone), and ABG
  - Patients are nearly always potassium depleted; however, chemistries may reveal pseudohyperkalemia caused by acidosis and lack of insulin
  - ABG may reveal metabolic acidosis (anion gap)
  - BUN and creatinine may be high due to osmotic diuresis and dehydration
- Consider ECG if cardiac ischemia may be the cause of hyperglycemia
- Evaluate for possible triggers of hyperglycemia, including physiologic stressors (e.g., MI, stroke, dehydration, trauma, pancreatitis) and medication noncompliance

Initial patient management

- Management of hyperglycemia includes identifying causative factors, correcting or reversing those factors, choosing appropriate medication(s) to promote euglycemia, ensuring hydration and nutrition, and correcting electrolyte imbalances
- Resist the temptation to order insulin without evaluating the patient
- Hyperglycemia in the absence of ketoacidosis will generally respond to insulin therapy (IV or SC) and fluids
- If treatment is necessary, insulin is often the most appropriate therapy for uncontrolled diabetes, DKA, hyperosmolar hyperglycemia, and patients with critical illnesses, either in place of or in addition to the patient's usual regimen
  - IV insulin may be required, particularly for patients with DKA (when given, fingerstick glucose monitoring should occur hourly until stable)

DIFFERENTIAL DIAGNOSIS

Diabetic ketoacidosis (DKA)
- A syndrome of hyperglycemia and metabolic acidosis that results from insulin deficiency, primarily in type 1 diabetics
  - Can also occur in type 2 diabetics who are very insulin-resistant
- Diagnosis requires blood glucose level of >250 mg/dL (often much higher), pH <7.3, and bicarbonate level of <18 mEq/L
- Most common precipitant of DKA is infection

Hyperosmolar hyperglycemic coma
- Systemic stress in type 2 diabetics results in hyperglycemia over days to weeks, leading to osmotic diuresis with severe dehydration, hyperosmolarity, and mental status changes
- Differentiated from DKA by absence of ketosis and acidosis
- Precipitants include infection, medication noncompliance, alcohol, and acute illness

Acute illness
- Acute illness (e.g., cardiac ischemia, stroke, infection) causes increased catabolism, gluconeogenesis, and lipolysis, resulting in elevated blood glucose
- Intensive IV insulin therapy is indicated in patients with MI or requiring intensive care; should be titrated to achieve a target blood glucose of 80–110 mg/dL

Medication error
- Type 1 diabetics require some basal insulin, even when not eating
- Hyperglycemia may occur when IV medications are given in a dextrose solution

Corticosteroid therapy
- Steroids affect blood glucose levels by inhibiting glucose uptake in peripheral tissues and increasing hepatic gluconeogenesis
- The major risk factors for steroid-induced hyperglycemia in nondiabetics are higher steroid doses, advanced age, and family history of diabetes
- In most cases, blood glucose elevations occur postprandially, because peripheral glucose utilization is impaired
- Recommended management is insulin rather than oral hypoglycemic medications
- IV insulin may be utilized to obtain rapid glucose control

Total parenteral nutrition (TPN) or enteral feeding
- Nearly all diabetics receiving TPN will require insulin therapy to maintain euglycemia
- Enteral feedings predispose to hyperglycemia of increased carbohydrate loads (45–90% of calories from carbohydrates) that exceed the recommended 12–15 daily carbohydrate servings for a typical diabetic diet
  - Enteral feedings can also predispose to hypoglycemia if discontinued abruptly when long-acting insulin has been administered

Postoperative
- Surgical patients are at increased risk for hyperglycemia from the stress of surgery
- Type 1 diabetics will become hyperglycemic if not given a basal insulin dose, even if they are not eating

Other
- Impaired fasting glucose
- Gestational diabetes
- Pancreatic disease (e.g., acute or chronic pancreatitis, pancreatectomy, pancreatic carcinoma, hemochromatosis, cystic fibrosis)
- Acromegaly
- Cushing's syndrome
- Pheochromocytoma
- Hyperthyroidism (thyroid storm)
- Glucagonoma
- Amyloidosis

Hypoglycemia

INTRODUCTION

Hypoglycemia is defined as a triad of (1) plasma glucose < 45–50 mg/dL, (2) neuroglycopenia and/or hyperadrenergic symptoms, and (3) resolution of symptoms on administration of glucose. It is common in diabetics. Maintaining appropriate blood glucose requires regulation of glucose influx into the circulation. The balance of glucose production in the liver with uptake and use in peripheral tissues is regulated by a complex network of hormones, neural pathways, and metabolic signals. As glucose becomes low, release of glucagon, growth hormone, and epinephrine occurs, which rapidly mobilizes hepatic glycogen to provide fuel. If untreated, it can result in diminished glucose delivery to the brain, which may cause irreversible neurologic dysfunction. Education of diabetic patients to coordinate the timing of medications, diet, and exercise is essential.

DIAGNOSTIC WORKUP & INITIAL MANAGEMENT

- Assess vital signs, airway, breathing, and circulation
- Suspect hypoglycemia in patients with signs of neuroglycopenia (sudden change in mental status, seizures, focal neurologic deficits) or hyperadrenergic symptoms (e.g., diaphoresis, tachycardia, palpitations, tremor)
- If patient is not mentating well (and not hypotensive), elevate the head of bed to 90° to keep the patient from aspirating
- If patient is asymptomatic but blood glucose is low, recheck to confirm
- Patients with long-standing type 1 diabetes may have hypoglycemic unawareness until they reach very low blood glucose levels
- Review medication records for oral hypoglycemics and insulin dosing

Initial patient management

- Treat hypoglycemia immediately
  - If patient is mentating well and protecting the airway, give 4–8 oz of fruit juice
  - If patient is obtunded or comatose and has IV access, give 0.5 amp of 50% dextrose solution; repeat as necessary to raise the glucose to >70 mg/dL
  - If no IV access and patient cannot take anything by mouth, give IM glucagon (1 mg), which should be stocked on the code cart
- Recheck blood glucose every 5 minutes until it stabilizes and symptoms improve
- If blood sugars continue to drop, start D5W IV drip; if inadequate, change to 10% solution; if necessary, place a central line to administer 20% solution
- If suspect adrenal insufficiency, measure cortisol level, then give 100 mg IV hydrocortisone

History and physical examination

- Detailed history should include medication history; timing of hypoglycemia relative to medications, meals, or exercise; alcohol intake; history of diabetes, liver or renal disease, or gastric surgery; family history of diabetes or MEN syndromes; signs or symptoms of hormonal excess or deficiencies (e.g., hypopituitarism); nutritional state; and recent illness or infection
- Physical exam should evaluate for signs of adrenal insufficiency (e.g., hypotension, hyperpigmentation) or sepsis (e.g., hypotension, fever, mental status changes)

Diagnostic testing

- Labs should be performed when the blood glucose is <50 mg/dL
  - Testing may include plasma glucose, insulin, proinsulin, C-peptide (produced during endogenous insulin production), sulfonylurea, and cortisol; these tests assess for factious hypoglycemia, insulinoma, and adrenal insufficiency
- Also check liver and renal function
- Initiate workup for infection (e.g., blood, urine, sputum cultures) if suspect sepsis
- CT or MRI may be necessary to evaluate for insulinoma

DIFFERENTIAL DIAGNOSIS

Medications
- Most cases of hypoglycemia occur in diabetics and can be attributed to insulin or sulfonylurea use (e.g., glipizide, glyburide)
  - Exogenous insulin administration is the most common cause overall; may occur with inadequate food ingestion or excessive exercise following an insulin dose; may also occur as a result of delayed absorption of food (e.g., diabetic gastroparesis)
- Alcohol is a common cause: Ethanol impairs gluconeogenesis so that hypoglycemia can be seen after hepatic glycogen stores are depleted (occurs after 8–12 hours of fasting)
- Renal insufficiency (decreased clearance of insulin) and liver failure (decreased gluco-neogenesis) predispose to hypoglycemia
- Assess for prescription errors (e.g., administration of wrong medication)
- Fluoroquinolones (especially gatifloxacin, which should be avoided in diabetics), β-blockers, quinine, warfarin, pentamidine, and haloperidol have also been implicated

Sepsis or severe infection
- Can result in blunted gluconeogenesis, resulting in hypoglycemia

Adrenal insufficiency
- Suspect the diagnosis in patients who are also hypotensive or have been in the ICU

Insulinoma
- A pancreatic beta-cell tumor; it can cause hypoglycemia because it is insensitive to blood glucose levels and can inappropriately secrete insulin during a period of fasting
- May be associated with MEN1 syndrome

IGF-2–secreting tumors
- Non–islet cell tumors (e.g., retroperitoneal fibrosarcoma, hepatocellular carcinoma, adrenocortical carcinomas, GI tumors, lymphoma, leukemia) have been associated with hypoglycemia

Severe nutritional deficiency
- Alcoholism, end-stage AIDS, and terminal cancers may result in severe nutritional defi-ciencies, leading to impaired gluconeogenesis

Reactive (postprandial) hypoglycemia
- Common after gastric surgery when there is rapid emptying of ingested food, causing overstimulation of vagal reflexes and mismatch of insulin and glucose levels
- Occult or early diabetes may cause a delay in 1st-phase insulin release at the beginning of a meal; the resultant hyperglycemia produces an exaggerated insulin release 4–5 hours after a meal that may result in hypoglycemia

Artifactual hypoglycemia
- In patients with leukemia or severe hemolytic disease, excess white blood cells or red blood cell precursors can take up glucose before the sample can be analyzed; consider putting another sample on ice in a gray-top tube

Other
- Attention-seeking behavior (factitious)
- Hypothyroidism
- Malnutrition/fasting
- Renal failure
- Sarcomas
- Pituitary insufficiency
- Congenital hormone or enzyme defects
- Severe hepatic dysfunction (e.g., hepatitis, hepatic toxins, hepatic necrosis)

Hyperkalemia

INTRODUCTION

Potassium is the major intracellular cation. It contributes to generation of membrane electropotentials responsible for facilitating muscular contraction, including cardiac muscle contraction. Potassium is primarily stored intracellularly and is excreted in the urine (>90%) and to a lesser extent in feces and perspiration. A major regulator of serum potassium concentration is aldosterone, which increases renal sodium reabsorption in exchange for potassium secretion into the urine. Ingested potassium is rapidly sequestered intracellularly (mediated in part by insulin) to prevent a harmful rise in serum concentration. Over 6–8 hours, aldosterone-mediated urinary excretion eliminates excess potassium from the body. Hyperkalemia (>5.5 mEq/L) may result in arrhythmias, ventricular fibrillation, or asystole.

DIAGNOSTIC WORKUP & INITIAL MANAGEMENT

- Intervention with IV calcium, sodium bicarbonate, insulin, β_2-agonists, sodium polystyrene resin, or dialysis is necessary if potassium exceeds 6.0 mEq/L, the rise is sudden, or ECG changes are present

History and physical examination
- May be completely asymptomatic
- Most often, the presentation is related to the underlying condition
- Most common symptoms of hyperkalemia are muscle weakness and cardiac conduction abnormalities
- Weakness typically begins in the lower extremities and then ascends; respiratory muscles and muscles innervated by the cranial nerves are usually spared
- Numbness, decreased reflexes, or irritability may also occur
- Hypoventilation is a late finding
- History may reveal excessive dietary potassium intake or medication-induced potassium retention or cellular shifts
- Unless the patient is hemodynamically unstable, cardiac toxicity most likely will be detected only by ECG

Initial diagnostic workup
- Address any hemodynamic or cardiovascular instability before extensive diagnostic evaluation; hyperkalemia can be rapidly fatal
- Rule out pseudohyperkalemia (e.g., hemolysis, WBC > 100,000/mm^3, platelets > 1,000,000/mm^3) by repeat potassium measurement and clinical presentation
- Rule out hyperkalemia from diabetic ketoacidosis, for which management differs
- All patients require an ECG, which shows classic progressive changes:
  - 5.5–6.5 mEq/L: Tall, peaked T waves and shortened QT interval
  - 6.5–7.5 mEq/L: 1st-degree AV block; flat, wide p waves; widened QRS complex
  - 7.5–8.5 mEq/L: Loss of p waves; left or right bundle branch block; ST elevation; ventricular tachycardia, ventricular fibrillation, or asystole
- Initial laboratory tests may include electrolytes including calcium, magnesium, and phosphate; BUN and creatinine, cortisol, creatine phosphokinase, and glucose
  - Assess underlying renal function and adequacy of urine output
- Consider ABG to evaluate for metabolic acidosis (every 0.1 decrease in pH causes an increase in plasma potassium of 0.5 mmol/L)
- Digoxin level, if applicable
- If renal function is normal and history is unrevealing, consider transtubular potassium gradient (TTKG) to evaluate for hypoaldosteronism (morning plasma renin and aldosterone, paired serum and urine osmolality, urine and plasma potassium)
- Discontinue possible offending medications (e.g., NSAIDs, ACE inhibitors, potassium-sparing diuretics)

DIFFERENTIAL DIAGNOSIS

Decreased urinary excretion of potassium
- Acute or chronic renal insufficiency
- Aldosterone resistant or deficient states
  - Primary adrenal insufficiency
  - Aldosterone resistance: Drugs (e.g., spironolactone, potassium-sparing diuretics, trimethoprim, pentamidine, cyclosporine), tubulointerstitial disease, type IV renal tubular acidosis
  - Secondary hypoaldosteronism: Drugs (e.g., ACE inhibitors, angiotensin-receptor blockers, heparin), AIDS, hyporeninemia (e.g., diabetes mellitus, NSAIDs, cyclosporine)
- Gordon's syndrome
- Ureterojejunostomy
- Marked effective circulating volume depletion (e.g., severe CHF)
- Missed dialysis

Increased potassium release from cells
- Pseudohyperkalemia
  - Prolonged use of tourniquet with or without repeated fist clenching
  - Hemolysis after blood is drawn
  - Marked leukocytosis and thrombocytosis (cells release potassium into the serum during clotting)
- Extracellular shifting of potassium in response to drugs
  - Nonselective β-blockers
  - Severe digitalis toxicity
  - Succinylcholine
  - α-Adrenergic agonists
  - Excessive potassium supplementation in a patient with impaired renal function
- Tissue breakdown
  - Intravascular hemolysis
  - Tumor lysis syndrome
  - Ischemia
  - Excessive exercise
  - Trauma
  - Rhabdomyolysis
- Metabolic acidosis
- Hyperosmolar states (e.g., hyperglycemia)
- Insulin deficiency
- Hyperkalemic periodic paralysis
- Depolarizing muscle paralysis

Excess intake of potassium
- Oral or IV potassium replacement
- Dietary excess (e.g., bananas, potatoes)

Hypokalemia

INTRODUCTION

Potassium is the major intracellular cation and is responsible for facilitating muscular contraction, including cardiac muscle function. Potassium is primarily stored intracellularly and is excreted in the urine (>90%) and also in feces and perspiration. Aldosterone is a major regulator of serum potassium concentration. It increases renal sodium reabsorption in exchange for potassium secretion into the urine. In general, loss of 200–400 mEq of potassium is necessary to lower the serum level from 4.0 to 3.0 mEq/L, and loss of another of 200–400 mEq will cause a drop to 2.0 mEq/L. Intracellular potassium will enter the extracellular fluid in an effort to maintain normal serum concentrations for as long as possible. Hypokalemia (<3.5 mEq/L) increases the risk for muscle weakness and cardiac arrhythmia.

DIAGNOSTIC WORKUP & INITIAL MANAGEMENT

History and physical examination

- May be asymptomatic; symptoms usually begin when potassium falls to <2.5 mEq/L
- Muscle weakness is the most common symptom
- Other initial symptoms include fatigue, myalgias, muscle cramps, constipation, respiratory muscle weakness, or paralysis
- Assess for etiologies of potassium loss (e.g., diarrhea, prolonged vomiting, diuretic usage, renal tubular acidosis, poor dietary intake)
- Assess for acid/base disturbances that could result in transcellular potassium shifts
- Cardiac abnormalities are common and include hypertension, life-threatening arrhythmias (e.g., ventricular tachycardia or fibrillation), potentiation of digoxin, and heart block
- Other presentations include rhabdomyolysis, dehydration from nephrogenic diabetes insipidus, hyperglycemia, ileus, or worsening of hepatic encephalopathy
- CHF patients are at higher risk for arrhythmias, even with mild hypokalemia
- Liver failure patients are at higher risk for hepatic coma, even with mild hypokalemia

Initial diagnostic workup

- Initial labs should include repeat potassium to ensure level is accurate, electrolytes (may reveal associated hypomagnesemia or hypophosphatemia), glucose (rule out diabetic ketoacidosis), and CBC
  - 40% of patients with hypokalemia are also hypomagnesemic
  - Pseudohypokalemia may occur with massive leukocytosis (e.g., leukemia)
- The fractional excretion of potassium in the urine is increased in cases of increased renal potassium loss
  - Urine sodium and creatinine concentrations can be useful
- ABG will reveal a decrease in plasma potassium of 0.5 mmol/L for every 0.1 increase in pH
- Progressive ECG changes occur as serum potassium level falls: Low-voltage QRS complexes, flattened T waves, depressed ST segments, prominent P and U waves (U waves follow the T wave), prolonged PR and QT intervals, wide QRS complexes, and ventricular arrhythmias
  - *Note that ECG changes do not correlate well with degree of hypokalemia*
  - ECG changes occur in 80% of patients with serum potassium of <2.7 mEq/L

Initial patient management

- Magnesium must be replaced before successful potassium repletion
- In asymptomatic, mild to moderate cases, oral potassium repletion is usually sufficient
- In severe or symptomatic cases, consider simultaneous IV and oral potassium repletion
- In cases of chronic hypokalemia, consider a daily potassium supplement (20–40 mEq/day) and a potassium-sparing diuretic (e.g., triamterene, spironolactone)
- Address the underlying cause(s) of potassium deficiency and treat as necessary

DIFFERENTIAL DIAGNOSIS

Increased potassium losses
Primarily via urinary or GI losses
- Medications (e.g., kayexalate, diuretics, high-dose penicillin, aminoglycosides, steroids, amphotericin B)
- Dialysis
- Vomiting
- Diarrhea
- Laxative abuse
- Nasogastric suction
- GI fistula
- Excessive sweating
- Geophagia
- Hyperaldosteronism
  - Consider mineralocorticoid excess states in patients who are resistant to repletion with appropriate doses of potassium or have marked hypokalemia with diuretic therapy
- Renal tubular acidosis type 1 or 2
- Osmotic diuresis from uncontrolled diabetes mellitus
- Magnesium deficiency
- Bartter's or Gitelman's syndrome
- Cushing's syndrome
- Liddle's syndrome
- Ureterosigmoidostomy

Intracellular redistribution from the serum
Transcellular shifts of potassium may transiently decrease (or increase) plasma potassium without altering total body potassium
- Medications (e.g., insulin, catecholamines, β-adrenergic agonists, caffeine, vitamin B_{12})
- Increased extracellular pH (alkalosis)
- Increased physiologic β-adrenergic activity (e.g., stress, ischemia)
- Hypokalemic periodic paralysis
- Digibind therapy (for digoxin toxicity)
- Barium or toluene ingestion
- Anabolic states or conditions of rapid cell multiplication (e.g., thyrotoxicosis)
- Hypothermia
- Chloroquine overdose

Decreased potassium intake
Rarely causes hypokalemia, because the kidneys are very efficient at conserving potassium
- Starvation
- Malabsorption
- Postoperative
- Administration of potassium-free IV fluids
- "Fad" diets (e.g., liquid protein)
- Clay ingestion (pica)

Other
- Pseudohypokalemia may result from metabolically active white blood cells (e.g., acute myelogenous leukemia) that take up serum potassium if the sample is not analyzed promptly

Hypernatremia

INTRODUCTION

Hypernatremia is a common clinical condition that occurs in ~1% of hospitalized elderly patients. Serum sodium may be increased by water deprivation, excessive water losses without sufficient repletion, or excessive sodium intake relative to water. The majority of cases result from a water deficit rather than a sodium excess. When evaluating a patient with hypernatremia, assess volume status to determine the etiology and subsequent treatment. As opposed to hyponatremia (in which patients can be either hypo- or hyperosmolar), all hypernatremic patients are hyperosmolar. Hypernatremia has been proposed as a marker of infection and perhaps neglect (i.e., dehydration) in elderly nursing home patients.

DIAGNOSTIC WORKUP & INITIAL MANAGEMENT

History and physical examination

- Hypernatremia is defined as a serum sodium concentration > 145 mEq/L
- Severity of symptoms relates to acuity and magnitude of the rise in sodium
- Common symptoms include increased thirst, weakness, hypertonia, ataxia, restlessness, tremulousness, irritability, confusion, headache, and lethargy
- Symptoms may progress to changes in mental status, focal neurologic deficits, seizures, coma, and cerebral hemorrhage (from severe neuronal dehydration, usually in infants)
- Note thirst and urination patterns, mental status, presence of diarrhea and vomiting, medications, access to oral fluids, IV fluid administration, and recent CNS surgery
- Assess vital signs for evidence of decreased circulating volume
- Dry mucous membranes and poor skin turgor may be present

Initial diagnostic workup

- History and exam are almost always diagnostic without need for extensive testing
- Studies include electrolytes, renal function, serum osmolality, urine sodium and osmolality
  - BUN:creatinine ratio > 20–40:1 may point to significant decrease in circulating volume (e.g., diuretics, diarrhea, impaired thirst)
  - Urine sodium level elevated in renal water loss (>20 mEq/L); decreased in GI, respiratory disease, and skin loss or poor oral intake (<10 mEq/L); normal in hyperaldosteronism
  - Urine osmolality is decreased in diabetes insipidus (DI); variable with diuretic usage; increased in GI disease, respiratory disease, skin loss, or poor oral intake
- Serum sodium of 150–170 mEq/L usually results from dehydration, 170–190 mEq/L is often from DI, and >190 mEq/L is usually from iatrogenic sodium administration
- DI is diagnosed by polyuria and urine osmolality > 250 mOsm/kg

Initial patient management

- Treat patients with severe dehydration and hypotension emergently with normal saline solution IV; change to more hypotonic fluid once hemodynamically stable
- Calculate the effect of 1 L of replacement fluid [($Na^+_{fluid} - Na^+_{serum}$)/(TBW + 1)], where TBW = weight × 0.6 (in men) or 0.5 (in women)
- Administer replacement fluids at a rate sufficient to reduce serum sodium by no more than 10–15 mEq/L per day (0.5 mEq/L per hour) in chronic hypernatremia and 1 mEq/L per hour in acute hypernatremia; account for ongoing losses as well
  - Overly rapid correction of serum sodium can precipitate seizures or cerebral edema
- Isovolemic hypernatremia: Replace fluid with D5W
- Hypovolemic hypernatremia: Replace fluid with normal saline until hemodynamically stable, then switch to half-normal saline or D5W as appropriate
- Hypervolemic hypernatremia: Administer D5W and loop diuretics concomitantly; ensure a net reduction in total body sodium and water; dialysis may be required in severe cases

DIFFERENTIAL DIAGNOSIS

Increased loss of water relative to sodium
- GI losses
  - Diarrhea
  - Vomiting
  - Intestinal fistula
- Drugs (e.g., diuretics, alcohol, amphotericin B, phenytoin, propoxyphene, lithium, demeclocycline)
- Excessive sweating
- Severe burns
- Fever
- Hyperventilation
- Diabetes insipidus (DI)
  - Central DI: Lack of antidiuretic hormone secretion by pituitary gland
  - Nephrogenic DI: Renal resistance to antidiuretic hormone
- Hyperglycemia (results from osmotic diuresis)
- Post-acute tubular necrosis diuresis
- Thyrotoxicosis
- Infection

Inadequate water ingestion relative to insensible losses and/or dietary sodium intake
- Poor oral intake (e.g., in the elderly)
- Inability to swallow water because of physical limitation (e.g., immobility, stroke)
- Lack of free access to fluids (e.g., infants, elderly, nursing home patients)
- Impaired thirst mechanism (e.g., hypothalamic lesion caused by stroke)
- Tube feeding or parenteral nutrition with inadequate free water
- Ventilated patients with insufficient fluid administration

Excessive sodium intake
- Ectopic ACTH
- Iatrogenic (e.g., hypertonic saline administration via enemas or resuscitation fluid)
- Seawater ingestion/drowning

Essential hypernatremia (reset osmostat)
- Mineralocorticoid excess
- Cushing's syndrome
- Some forms of congenital adrenal hyperplasia

Hyponatremia

INTRODUCTION

Hyponatremia is the most common electrolyte abnormality and is defined as plasma sodium concentration < 135 mmol/L. The etiology is classified by serum osmolality (hyperosmotic, isosmotic, or hyposmotic) and volume status. Hyponatremia results from an excess of water relative to sodium, regardless of the volume status. A hyponatremic patient can be hypovolemic, euvolemic, or hypervolemic. Hyponatremia is quite common among patients in chronic care facilities and intensive care settings. The mortality rate varies from 5–50%, depending on the severity and acuity of onset. About 7% of healthy elderly individuals have a serum sodium level < 137 mmol/L.

DIAGNOSTIC WORKUP & INITIAL MANAGEMENT

History and physical examination
- Severity of clinical presentation depends on rapidity and magnitude of fall in serum sodium
- Symptoms and clinical signs become most apparent when sodium falls to <120 mEq/L
- Early clinical symptoms include change in mental status, apathy, agitation, headache, ataxia, focal weakness or hemiparesis, and altered level of consciousness
- May progress to seizures and coma
- Clinical symptoms of the underlying etiology may be present (e.g., pulmonary and pedal edema in cases of CHF)
- Evaluate volume status by physical exam (dry mucous membranes, decreased urine output, and skin tenting suggests hypovolemia; edema suggests hypervolemia)

Initial diagnostic workup
- Initial labs include serum electrolytes, osmolality, BUN and creatinine, calcium, magnesium, TSH, glucose, and urine sodium, creatinine, and osmolality
- Assess plasma osmolality:
  - Hyperosmotic (plasma osmolality >295): Assess for hyperglycemia (sodium decreases 1.6 for every 100 mg/dL increase in glucose) or hypertonic infusions (e.g., mannitol, glycine)
  - Isosmotic (plasma osmolality 275–295): Consider pseudohyponatremia and isotonic infusions that do not contain sodium
  - Hyposmotic (plasma osmolality <275): Assess volume status and check BUN, creatinine, urine sodium and osmolality:
    - Hypervolemic: Urine sodium is <10 mmol/L in CHF, cirrhosis, or nephrosis; urine sodium may be >20 mmol/L in renal failure
    - Hypovolemic: Urine sodium is <10 mmol/L in extrarenal losses (e.g., vomiting, diarrhea, 3rd-spacing); urine sodium is >20 mmol/L in renal losses (e.g., diuretics, Addison's disease, salt wasting nephropathy)
    - Euvolemic: Usually from SIADH, adrenal insufficiency, hypothyroidism, or psychogenic polydipsia; urine sodium is often >20 mmol/L; clinical history guides workup; in SIADH, urine osmolality > serum osmolality
- If typical etiologies of SIADH are not readily identifiable, a malignancy workup may be indicated to evaluate for an ADH-secreting tumor

Initial patient management
- Treat severe hyponatremia (serum sodium <115 mEq/L; rapidly developed hyponatremia; *or* hyponatremia with serious CNS symptoms) with hypertonic (3%) saline at 25–100 mL/hour until sodium is 120 mEq/L; consider nephrology and ICU consultation
- If the patient is stable, correct serum sodium gradually (especially in chronic cases) to avoid osmotic demyelination syndrome; serum sodium should not rise faster than 0.5–1 mEq/L per hour or 12mEq/L in a 24 hour period (even if the patient is symptomatic)
- Treatment of mild-moderate hyponatremia is guided by the underlying disease process

DIFFERENTIAL DIAGNOSIS

Hyperosmotic hyponatremia (increased serum osmolality)
- Hyperglycemia
- Hypertonic infusions (e.g., mannitol, glycine, sorbitol)

Isosmotic hyponatremia (normal serum osmolality)
- Pseudohyponatremia (lab error because of marked hyperlipidemia or hyperproteinemia)
- Isosmolar infusions that do not contain sodium

Hyposmotic hyponatremia (decreased serum osmolality)
Hypovolemic
Loss of proportionately more sodium than water, resulting in a total body water deficit plus a larger total body sodium deficit
- Vomiting
- Diarrhea
- 3rd-spacing (e.g., pancreatitis, burns)
- Addison's disease
- Renal tubular acidosis
- Renal losses (e.g., diuretics, renal disease)

Euvolemic
Mild increase in total body water that still appears euvolemic (e.g., no edema)
- SIADH secretion
  - Common cause of hyponatremia
  - 6 criteria must be present for diagnosis: euvolemia; hyposmolar hyponatremia; urine osmolality >200 mEq/L; urine Na^+ >20 mmol/L; normal organ function; improvement with water restriction
  - May result from pain, nausea, emotion, medications (e.g. antipsychotics, chlorpropamide), pulmonary disease, malignancy, idiopathic
- Renal failure
- Hypothyroidism
- Adrenal insufficiency
- Psychogenic polydipsia

Hypervolemic
Excess total body sodium plus a proportionately greater excess of total body water from impaired ability to excrete water
- Cirrhosis
- CHF
- Acute or chronic kidney disease
- Nephrotic syndrome

Hyperpigmentation

INTRODUCTION

Disorders of skin hyperpigmentation can be focal or diffuse. In diffuse hyperpigmentation, it is important to search carefully for an underlying endocrine or systemic disease or a history of medications or heavy metals that may explain the findings. Refer to the *Skin Lesions: Pigmented* entry for a discussion of focal hyperpigmentation.

DIAGNOSTIC WORKUP & INITIAL MANAGEMENT

History and physical examination

- Assess onset, associated symptoms, history of previous rash or inflammation in the affected area, medical history, and family history
- Review the patient's medication list to rule out drug-induced pigmentation or melasma
- Note whether rash, erythema, or scale preceded the hyperpigmentation
- Heavy or irregular menses, hirsutism, and/or obesity may suggest polycystic ovarian syndrome

Initial diagnostic workup

- Diffuse hyperpigmentation must be evaluated for an underlying endocrine disorder; initial laboratory testing includes CBC, liver function tests and iron profile (rule out hemochromatosis), fasting glucose (rule out diabetes), ACTH level (rule out Addison's disease), and cosyntropin stimulation tests (rule out Cushing's disease)
- Trunk and chest lesions should have a KOH preparation performed (round "spores" and short, nonbranching, blunt hyphae suggest tinea versicolor)
- Age-appropriate malignancy screening is warranted in patients with acanthosis nigricans without evidence of endocrine dysfunction or obesity

Initial patient management

- Acanthosis nigricans improves with adequate treatment of the underlying endocrine disorder; treatments may include weight loss, dietary/medication control of insulin resistance, and topical exfoliants (e.g., lactic acid, tretinoin, urea-based medications)
- Tinea versicolor: Topical antifungals (e.g., ketoconazole) or oral antifungals (e.g., fluconazole) may be used
  ○ Normalization of pigmentation may take many months
  ○ Long-term maintenance therapy is necessary to prevent recurrence
- Melasma often improves spontaneously after pregnancy or discontinuation of oral contraceptives
  ○ Strict sun avoidance is essential; topical retinoids and hydroquinones facilitate normalization of skin pigment
  ○ Chemical peels or laser procedures may help to restore normal pigmentation
- Avoid offending medications
- Adjuvant laser therapy may be necessary to remove or destroy residual drug particles, hemosiderin, or excess melanin in the skin

DIFFERENTIAL DIAGNOSIS

Acanthosis nigricans
- Velvety, hyperpigmented thickening of skin folds (e.g., axillae, groin, neck, and inframammary regions)
- Associated with insulin resistance (e.g., diabetes mellitus, Cushing's disease, hypothyroidism, obesity, polycystic ovarian syndrome, exogenous corticosteroids)

Tinea versicolor
- Mottled macular hyperpigmentation (and/or hypopigmentation) with fine scale; often presents on the upper trunk and shoulders
- Caused by *Pityrosporum ovale* (*Malassezia furfur*), which look like "spaghetti and meatballs" on KOH preparation
- May be pruritic during the acute phase, particularly in warm environments that encourage growth of the fungus

Post-inflammatory hyperpigmentation
- Patchy, transient hyperpigmentation following resolution of inflammatory rashes
- In darker skin tones, it may take months to years to resolve

Melasma (chloasma, "mask of pregnancy")
- Gradual, blotchy, macular hyperpigmentation, especially of the malar surfaces, chin, and forehead
- Occurs with oral contraceptive use, during pregnancy, or may be idiopathic
- May fade postpartum or after discontinuing oral contraceptives and recur if either returns

Gray or blue hyperpigmentation
- May result from medications: Amiodarone, minocycline, imipramine, chemotherapeutic drugs (e.g., bleomycin, doxorubicin), antimalarials, AZT
- May result from heavy metal poisoning

Incontinentia pigmenti
- A genetic disorder with associated systemic abnormalities
- The final stage of skin disease can present as linear and whorled streaks of hyperpigmentation

Hemochromatosis
- Diffuse hyperpigmentation

Diabetic dermopathy
- Hyperpigmented, round, atrophic lesions located on the shins of diabetics

Confluent and reticulated papillomatosis of Gougerot and Carteud
- Dark-brown, often velvety plaques on the neck, chest, and back
- More diffuse than acanthosis nigricans
- Usually responds well to minocycline and topical keratolytics

Mongolian spots
- Benign, irregular, flat, congenital birthmarks common in persons of East Asian descent
- Normally disappear several years after birth

Chronic arsenic exposure
- Associated with hyperkeratosis
- Does not spare the hands and feet

Hypopigmentation

INTRODUCTION

Distinguishing between hypopigmentation and depigmentation is crucial to narrowing the differential diagnosis. Hypopigmentation is a decrease in the level of pigmentation of the skin, whereas depigmentation is a total loss of skin pigment. Both can be either localized or generalized, which also helps to narrow the differential. Skin biopsies are rarely helpful in this scenario. Hypopigmentation may be of significant cosmetic concern, especially patchy lesions in exposed areas on dark-skinned individuals. Unfortunately, some hypopigmentation conditions are difficult to treat.

DIAGNOSTIC WORKUP & INITIAL MANAGEMENT

History and physical examination
- Determine whether the skin is completely depigmented (chalk white) or merely hypopigmented (lighter than surrounding skin but with residual pigmentation)
  - Wood's lamp exam is helpful in this situation
- Assess onset, duration, and progression
- Assess medical history, including medication use, family history of hypopigmentation or neurocutaneous disorders, and personal history of thyroid disease or other endocrine disorders, diabetes, or exposure to chemicals
- History of allergies, hay fever, or asthma may support the diagnosis of post-inflammatory hypopigmentation caused by atopic dermatitis
- History of erythema or rash at the hypopigmented spot suggests pityriasis alba or post-inflammatory hypopigmentation
- Vitiligo is easily diagnosed on clinical exam alone
- Eye exam to rule out strabismus or iris translucency that can be present in albinism

Initial diagnostic workup
- Wood's lamp exam can be used to highlight the borders of hypopigmented and depigmented patches
- Skin biopsy can support the diagnosis of vitiligo but is not specific
- Check thyroid function tests in patients with recent-onset vitiligo, and consider fasting glucose or ACTH stimulation test to rule out diabetes and Addison's disease
- CBC (anemia, macrocytosis) may be indicated if suspect pernicious anemia in patients with vitiligo

Initial patient management
- Topical steroids may stimulate repigmentation of vitiligo and pityriasis alba
- Sunscreen is crucial to protect vulnerable skin
- Avoid trauma in patients who develop vitiligo (Koebner's effect)
- Repigmentation may be facilitated by phototherapy, either with PUVA or narrow-band UVB light
- Punch minigrafting from normal donor skin areas to vitiligo areas stimulates melanocyte repopulation
- Patients with diffuse or unresponsive vitiligo may diffusely and irreversibly depigment their skin via application of monobenzylether or hydroquinone
- Treatment of any associated thyroid or endocrine disorder often does not alter or improve the course of the associated vitiligo
- Oral β-carotene can be taken by patients with diffuse vitiligo or albinism and may impart a more "normal" skin color

DIFFERENTIAL DIAGNOSIS

Vitiligo
- Common; affects 1% of the population
- Begins as a focal or diffuse (more common) hypopigmented patch that progresses to total loss of pigmentation of the affected skin (chalk white)
- Usually symmetric; often on tops of hands, perioral, and periorbital skin, knees, elbows
- May be associated with thyroid disease

Pityriasis alba
- Very common, especially in dark-skinned children
- Less distinct borders than in vitiligo; does not result in complete depigmentation
- Hypopigmentation occurs on the face; plaques may appear lighter than surrounding skin and may be scaly
- Often occurs following mild inflammation (e.g., tinea versicolor or atopic eczema)
- Completely reversible; does not cause permanent hypopigmentation

Piebaldism
- Congenital, permanent, and irreversible
- Newborns often have a patch of white scalp hair and depigmented patches on the trunk, with normally pigmented patches within these larger depigmented areas

Chemical leukoderma (depigmentation)
- May be caused by phenols, germicides, and many other caustic chemicals
- Results in confetti-like macules of depigmentation in exposed skin

Post-topical steroid hypopigmentation
- Topical steroids, particularly fluorinated ones, may cause thinning, atrophy, and hypopigmentation with prolonged use
- More common on the face and perineum

Post-inflammatory hypopigmentation
- May occur after any type of cutaneous inflammation and last weeks to months
- More obvious in dark-skinned individuals

Albinism
- A congenital disorder of melanin synthesis with several phenotypes, ranging from complete lack of pigmentation (white hair and translucent or "red" iris) to the more common, diffuse hypopigmentation or "yellow" albinism that is prevalent in the black population
- Affects the skin, hair, and eyes
- Patients may have photophobia, decreased visual acuity, strabismus, and increased risk of skin cancer

Congenital birthmarks (e.g., nevus anemicus, nevus depigmentosis)
- Isolated patches of hypo- or depigmentation that remain unchanged over time

Tuberous sclerosis
- An inherited neurocutaneous disorder that results in hypopigmented macules in the shape of an "ash leaf" on the trunk and confetti-type depigmented macules on the arms/legs
- May affect the brain, eyes, kidneys, skin, and heart; mental retardation and seizures are common

Waardenburg's syndrome
- Associated with facial dysmorphism, a white forelock, and hypopigmentation
- May be accompanied by hearing deficit

Hyperreflexia

INTRODUCTION

Deep tendon reflexes are routinely tested on neurologic examination and can be helpful in localizing neurologic lesions. Hyperreflexia often reflects a CNS problem and can be a localizing sign for a focal injury. It suggests upper motor neuron dysfunction; thus, it is usually associated with spasticity and a positive Babinski sign. After an acute upper motor neuron lesion, hyperreflexia usually develops over a period of days to weeks rather than appearing immediately. Alone, hyperreflexia usually causes little specific disability; however, it is often associated with spasticity, which can be disabling. Reflexes are graded as follows: (0) no reflex even with reinforcement procedures, (1) reflex occurs with reinforcement procedures, (2) normal reflex, (3) brisk reflex with spread to other muscles, and (4) sustained clonus.

DIAGNOSTIC WORKUP & INITIAL MANAGEMENT

History and physical examination

- Assess present illness, time course of symptoms (acute vs. chronic), history, family history of neurologic diseases, and medications
- Perform complete neurologic history and exam; note other associated neurologic findings and deficits (e.g., weakness, sensory level, bladder or bowel compromise, Babinski)
- On musculoskeletal exam, examine for contractures, increased tone, spasticity, deformity
- Assess deep tendon reflexes while limbs are in a relaxed, symmetric position; if a reflex cannot be elicited, use reinforcement procedures (gritting teeth, pressing hands together)
- Hyperreflexia is an indication of upper motor neuron dysfunction; the etiology is usually suggested by the distribution of the hyperreflexia and associated physical findings
  - Hemihyperreflexia involving both the upper and lower extremities is most likely caused by a lesion of the brain or brainstem
  - Symmetric hyperreflexia involving only the lower extremities suggests a lesion of the thoracic or cervical spine
- Lower motor neuron lesions are often associated with weakness, muscle atrophy, fasciculations (visible contractions), and hypotonia, in addition to hyporeflexia
- Upper motor neuron lesions are often associated with weakness, hyperreflexia, hypertonia, and extensor plantar responses

Initial diagnostic workup

- Initial laboratory testing may include electrolytes, calcium, magnesium, thyroid function tests, BUN and creatinine, urine studies, parathyroid hormone (PTH) and vitamin D, and drug screen; consider also serologies for HTLV, HIV, and syphilis
- Head CT for emergent evaluation of suspected intracranial lesions; however, MRI is a better choice for most suspected brain and spinal causes of hyperreflexia
- EMG and nerve conduction studies if suspect amyotrophic lateral sclerosis
- Lumbar puncture with CSF analysis if suspect multiple sclerosis (oligoclonal bands, elevated IgG index) and some other etiologies

Initial patient management

- Hyperreflexia alone usually causes little disability; if associated with spasticity and hypertonicity, consider a combination of physical therapy, bracing, antispasticity agents (e.g., baclofen, tizanidine, dantrolene), botulinum toxin, and possibly surgical tendon release
- Manage endocrine, electrolyte, and treatable neurologic disorders as appropriate
- Multiple sclerosis is treated with steroids (for acute exacerbations), interferon, glatiramer acetate, and mitoxantrone
- Compressive myelopathies usually require surgical intervention to relieve the compression
- Traumatic spinal cord injury frequently requires surgical stabilization; high-dose steroid infusion during the initial 24 hours following trauma has been shown to improve outcome
- Some congenital conditions (e.g., neural tube defect, tethered cord) are treated surgically

DIFFERENTIAL DIAGNOSIS

Cerebral lesions
- Stroke
- Cerebral hemorrhage
- Tumors or other mass lesions
- Demyelinating disease (e.g., multiple sclerosis)
- Congenital processes (e.g., cerebral palsy, neural tube defects, tethered cord)
- Traumatic brain injury

Brainstem lesions
- Stroke
- Tumors
- Abcesses
- Demyelination

Spinal cord lesions
- Degenerative disk disease
- Transverse myelitis
- Traumatic spinal cord injury
- Spinal cord infarction
- Epidural abscess
- Compressive myelopathy caused by cervical or thoracic spondylosis and/or osteoarthritis
- Infectious or inflammatory causes (e.g., viral myelitis, such as HIV and HTLV-1; vasculitis)
- Syringomyelia (these patients frequently exhibit hyporeflexia at the level of the syrinx and hyperreflexia in segments below the level of the lesion)
- Spinal cord tumors (e.g., neuroblastoma, Ewing's sarcoma, astrocytoma, ependymoma)
- Tethered spinal cord

Motor neuron disease
- Amyotrophic lateral sclerosis (these patients have a combination of upper and lower motor neuron signs, such as hyperreflexia in a weak, atrophic limb with frequent fasciculations)
- Primary lateral sclerosis (hyperreflexia is accompanied by slowly progressive weakness and spasticity)

Other
- Almost any disorder of the brain or spine
- Normal variant (no other neurologic signs)
- Alcohol withdrawal
- Electrolyte disorders (e.g., hypocalcemia, hypomagnesemia)
- Tetanus
- Hyperthyroidism/thyrotoxicosis
- Hyperparathyroidism
- Anxiety
- Lithium overdose
- Monoamine oxide inhibitor overdose
- Serotonin syndrome
- Familiar spastic paraplegia
- Acute disseminated encephalomyelitis
- Rett's syndrome
- Pelizeus-Merzbacher syndrome
- Syringobulbia
- Spinocerebellar ataxia
- Cerebral palsy
- Hypoxic ischemic encephalopathy

Hyporeflexia

INTRODUCTION

Deep tendon reflexes are routinely tested on neurologic exam and, although nonspecific, can help in localizing neurologic lesions. They can be decreased by any process that affects the reflex arc (lower motor neuron, muscle, sensory neuron), by acute upper motor neuron lesions, and by mechanical factors (e.g., joint disease). Hyporeflexia is usually a general indicator of lower motor neuron dysfunction, which may result from a lesion anywhere in the anterior horn cell, spinal motor nerve or nerve root plexus, peripheral nerve, neuromuscular junction, or muscle. Hyporeflexia alone, in the absence of pathology, generally causes no disability and requires no treatment. Reflexes are graded as: (0) no reflex, (1) reflex with reinforcement procedures, (2) normal reflex, (3) brisk reflex with spread to other muscles, (4) sustained clonus.

DIAGNOSTIC WORKUP & INITIAL MANAGEMENT

History and physical examination

- Assess present illness, time course of symptoms (acute vs. chronic), past history, family history of neurologic diseases, and medications
- Perform a complete neurologic history and exam, and note other associated neurologic findings and deficits (e.g., weakness, sensory level, Babinski's sign)
- Musculoskeletal exam for muscle bulk, consistency, tenderness, and tone
- Assess deep tendon reflexes while limbs are in relaxed and symmetric position; if a reflex cannot be elicited, use reinforcement procedures (grit teeth, press hands together)
- Etiology (e.g., neuropathy or myopathy) may be specified by associated signs on physical exam (e.g., symmetric stocking-glove territory sensory loss in association with hyporeflexia suggests peripheral neuropathy; isolated loss of an ankle jerk with associated weakness of ankle plantar flexion suggests S1 radiculopathy)
- Lower motor neuron lesions are associated with weakness, muscle atrophy, fasciculations (visible contractions), and hypotonia, in addition to hyporeflexia; upper motor neuron lesions are associated with weakness, hyperreflexia, hypertonia, and extensor plantar responses

Initial diagnostic workup

- Nerve conduction studies and EMG are useful in evaluating suspected peripheral polyneuropathy, single or multiple mononeuropathies, radiculopathy, or myopathy
- MRI of the spine may help to diagnose radiculopathy
- Consider muscle and/or nerve biopsy
- If suspect Guillain-Barré syndrome or chronic inflammatory demyelinating polyneuropathy, CSF analysis may show elevated protein levels; reflexes will be diffusely absent or absent in lower extremities first
- For generalized peripheral neuropathy, further labs include CBC, electrolytes, glucose, calcium, SPEP, UPEP, ESR, ANA, RF, HIV, RPR, vitamin B_{12}, creatine phosphokinase, thyroid function tests, Hb_{A1c}, and heavy metal screen
- Consider cardiac evaluation (cardiomyopathy may coexist)

Initial patient management

- Hyporeflexia alone is not an indication for treatment; no disability may be associated with hyporeflexia, but treatment varies depending on underlying cause
- Weakness and hypotonia may require physical therapy and bracing
- Treat identified causes of peripheral neuropathy (e.g., thyroid disease, vitamin B_{12} deficiency)
- Guillain-Barré syndrome has improved outcome if treated with plasmapheresis or IVIG within 2 weeks of the onset of symptoms
- Radiculopathy may be treated conservatively with physical therapy and medications (e.g., NSAIDs), more aggressively with epidural steroid injections, or surgically
- Other causes of focal hyporeflexia (e.g., traumatic nerve injury) are treated individually, but usually the only option is supportive care while awaiting spontaneous recovery or surgery

DIFFERENTIAL DIAGNOSIS

Peripheral neuropathy
- Most common cause of symmetric hyporeflexia (polyneuropathy or mononeuropathy)
- May present with symmetric sensory complaints or weakness with distal muscular atrophy
- Most frequently associated with diabetes; other etiologies include hypothyroidism, syphilis, vitamin B_{12} deficiency, CIDP, and others

Isolated peripheral nerve injury/dysfunction
- Trauma
- Postsurgical
- Tumor compression

Radiculopathy
- Isolated loss of a single reflex may suggest dysfunction of that nerve root (ankle reflex, S1,2 nerve root; knee jerk, L3,4; biceps, C5,6; triceps, C7,8)
- Associated symptoms may include dermatomal sensory loss or pain and weakness of muscles in the territory of the affected root

Guillain-Barré syndrome
- Results from inflammatory demyelination (likely viral) of peripheral nerves
- Produces subacute onset of progressive weakness (hours to days) and hypo- or areflexia
- Patients may experience respiratory compromise or autonomic dysfunction

Brachial or lumbosacral plexopathy
- May be spontaneous or secondary to trauma
- Usually associated with severe pain in shoulder and arm (brachial plexopathy) or hip and leg (lumbosacral plexopathy)

Lambert-Eaton myasthenic syndrome
- Presynaptic neuromuscular disease associated with small cell carcinoma of the lung

Multifocal motor neuropathy
- May mimic amyotrophic lateral sclerosis but without upper motor neuron signs

Myopathy
- Patients present primarily with weakness but may also exhibit hyporeflexia
- Muscular dystrophy
- Myotonic dystrophy

Motor neuron disease
- Poliomyelitis
- Amyotrophic lateral sclerosis

Acute spinal cord injury ("spinal shock")
- Spinal cord compression or infarction
- Disk herniation
- Transverse myelitis
- Occult spina bifida

Other
- Toxins (antineoplastics, antiretrovirals, isoniazid, metronidazole, phenytoin, pyridoxine)
- Normal variant (obese or muscular patients may have quiet reflexes without pathology)
- Cauda equina syndrome
- Spinal muscular atrophy
- Charcot-Marie-Tooth syndrome
- Endocrine/electrolyte disorder (hypokalemia, hypoparathyroidism, vitamin E deficiency)
- Acute stroke
- Friedreich's ataxia
- Miller-Fischer syndrome
- Tick paralysis
- Xeroderma pigmentosa

Hypersomnia

INTRODUCTION

Hypersomnia is a symptom that may occur as a normal response to sleep deprivation, secondary to medications, or secondary to serious underlying brain pathology. It is also a common presenting symptom of many sleep disorders. A careful history of sleep habits, including the time spent in bed or trying to sleep elsewhere, bed mate, noise level, safety, and interruptions, is imperative for diagnosing and treating sleep disorders.

DIAGNOSTIC WORKUP & INITIAL MANAGEMENT

History and physical examination

- Acute onset of hypersomnia suggests acute illness or toxic effect
- Chronic hypersomnia is more likely to be related to sleep disorders, depression, or chronic use of sedating medication
- Obtain a detailed sleep history; a sleep log or diary may be useful
- Review medication use
- Screen for symptoms of depression
- Physical exam should be directed toward identifying evidence of focal neurologic, psychiatric, and/or other organ system dysfunction (e.g., hepatic or renal failure)
- Note body habitus (e.g., central obesity in patients with obstructive sleep apnea)

Initial diagnostic workup

- Laboratory testing may include CBC, monospot test, metabolic evaluation, and drug screen
- Neuroimaging and EEG may be indicated for patients with acute onset of hypersomnia without clear cause or with focal neurologic abnormalities on exam
- Polysomnography is often useful
- Multiple sleep latency testing is especially useful in cases of suspected narcolepsy
- CSF exam if suspect a CNS infectious cause

Initial patient management

- Improve sleep hygiene: Maintain regular sleep hours; avoid caffeine, alcohol, and other substances that may interfere with natural sleep; avoid exertion at bedtime
- Obstructive sleep apnea: Nasal CPAP at night is very helpful but cumbersome to use consistently; weight loss often improves symptoms; surgical elimination of redundant tissue (uvulopalatopharyngoplasty) may be necessary in severe cases
- Correct metabolic abnormalities as necessary
- Treat infectious causes (e.g., acyclovir for herpes simplex encephalitis, appropriate antibiotics for bacterial meningitis, supportive care for mononucleosis)
- Narcolepsy may be treated with stimulants and antidepressants, which limit REM sleep
- Structural brain lesions may require surgical resection or other specifically directed treatment
- Periodic limb movements of sleep and restless legs syndrome may be treated with dopaminergic agents, benzodiazepines, or opiates

DIFFERENTIAL DIAGNOSIS

Sleep disorders
- Poor sleep hygiene (e.g., going to bed too late, frequently changing sleep patterns secondary to shift work)
- Sleep apnea
- Narcolepsy
  - A disorder of wakefulness characterized by attacks of irresistible sleepiness (REM sleep), cataplexy, hypnagogic hallucinations, and/or sleep paralysis
- Periodic limb movements of sleep
  - Patients have repetitive movement of the extremities (usually legs) during sleep that may result in frequent arousals
- Restless legs syndrome
  - Patients experience uncomfortable feelings in the lower extremities at rest that are improved with movement, causing difficulty in remaining still to fall asleep

Depression
- Frequently causes disturbances of sleep, including hypersomnia, insomnia, or excessive daytime sleepiness

Medications
- Sedating cold and allergy medications
- Certain antidepressants (e.g., paroxetine, tricyclic antidepressants, bupropion)
- Benzodiazepines
- Narcotics
- Tramadol
- Certain antiepileptics (e.g., gabapentin, topiramate, valproate)

Encephalopathy
- Metabolic (e.g., hepatic or uremic encephalopathy)
- Toxic (e.g., sedating medications, alcohol, illicit sedating drugs)

Structural brain lesions
- Lesions involving the reticular activating system of the brainstem
- Large lesions
- Bihemispheric lesions

Infection
- Mononucleosis
- Encephalitis
- Chronic meningitis (e.g., fungal)

Complex partial status epilepticus
- Frequently results in waxing and waning levels of alertness

Idiopathic hypersomnia
- Similar to narcolepsy but with attacks of non-REM sleep

Trypanosomiasis (African sleeping sickness)
- A parasitic illness carried by the tsetse fly

Carbon dioxide retention
- COPD
- Metabolic

Hypertension

INTRODUCTION

Hypertension is the most common primary diagnosis in the U.S., accounting for 35 million office visits. It is defined by blood pressure (BP) > 140/90 mm Hg on 2 separate measurements. Hypertension is an independent risk factor for cardiovascular disease and stroke and the second most common cause of end-stage renal disease. Most (95%) cases are idiopathic (essential hypertension), which may be familial but can also be associated with excessive alcohol, obesity, older age, and African-American race. Hypertensive urgency is characterized by asymptomatic, severe hypertension (systolic > 220 mmHg or diastolic > 125 mmHg). Hypertensive emergency is characterized by any BP associated with acute end-organ damage (pulmonary edema, renal failure, chest pain, visual changes).

DIAGNOSTIC WORKUP & INITIAL MANAGEMENT

- Suspected hypertensive urgency or emergency requires immediate therapy
  - Hypertensive emergency requires IV antihypertensives and arterial line to monitor mean arterial pressure (do not lower by more than 20%–25% within 24 hours)
  - Hypertensive urgency requires BP to be reduced over several hours; if no evidence of end-organ damage, oral agents are preferred (these agents have a longer duration of action and can be transitioned to outpatient use)

History and physical examination

- Preferably, use a properly calibrated and validated mercury sphygmomanometer; ensure proper cuff size and cuff bladder encircling 80% of the arm; patient should be comfortably seated for at least 5 minutes before measurement
- Establish the patient's baseline BP; measure BP in both arms to exclude subclavian stenosis or aortic dissection as a cause for blood pressure underestimation
- Review the medication list, and note missed medications or those that may result in elevated BP (e.g., NSAIDs, cyclosporine, erythropoietin)
- Note sources of pain, infection, or emotional triggers that may elevate BP
- Assess risk factors (e.g., history of diabetes, heart disease, or stroke; smoking; dyslipidemia; drug use; stress; pain; obesity)
- Evaluate for target organ disease (e.g., angina, CHF, aortic dissection, stroke or transient ischemic attack, renal dysfunction, retinal hemorrhage)
- Note withdrawal from alcohol, clonidine, nicotine, or opiates

Initial workup and management

- Initial testing includes urinalysis, metabolic panel, calcium, lipids, ECG, chest x-ray, and echocardiography; consider head CT if neurologic or mental status changes are present
- Consider secondary causes of hypertension if sudden onset of hypertension, severe refractory hypertension (>3 medications used), rapid renal dysfunction with ACE inhibitors, younger age (<30 years), or family history of early hypertension
  - Renal duplex ultrasound, abdominal MRA or CT, and additional blood and urine tests may be needed for diagnosis
  - Clinical findings may suggest the underlying cause of secondary hypertension [e.g., flank bruits suggest renal artery stenosis; Cushing's syndrome is associated with osteoporosis, obesity, muscle weakness, moon facies, hirsutism, dyslipidemia, hyperglycemia, and hypokalemia; pheochromocytoma is associated with extremely labile BP (episodic or paroxysmal hypertension), headaches, palpitations, and diaphoresis; primary hyperaldosteronism is associated with isolated hypokalemia]
- Lifestyle changes (e.g., smoking cessation, dietary changes, exercise, moderate alcohol) are usually the initial and long-term interventions for essential hypertension
- Medications are often necessary, including diuretics, β-blockers, and ACE inhibitors (the latter is especially useful in diabetes, left ventricular dysfunction, vascular disease)

DIFFERENTIAL DIAGNOSIS

Essential hypertension
- Often associated with obesity, sedentary lifestyle, tobacco use, African-American race, and diets high in sodium or low in potassium

Extracellular volume overload
- Excess sodium intake
- Inadequate diuretic therapy
- Fluid retention caused by kidney or cardiac disease or missed dialysis

Drug- or toxin-induced
- Excessive alcohol intake
- Alcohol withdrawal
- Cocaine
- NSAIDs
- Sympathomimetics
- Steroids
- Oral contraceptives
- Cyclosporine
- Erythropoietin
- Pseudoephedrine or ephedrine
- Black licorice ingestion

Secondary hypertension
- Chronic renal disease
- Renal vascular disease (e.g., renal artery atherosclerosis, fibromuscular dysplasia)
- Cushing's disease
- Pheochromocytoma
- Primary hyperaldosteronism
- Hyperthyroidism
- Coarctation of aorta

Other
- "White coat" hypertension
- Nonadherence to medication regimen
- Improper measurement
- Elevated BP associated with pain, stress, or exercise
- Obstructive sleep apnea
- Isolated systolic hypertension
- Malignant hypertension
- Preeclampsia or eclampsia
- Pregnancy-induced hypertension
- Hyperthyroidism
- Hypercalcemia
- Increased intracranial pressure
- Congenital adrenal hyperplasia

Hypotension

INTRODUCTION

Hypotension is defined as systolic pressure < 90 mm Hg or a drop in pressure by >40 mm Hg below baseline. Chronic low blood pressure is generally benign and may occur in those with small body habitus, athletes, end-stage liver disease, or severe left ventricular dysfunction. Shock is a physiologic state of tissue hypoperfusion that presents as altered function of the brain, heart, and/or visceral organs. A sudden, precipitous drop in pressure may signal a serious condition (e.g., cardiac dysfunction, severe infection, cardiac tamponade, pulmonary embolism (PE), tension pneumothorax, anaphylaxis, severe neurologic disease, adrenal crisis, ruptured aortic aneurysm, drug overdose, volume depletion). Mean arterial pressure (2/3 × diastolic BP + 1/3 × systolic BP) is a useful guide of organ perfusion.

DIAGNOSTIC WORKUP & INITIAL MANAGEMENT

- Immediately assess airway, breathing, and circulation, and evaluate for end-organ hypoperfusion: waning mental status, ischemia (chest pain, cool extremities), oliguria
- Address immediate concerns (e.g., lay patient flat, secure airway, administer supplemental oxygen, control bleeding, ensure venous access, consider arterial access for BP monitoring, address arrhythmias)

History and physical examination

- Obtain a manual BP in both arms (to exclude subclavian stenosis) with an appropriate sized cuff; also measure orthostatic vital signs (drop in systolic pressure of >20 mm Hg or increase in heart rate by >10 bpm within 2–5 minutes of standing is significant and may indicate volume depletion)
- Review baseline BP and heart rate (i.e., a patient with baseline systolic pressure of 180 mm Hg may be relatively hypotensive with systolic pressure of 100 mm Hg)
  - Absence of reflex-induced increase in heart rate as BP falls suggests autonomic failure in the absence of obvious pharmacologic cause (e.g., β-blockers)
- Physical exam with close attention to cardiovascular, pulmonary, neurologic, and abdominal systems (intra-abdominal catastrophe can be subtle in elderly patients)
- Review medications and medication allergies

Initial workup and management

- Testing should be guided by differential diagnosis and may include chemistries, CBC, cardiac enzymes, pancreatic enzymes, lactate, cultures (blood, urine, effusion), toxicology screen, ABG, urinalysis, urine electrolytes, and cortisol stimulation test
- Radiologic studies may be necessary in some cases (e.g., chest radiography to rule out pneumothorax, CT to rule out pulmonary embolism or intra-abdominal process)
- ECG may help to assess underlying rhythm and myocardial ischemia or infarction
- Echocardiography may help to assess cardiac function and pericardial disease
- Initiate IV fluid challenge with 0.9% isotonic saline based on clinical judgment; use caution in those with CHF or end-stage renal disease (250–500 mL may be appropriate); CHF and MI patients may require diuresis or balloon pump for support rather than volume infusion
- Use packed RBCs rather than IV fluids in active blood loss
- Inotropes may be indicated in some patients
- Use vasopressors after appropriate volume resuscitation; may be helpful for hemodynamic stabilization
- Subcutaneous epinephrine may be needed to treat anaphylaxis
- Swan-Ganz catheterization may help if volume status is questionable
- Consider prompt antibiotic therapy and cardiology, surgery, neurology, or GI consultations; ICU admission is often necessary
- Hold and/or discontinue antihypertensive medications, as appropriate

DIFFERENTIAL DIAGNOSIS

Orthostatic hypotension
- Most common in the elderly; may result in syncope or presyncope on standing

Hypotension secondary to medications
- Common in elderly patients
- Consider excessive doses of antihypertensive medications
- Other medications with little known antihypertensive effects: Opiates, diuretics, benzodiazepines, tricyclics, dopaminergic compounds (e.g., amantadine, levodopa)

Hypovolemia/volume depletion
- Often caused by hyperglycemia, dehydration, vomiting or diarrhea, pancreatitis, extensive burns, infection, hyperthermia (increased insensible losses), diuretic use
- Hemorrhage may result from ruptured ectopic pregnancy, splenic rupture, aortic aneurysm rupture, GI bleeding, trauma, or postoperative

Myocardial ischemia and cardiac pump failure
- Can result in hypotension and cardiogenic shock from acute or progressive ventricular failure; mechanical complications of MI (e.g., mitral regurgitation, ventricular rupture) can also present as hypotension
- In particular, right ventricular MI often presents with hypotension and preload dependence in inferior MI; may require vigorous volume resuscitation

Autonomic dysfunction and postural hypotension
- Occurs when the vasculature is unable to quickly vasoconstrict on abruptly standing
- Etiologies include Parkinson's disease, cerebellar disorders, hypothalamic disorders (e.g., hypopituitarism), neuropathies (e.g., diabetes), Shy-Drager syndrome, toxins or acute poisoning (e.g., botulinum, organophosphates), malignancy, and α-blockade

Postprandial hypotension (within 75 minutes of eating)
- Very common in elderly because of blood redistribution

Adrenal insufficiency/crisis
- Can be primary (rare) or secondary (generally from long-term steroid use)
- Normally, endogenous glucocorticoids and mineralocorticoids enhance the effect of catecholamines on the vascular endothelium, allowing for vascular tone (i.e., vessels are able to respond appropriately to standing or volume loss by constricting)
- Hospitalized patients (especially ICU patients) are susceptible to stressors (e.g., cardiac ischemia, sepsis) that may potentiate adrenal insufficiency
- An inappropriately blunted response to stressors may be seen in those on chronic steroids, producing a similar scenario

Sepsis
- Septic shock often develops over hours to days as the inflammatory response to an infection builds
- Elderly patients may not manifest fever or elevated white blood cell count; a careful history and physical exam is mandatory to uncover possible sources
- A high-output state can be created by inadequate peripheral oxygen delivery

Anaphylaxis
- Inflammatory response to offending antigen (e.g., drug, bee sting, contrast, latex)
- Cardiovascular collapse is a late manifestation of anaphylaxis and may be preceded by urticaria, stridor, angioedema, or airway compromise

Other
- Hepatitis or pancreatitis
- Hemodialysis
- Pulmonary embolus
- Pericardial tamponade
- Valvular heart disease
- Sildenafil use with nitrates
- Traumatic brain injury
- Arrhythmias
- Tension pneumothorax
- Excessive PEEP in ventilated patients
- Hypertrophic cardiomyopathy

Hypesthesia (Numbness)

INTRODUCTION

Sensory loss (hypesthesia, or decreased sensation, most commonly noticed in response to painful or touch stimuli) can occur secondary to a problem anywhere in the nervous system. It is often accompanied by paresthesia (an abnormal sensation, such as numbness or tingling). The etiology of hypesthesia is usually suggested by the distribution of the finding and the associated symptoms.

DIAGNOSTIC WORKUP & INITIAL MANAGEMENT

History and physical examination

- Tempo of onset may suggest the etiology (e.g., acute onset of sensory loss suggests a vascular event, migraine, acute nerve injury, or seizure)
- Distribution of numbness or sensory loss will help to localize the lesion
  - Distal symmetric sensory loss suggests peripheral neuropathy
  - Sensory loss in the distribution of a single peripheral nerve or nerve root suggests a mononeuropathy or radiculopathy
  - A sensory level beginning at one dermatome and extending caudally suggests a spinal cord lesion
  - Hemisensory loss suggests a brainstem or hemispheric cerebral lesion

Initial diagnostic workup

- EMG and nerve conduction studies are used to evaluate suspected peripheral neuropathy, mononeuropathy, or radiculopathy
- Initial laboratory testing may include screening for causes of neuropathy, including CBC, serum electrophoresis, rheumatoid factor, antinuclear antibody, HIV and syphilis testing, vitamin B_{12} and folate levels, thyroid function tests, Hb_{A1c}, and testing for heavy metals
- CT is a useful initial screen for suspected brain lesions
- MRI is usually the best imaging choice for lesions of the brain or spinal cord
- Genetic testing is available for some forms of inherited neuropathy

Initial patient management

- Few measures exist to restore feeling to numb areas; treatment generally consists of identifying and treating the underlying etiology
- General measures that may help to ameliorate painful dysesthesias include tricyclic antidepressants (e.g., amitriptyline), anticonvulsants (e.g., gabapentin), and topical preparations (e.g., capsaicin cream)
- Treat the underlying etiology of peripheral neuropathies
- Mononeuropathies will frequently improve if the offending cause is alleviated (e.g., treat carpal tunnel syndrome with wrist splints or surgery)
- Radiculopathy may be treated conservatively with physical therapy and medications, more aggressively with epidural injections, or surgically
- Compressive myelopathies often require surgical intervention to alleviate the compression

DIFFERENTIAL DIAGNOSIS

Peripheral neuropathy
- Metabolic (e.g., diabetes mellitus)
- Toxic (e.g., alcohol, heavy metal poisoning)
- Inflammatory (e.g., chronic inflammatory demyelinating polyneuropathy)
- Deficiency states (e.g., vitamin B_{12})
- Inherited (e.g., Charcot-Marie-Tooth)

Mononeuropathy
- Median nerve compression at the wrist, producing carpal tunnel syndrome
- Diabetic mononeuropathy
- Traumatic or compressive nerve injury

Radiculopathy
- Results in dermatomal sensory loss in the territory of the affected nerve root
- May be due to compressive disk disease or herpes zoster

Myelopathy
- May result in sensory loss beginning at the dermatomal level of the lesion and progressing caudally

Brainstem lesion
- May cause both facial numbness (ipsilateral to the lesion) and hemicorporal sensory loss (commonly contralateral to the lesion)

Subcortical lesions
- Cerebrovascular infarct or hemorrhage
- Multiple sclerosis
- Tumor

Cortical lesion
- Specific types of sensory loss (e.g., diminished graphesthesia or stereognosis) help to immediately localize the problem to the contralateral cerebral cortex, usually the parietal lobe
- Cerebrovascular causes (e.g., cerebral infarct or hemorrhage)
- Tumor

Syringomyelia
- Results in a suspended area of sensory loss in the affected dermatomes with normal sensation elsewhere

Other
- Transient ischemic attack
- Cerebral abscess
- Paraneoplastic neuropathy
- Simple partial seizure
- Aura of migraine (produces transient numbness or paresthesia)
- Plexopathy (usually produces a polyradicular pattern of sensory loss in addition to motor findings)
- Cauda equina syndrome

Hypothermia

INTRODUCTION

Hypothermia is defined as core body temperature of <95°F (35°C) and can be further defined as mild (90–95°F, or 32–35°C), moderate (82–90°F, or 28–32°C), or severe (<82°F, or 28°C). Accidental hypothermia from environmental exposure is the most common cause of severe hypothermia; other causes include impaired thermoregulation (e.g., stroke), decreased thermogenesis, and diminished ability to respond appropriately to the cold (e.g., mental status change). High-risk patients include the elderly (impaired thermoregulation, mental status changes), neonates (large body surface area), and drug/alcohol abusers. Severe hypothermia protects organs from ischemia, and return of spontaneous circulation has been documented from temperatures as low as 57.6°F (14.2°C) in infants and 56.7°F (13.7°C) in adults.

DIAGNOSTIC WORKUP & INITIAL MANAGEMENT

Initial treatment

- Asymptomatic mild hypothermia only requires a workup to define/treat underlying causes
- For symptomatic hypothermia, initial treatment may include passive rewarming to prevent further heat loss (e.g., remove wet clothes, cover with blankets), active external rewarming (e.g., radiant warmers, heating blankets), and/or active core rewarming (e.g., warmed IV fluids, pleural lavage, dialysis)

History and physical examination

- Complete history and physical exam are essential; assess for environmental cold exposure
- Careful exam of extremities and dependent body parts for signs of frostbite
- Assess core temperature (rectal temperature preferred) using a low-temperature thermometer; most thermometers only read to 34.4°C, so a specialized, low-reading thermometer may be required
  - 30–35°C: Increased metabolic output with tachycardia, hypertension, tachypnea
  - 24–30°C: Slowing of body functions, decreased oxygen demand, altered mental status, bradycardia, hypotension, arrhythmias
  - <24°C: Most organ systems shut down; may have asystole, ventricular fibrillation

Initial workup and management

- ECG may reveal Osborne waves (J waves) if temperature is <91.4°F (33°C)
  - These waves appear as a hump at the junction of the QRS and ST segments
  - Other findings may include T wave inversions; prolongation of PR, QRS, or QT waves; or arrhythmias (e.g., bradycardia, atrial fibrillation or flutter, ventricular fibrillation, asystole)
  - A severely hypothermic myocardium is very irritable and often refractory to conventional therapy (i.e., simple maneuvers, such as placing a central line, CPR, or even simply moving the patient, may cause refractory ventricular fibrillation)
- Labs may include CBC, electrolytes, renal function (for acute tubular necrosis), glucose, calcium, LFTs, coagulation studies, CPK and urinalysis for rhabdomyolysis, TSH, and free T_4
  - CBC may show increased hemoglobin because of hemoconcentration
  - Coagulation studies (PT/PTT) may be normal despite the presence of a clinical coagulopathy (normal coagulation function may occur in lab as blood is warmed)
- Chest radiography, blood and urine cultures, and plasma cortisol levels may be indicated to assess for infection in cases of suspected sepsis
- Head CT to assess for altered mental status
- ABG reveals metabolic acidosis with either respiratory acidosis (decreased ventilation) or alkalosis (decreased CO_2 production)
- Hydrocortisone, thiamine, and antibiotics are standard therapy until the cause is found
- Treat identified causes as appropriate (e.g., IV thyroxine and IV hydrocortisone for hypothyroid patients with myxedema coma; antibiotics, fluids, and vasopressors for sepsis)
- Bretylium may be used for ventricular fibrillation due to hypothermia

DIFFERENTIAL DIAGNOSIS

Environmental exposure
- Alcohol intake is a common risk factor; it both alters thermoregulation and promotes risk-taking behavior; consider the possibility of abuse
- Shivering, amnesia, ataxia, and dysarthria occur with mild hypothermia (>89.6°F, or >32°C)
- Stupor, absence of shivering, atrial fibrillation, and/or bradycardia occur with moderate hypothermia (82–90°F, or 28–32°C)
- Coma, ventricular fibrillation, apnea, asystole, and/or areflexia occur with severe hypothermia (<82.4°F, or <28°C)

Sepsis
- Mild hypothermia is common in sepsis, especially as a result of infections with Gram-negative rods (e.g., *E. coli*) and in the elderly

Hypothyroidism and/or myxedema coma
- Up to 10 times more common in females
- May be of autoimmune, postsurgical, or pituitary etiology (e.g., hypopituitarism)
- Symptoms include hypothermia, hair loss, dry skin, pretibial myxedema, weight gain, constipation, and prolonged relaxation phase of deep tendon reflexes

Stroke or other CNS insult
- Hypothermia may result from altered cerebral thermoregulation

Hypovolemic shock
- Poor peripheral perfusion often results in mild hypothermia

Massive blood transfusion
- Hypothermia from refrigerated blood that is rapidly transfused without warming

End-stage liver disease
- Consider spontaneous bacterial peritonitis and sepsis in patients with ascites

Large surface area burns
- Hypothermia results from the damaged skin's inability to avoid heat loss

Wernicke's encephalopathy
- A triad of ataxia, ophthalmoplegia, and acute mental confusion caused by thiamine deficiency
- Often seen in patients with alcoholism or malnutrition

Other
- Hypoadrenalism
- Hypoglycemia

Infertility

INTRODUCTION

Infertility is defined as the failure to conceive after 1 year of regular, unprotected intercourse. It affects 1 in 6 couples and is more common with increasing age. Female factors account for 30%–40% of cases, male factors for 20%, and combined male and female factors for 20%. The remaining 20% are unexplained. Fecundity is the probability of pregnancy in 1 menstrual cycle; normal fecundity is 20% at each cycle, 50% at 3 months, and 85% at 1 year. An age-related decrease in fecundity begins at age 35 years and is exacerbated after age 40. Most clinicians initiate a workup for inability to achieve pregnancy after 6 months in women ≥35 years. In 2002, 1% of live births in the United States were conceived through assisted reproductive techniques.

DIAGNOSTIC WORKUP & INITIAL MANAGEMENT

History and physical examination

- Complete history and physical exam looking for risk factors that impact fertility
- Male infertility may present with lack of sexual hair growth, gynecomastia, varicocele, scars of previous surgery (e.g., hernia repair) or trauma to genitals, or hypogonadism
- Female infertility may present with dysmenorrhea or cyclic pelvic pain, dyspareunia, and menstrual irregularity outside the normal range (22–35 days); hirsutism, obesity, galactorrhea, or signs of virilization; heavy bleeding and pain; signs of thyroid disease; or history of previous gynecologic procedures (e.g., cryotherapy, conization, cervical dilations) or sexually transmitted infections (e.g., pelvic inflammatory disease)

Initial diagnostic workup

- Tests for male infertility may include semen analysis (sperm count, volume, motility, pH, morphology, WBC count) and endocrine tests (e.g., FSH, testosterone, TSH, prolactin)
  - Less common tests include postejaculatory urinalysis (if semen volume < 1.0 mL) to assess for retrograde ejaculation and postcoital testing to examine the interaction between sperm and the cervical mucus
- Tests for female infertility include basal body temperature charts, FSH on day 21 of menstrual cycle, urine LH surge, TSH, prolactin, and cervical culture
  - In women ≥35 years, test for FSH on day 3 of the cycle to assess ovarian reserve
  - Hysterosalpingography may be indicated to assess uterine cavity/fallopian tubes
  - Peritoneal exam via laparoscopy may be indicated
- No apparent cause for infertility is found in 15%–20% of couples

Initial patient management

- Correction of apparent endocrine disorders generally restores fertility
- Male infertility:
  - Limit intercourse to once every 2 days
  - Repair anatomic defects (e.g., varicocele), if present
  - Consider washed sperm for intrauterine insemination or intracytoplasmic sperm injection (ICSI)
  - In refractory cases, may attempt artificial insemination with donor sperm
- Female infertility:
  - Intrauterine insemination
  - Ovulation induction with clomiphene citrate or gonadotropins
  - In-vitro fertilization (IVF) or gamete intra-fallopian transfer (GIFT)
  - In refractory cases, may attempt egg or embryo donation, gestational surrogacy, or adoption
  - Group psychotherapy may improve pregnancy rate

DIFFERENTIAL DIAGNOSIS

Female factors

Peritoneal factors
- Pelvic adhesions from previous surgery
- Endometriosis
- Chronic pelvic inflammatory disease

Ovulatory factors
- Polycystic ovarian syndrome
- Thyroid dysfunction
- Premature ovarian failure

Uterine-tubal factors
- Tubal occlusion
- Fibroids
- Endometriosis
- Asherman's syndrome

Recurrent implantation failure
- Poor embryo transfer technique
- Uterine cavity lesion
- Hydrosalpinx
- Fibroids
- Endometriosis

Cervical factors
- Structural abnormalities
- Mucus abnormalities

Age
- Poor ovarian reserve and/or poor response to stimulation
- Increase in ovum aneuploidy

Male factors

Endocrine disorders
- Pituitary or hypothalamic dysfunction
- Adrenal hyperplasia
- Thyroid disease
- Testosterone deficiency
- Andropause

Abnormal spermatogenesis
- Mumps orchitis
- Varicocele
- Cryptorchidism

Abnormal sperm motility
- Antisperm antibodies
- Immotile cilia syndrome

Sexual dysfunction
- Retrograde ejaculation
- Impotence
- Ductal obstruction

Other (e.g., occupational heat exposure, medications)

Male and/or female factors
- Sexual dysfunction, celiac disease, subclinical bulimia nervosa, carcinoma

Idiopathic/unexplained

Insomnia

INTRODUCTION

Insomnia is a common disorder of insufficient or poor-quality sleep that can result in adverse daytime consequences (e.g., fatigue, diminished energy, memory impairment, difficulty concentrating, low motivation, loss of productivity, interpersonal difficulties, irritability, increased worrying, anxiety, depression). It may be a primary diagnosis or a complaint or symptom secondary to an underlying acute or chronic disorder. It can present as trouble falling asleep, trouble staying asleep, or feelings of insufficient or nonrefreshing sleep. Chronic sleep loss is a major risk factor for fatigue-related accidents, job loss, marital and social problems, major depression, impaired weight control, and heart disease. A careful history of sleep habits is imperative.

DIAGNOSTIC WORKUP & INITIAL MANAGEMENT

History and physical examination

- Many patients have insomnia but do not tell their doctors, so questions about sleep quality should be asked during health maintenance visits
- History should be elicited from the patient and his/her bed partner, if possible
- Careful attention to age of onset, predisposing factors/traits, precipitating events, duration, specific characteristics (e.g., nightly vs. intermittent vs. situation-specific)
- Review medications: Stimulant medications (e.g., methylphenidate), over-the-counter drugs (e.g., caffeine, pseudoephedrine), herbal or alternative agents (e.g., ephedra, nicotine)
- A sleep log or diary is useful to identify circadian rhythm disorders and determine severity
  - Should be recorded each morning
  - Include time in bed, time asleep, estimate of sleep quality, awakenings, noise level, safety, interruptions, associated symptoms (e.g., pain, dyspnea, urinary frequency)
- In cases of secondary insomnia, symptoms of the underlying disorder may be present (e.g., snoring and hypertension in patients with sleep apnea, crackles and decreased exercise tolerance in patients with CHF, wheezing in patients with asthma, "heartburn" in patients with GERD)
- A focused physical exam to evaluate cardiovascular, pulmonary, and neurologic systems and mental status will improve diagnostic accuracy
- Insomnia may be transient (e.g., related to stress, travel, or illness) or chronic (defined as occurring nightly for at least 6 months)

Initial diagnostic workup

- "Insomnia" is a self-reported condition; labs or other testing is often unnecessary unless suspect underlying medical conditions
- Labs may include CBC, complete metabolic panel, and thyroid studies
- Urine toxicology screen may be indicated to detect illicit use of stimulant drugs (e.g., amphetamines, cocaine)
- Psychological screening (e.g., Beck Depression, Beck Anxiety) may identify presence and severity of depression or other psychiatric disorders
- Polysomnography (sleep study) may be indicated to diagnose organic sleep disorders (e.g., obstructive sleep apnea, periodic limb movement disorders, restless legs syndrome
- Further testing may be indicated, depending on suspected underlying disorders (e.g., ECG, chest radiography, echocardiography, or pulmonary function tests if suspect undiagnosed cardiac or pulmonary disease; EEG if suspect undiagnosed seizure disorder; TSH and free T_4 if suspect thyroid disease; iron studies if suspect restless legs syndrome or periodic limb movement disorder (iron deficiency and renal failure are risk factors for both); blood alcohol level, liver function tests, and toxicology screen if suspect alcohol or illicit drug abuse)

DIFFERENTIAL DIAGNOSIS

Acute, transient insomnia
- Situational stress (most common)
- Acute illness or injury
- Medications or drugs (e.g., nonsedating cold medications, oral contraceptives, antidepressants, bronchodilators, pseudoephedrine, cocaine, nicotine)
- Caffeine
- Alcohol
- Change in sleep environment or hours (e.g., travel, shift work)

Chronic insomnia

Primary insomnia
- Hypothesized to be a disorder of hyperarousal, either from stress or lifestyle

Conditioned insomnia
- Acute insomnia progresses to chronic insomnia from distorted sleep cognitions

Primary sleep disorders
- Restless legs syndrome
  - "Creepy-crawly," unpleasant sensations in the legs and/or feet
  - Temporarily relieved by moving limbs
- Periodic limb movement disorder
  - Arms and/or legs jerk during sleep
  - May be a primary disorder or secondary to uremia, neuropathy, or iron deficiency
- Sleep-related breathing disorder (e.g., REM-behavior disorder)
- Narcolepsy
- Prion fatal familial insomnia

Insomnia secondary to medical comorbidities
- Obstructive sleep apnea
- CHF
- COPD
- Asthma
- Chronic pain syndromes
- Hyperthyroidism
- GERD or peptic ulcer disease
- Angina
- Benign prostatic hypertrophy
- Urinary tract infection (UTI)
- Inflammatory bowel disease (IBD)
- Uremia
- Diabetes mellitus
- Pruritis syndromes
- Seizures

Psychological disorders
- Mood disorder/depression
- Anxiety
- Dementia
- Psychosis
- Mania
- Posttraumatic stress disorder

Other
- Unnecessary concern about deviation from "normal" sleeping patterns
- Caretaker insomnia
- Pregnancy
- Perimenopause

Jaundice

INTRODUCTION

Jaundice in an adult patient can be benign or life-threatening. The classic definition of jaundice is yellow staining of the skin, sclera, and mucous membranes, which usually occurs when serum bilirubin exceeds 2.5–3 mg/dL (normal is <10 mg/dL; of this, <5% is present in conjugated form). Bilirubin is the major breakdown product of hemoglobin that is released from dying or damaged erythrocytes. Evaluation of jaundice generally requires a careful history and physical examination as well as additional tests of liver injury, including AST, ALT, alkaline phosphatase, γ-glutamyl transferase, and fractionated bilirubin. Pseudojaundice can occur with excessive ingestion of foods rich in β-carotene (e.g., carrots, squash, melons); in the case of pseudojaundice, hyperbilirubinemia is absent.

DIAGNOSTIC WORKUP & INITIAL MANAGEMENT

History and physical examination

- Evaluate onset (acute vs. chronic), duration, associated symptoms (e.g., fever, chills, arthralgias, myalgias, anorexia, weight loss, pruritis, abdominal pain, fatigue, changes in urine and stool color, skin hyperpigmentation, xanthomas, Kayser-Fleischer rings), medications (prescribed drugs, over-the-counter drugs, and herbal preparations), drug and alcohol use, medical history, and family history of liver disease
- Physical exam should evaluate for hepatomegaly, splenomegaly, palpable gallbladder, and signs of chronic liver disease (e.g., bruising, gynecomastia, testicular atrophy, palmar erythema, spider telangiectasias, ascites)
  - Jaundice is best seen in the periphery of ocular conjunctivae and oral mucous membranes
  - Yellow skin discoloration without icterus may occur with elevated serum carotene level

Initial diagnostic workup

- Assess liver function by measuring aminotransferases (AST, ALT), alkaline phosphatase, γ-glutamyl transferase, bilirubin, prothrombin time, albumin level, and serum ammonia
  - AST and ALT are the most sensitive tests for acute hepatocellular injury; the greatest elevations occur with viral hepatitis and drug injury
  - Alkaline phosphatase is the best indicator for biliary obstruction
  - Bilirubin level corresponds to hepatic uptake, metabolic, and excretory functions
- Evaluate the etiology of abnormal liver function tests if significant probability of underlying hepatobiliary disease; check direct and indirect bilirubin if total bilirubin is high
- If suspect hepatocellular injury, obtain further serologic tests to support or exclude likely diagnoses; tests may include CBC, viral hepatitis serologies, acetaminophen level, serum iron and total iron-binding capacity, serum protein electrophoresis, ceruloplasmin, ANA, anti-SM antibody, liver–kidney microsomal antibody, and α_1-antitrypsin level
- If suspect cholestasis, assess the biliary tree with a right upper quadrant ultrasound
- Abdominal CT or ERCP is often needed to identify the cause of biliary obstruction
- Liver biopsy may be required for definitive diagnosis

Initial patient management

- Medical emergencies include massive hemolysis, acetaminophen toxicity, acute liver failure, and ascending cholangitis; definitive therapy is based on the underlying etiology
  - Treat acetaminophen toxicity with activated charcoal and N-acetylcysteine, which reduces the production of toxic metabolites and acts as an anti-inflammatory and antioxidant agent
  - Treat ascending cholangitis with broad-spectrum antibiotics and biliary drainage
- Further management should be aimed at controlling symptoms (e.g., ascites, portal hypertension) and preventing progression to cirrhosis or fulminant hepatic failure
- Patients with chronic liver disease should receive hepatitis A and B immunizations
- Liver transplant may be necessary in severe cases when other treatment options fail

DIFFERENTIAL DIAGNOSIS

Prehepatic disease

- Due to hemolysis caused by excess heme production and resulting in elevated unconjugated (indirect) bilirubin
- Sickle cell disease
- Glucose-6-phosphate dehydrogenase deficiency
- Spherocytosis
- Hemoglobinopathies
- Intravascular hemolysis
- Hypersplenism
- Sepsis
- Infections (e.g., malaria, babesiosis)
- Hemolytic-uremic syndrome
- Lead toxicity
- ABO compatibility

Intrahepatic disease

- Pathophysiology of intrahepatic disease includes direct liver cell injury (leading to elevated AST and ALT), defective conjugation of bilirubin (resulting in increased unconjugated [indirect] bilirubin), intrahepatic cholestasis (resulting in elevated conjugated bilirubin), or infiltrative diseases (resulting in elevated alkaline phosphatase)
- Acute ischemic liver injury
- Hepatitis (e.g., viral, alcoholic, autoimmune)
- Medications (e.g., NSAIDs, acetaminophen, antibiotics, isoniazid, estrogens, chlorpromazine, erythromycin, nitrofurantoin, rifampin, Kava)
- Gilbert's syndrome
- Infiltration (fatty liver, lymphoma, tuberculosis, tumors, sarcoidosis, fungal)
- Hemochromatosis
- Wilson's disease
- Primary biliary cirrhosis
- α_1-Antitrypsin deficiency
- Celiac sprue
- Muscle injury
- Pregnancy

Posthepatic disease (extrahepatic cholestasis)

- Posthepatic disease results in elevated γ-glutamyl transferase and conjugated bilirubin (high alkaline phosphatase also occurs in bone disorders and pregnancy, but concomitrant increase in γ-glutamyl transferase only occurs in liver disease)
- Crigler-Najjar syndrome
- Choledocholithiasis
- Biliary tract tumors
- Primary sclerosing cholangitis
- Parasitic infections
- Ascending cholangitis

Pseudojaundice

- May result from excessive foods rich in β-carotene (e.g., carrots, squash, melons)
- Hyperbilirubinemia is absent

Other

- Cholecystitis
- Malignancy (liver, pancreas, gallbladder, common bile duct, metastatic)
- Total parenteral nutrition (usually requires ≥ 2 weeks of therapy)
- Cholangitis
- Intrahepatic cholestasis of pregnancy
- Hereditary cholestatic disorders (e.g., Dubin-Johnson syndrome, Rotor's syndrome)
- Physiologic jaundice of newborn; breast-feeding and breast milk jaundice

Jaw Pain

INTRODUCTION

Jaw pain is a common presenting or incidental complaint; its etiology is often identified by a careful history and physical examination. In many cases, consultation with a dentist will aid in the diagnosis and treatment. In older patients, rule out serious causes, such as temporal arteritis, malignancy, angina, and MI. Note that cranial nerves V, VII, IX, and X and cervical nerves C2, C3, and C4 all have input to orofacial sensation.

DIAGNOSTIC WORKUP & INITIAL MANAGEMENT

History and physical examination

- Review onset, character, and pattern of pain; medical and surgical history; associated symptoms (e.g., weight loss, sinus pain, skin complaints); and complete review of systems, including screening for local and systemic pathology and a cervical evaluation for muscle, neural, or skeletal referred pain
- Perform a thorough oral exam of the buccal mucosa, lips, hard palate, soft palate, posterior pharynx, floor of mouth, and top, sides, and undersurface of tongue
- Perform head, neck, ear, nose, cardiac, pulmonary, and lymphatic exams
- Suspect dental pathology until proven otherwise

Initial diagnostic workup

- Initial workup is aimed at assessing the mouth and jaw for dental, periodontal, or temporomandibular joint (TMJ) disorders
- Appropriate laboratory studies are based on the suspected diagnosis (e.g., CBC and ESR when suspect temporal arteritis)
- Imaging studies may include Panorex films, sinus radiography, CT, and/or MRI
- Temporal artery biopsy is indicated if ESR is elevated
- Biopsy any suspicious lesions
- Referral to a dental or medical specialist may be necessary

Initial patient management

- A therapeutic trial of medications (e.g., NSAIDs) may be helpful
- Dental or periodontal pathology, oral lesions, salivary pathology, and oral neoplasms require specialized treatment by dental specialist or oral surgeon
- TMJ syndrome is treated with pain management, bite block, cold or warm compresses, intra-articular steroid or lidocaine injections, and avoidance of jaw clenching and gum chewing
  - Intraoral manipulation may be helpful to manage pain
- Temporal arteritis requires temporal artery biopsy and high-dose steroids
- Treat headache syndromes as appropriate (refer also to the *Headache* entry)
- Neuralgia and neuropathies may be treated with NSAIDs, anticonvulsants (e.g., valproic acid, gabapentin), medical pain management, and/or directed therapy (e.g., nerve block)
- Treat underlying systemic etiologies and behavioral disease as necessary

DIFFERENTIAL DIAGNOSIS

Dental or periodontal pathology
- Associated with temperature sensitivity and pain on biting

Temporomandibular joint disorders
- Associated with unilateral or bilateral achy pain and diffuse tenderness of the masseter and temporalis muscles
- Exaggerated by jaw use
- Joint may be tender to palpation; "clicking" sounds are often present

Giant cell (temporal) arteritis
- Presents as unilateral pain in older patients
- May be accompanied by headache, jaw claudication, and vision loss
- A tender, visible temporal artery may be seen

Mucosal lesions (buccal mucosa, hard and soft palate, floor of mouth, oropharynx)
- Aphthous ulcers
- Herpes simplex or coxsackievirus B
- Cancer
- Tongue or lip lesions

Paranasal sinus pathology
- Most common pathology is maxillary sinusitis secondary to viral upper respiratory infection
- Pain is often referred to the upper molars

Salivary gland pathology
- Inflammation (e.g., parotiditis)
- Ductal stone (pain is worse with eating, especially acidic foods)
- Neoplasm

Other etiologies
- Headache with radiation to the jaw
- Referred pain from cardiac, cervical spine, pulmonary, or throat disease
- Neuralgias (e.g., trigeminal, glossopharyngeal)
- Neuropathies
  - Systemic neuropathies (e.g., HIV infection, diabetes)
  - Dental or alveolar neuropathies, usually subsequent to extrinsic trauma (e.g., blow to face, dental surgical intervention)
- Behavioral disorders (e.g., bruxism)
- Primary neoplasms of the maxilla, mandible, or major salivary gland
- Metastases to the mandible, maxilla, or TMJ
- Herpes zoster or postherpetic neuralgia
- Fibromyalgia
- Rheumatologic disease (e.g., Sjögren's syndrome)
- Systemic arthritis (e.g., rheumatoid arthritis)

Joint Pain and Swelling, Ankle

INTRODUCTION

Ankle sprains, most commonly resulting from traumatic inversion injury, are the most common cause of ankle pain. Following ankle injury, radiography is indicated if tenderness exists around the malleoli or if the patient is unable to bear weight. Bilateral ankle swelling suggests cardiovascular etiologies, such as congestive heart failure or venous insufficiency, rather than intrinsic ankle disease. Unilateral ankle swelling may suggest the presence of deep venous thrombosis.

DIAGNOSTIC WORKUP & INITIAL MANAGEMENT

History and physical examination

- The ankle joint is composed of the tibia, fibula, talus, and three groups of stabilizing ligaments:
  - Lateral ligaments: anterior talofibular (ATFL), posterior talofibular (PTFL), and calcaneofibular (CFL) limit ankle inversion and prevent lateral subluxation of the talus
  - Medial ligaments: Deltoid ligaments limit eversion and talar subluxation
  - Anteroposterior ligaments: Tibiofibular ligaments limit bony displacement
- Assess the ankle, foot, and lower leg
- Evaluate neurovascular status, including pulses, color, and capillary refill
- Observe the bones and soft tissues, including color changes and swelling
- Anterior drawer (for ATFL) and posterior drawer (for PTFL) tests to evaluate for instability: Hold the ankle in one hand and provide anterior and posterior force on the lower tibia
- Assess range of motion both actively and passively (grinding or popping suggests degenerative joint disease) and muscle strength
- The Ottawa ankle rules determine the need for radiography following acute trauma:
  - Tenderness of the distal 6 cm of the fibula or tibia
  - Tender navicular area
  - Tender proximal 5th metatarsal
  - Cannot bear weight (unable to walk more than 4 steps)

Initial diagnostic workup

- If indicated by Ottawa rules, radiography may include standard three-view ankle radiographs, stress views (inversion or eversion), and foot or lower leg series
- Lateral radiography with the foot held in plantar- or dorsiflexion may help to evaluate for anterior or posterior impingement
- CT or MRI may be indicated to clarify findings on plain-film radiographs and to evaluate cartilage, nerves, tendons, and ligaments

Initial patient management

- General injury management includes "PRICE" and pain control (NSAIDs and/or narcotics):
  - P = protection from additional strain or injury
  - R = relative rest (stretching is okay), which may include use of crutches
  - I = ice application for the initial 24–48 hours after trauma
  - C = compression dressing (elastic wrap or ankle support)
  - E = elevation of the foot (higher than the pelvis)
- Casting is often indicated for fractures and significant ankle sprains
- Splinting or bracing for ligament sprains
- Immediate reduction and orthopedic consultation for ankle dislocation
- Surgery may be indicated (e.g., bimalleolar or trimalleolar fracture, Achilles tendon rupture)
- Physical therapy referral to improve strength, range of motion, and proprioception

DIFFERENTIAL DIAGNOSIS

Inversion sprain (85% of ankle sprains)
- Results in pain, swelling, and ecchymosis of the lateral malleolar area
- Damage occurs to the 3 ligaments of inferior fibula (anterior and posterior talofibular and calcaneofibular ligaments) and peroneal muscle

Degenerative joint disease
- Pain is worse toward the end of the day and is not relieved with activity

Inversion or eversion injury of subtalar joint
- Results in pain while walking on uneven ground

Syndesmosis injury ("high ankle sprain")
- Not a true ankle sprain; results from excessive stretching of the interosseous membrane between the tibia and fibula
- Results in pain at the lower leg

Fracture
- Unimalleolar fracture of the lateral or medial malleolus
- Bimalleolar fracture
- Trimalleolar fracture (bimalleolar fracture plus fracture of lateral aspect of distal tibia)
- Plafond fracture (fracture of anterior tibia)
- Pilon fracture (comminuted high-energy distal tibial fracture)
- Maisonneuve fracture (proximal fibula fracture, disruption of the interosseous membrane, medial malleolus fracture)
- Talar dome fracture (bone and cartilage damage that may be missed on initial radiographs)
- Avulsion fracture of the distal fibula

Achilles tendon rupture
- Caused by excessive forced dorsiflexion (e.g., landing from a jump)

Other
- Ankle dislocation
- Peroneal tendon injury
- Repetitive injury with disruption of the ankle retinaculum
- Poor shoe alignment
- Neoplasm
- Peroneal nerve entrapment
- Diabetic (Charcot's) arthropathy
- Deep venous thrombosis
- Edema (usually bilateral) caused by a systemic etiology (e.g., congestive heart failure, cirrhosis, nephrosis)

Joint Pain and Swelling, Elbow

INTRODUCTION

The elbow joint is formed by the radius, ulna, and distal humerus. Overuse can lead to epicondylitis. Lateral epicondylitis, commonly known as "tennis elbow," and medial epicondylitis, commonly known as "golfer's elbow," reflect the types of repetitive motions that lead to these injuries. Entrapment of the ulnar nerve at the elbow can lead to pain that projects from the elbow down to the 4th and 5th digits of the hand. In addition to fracture, falling on an outstretched hand may lead to injury of the axillary, radial, ulnar, or median nerve. The elbow is the 3rd most commonly dislocated large joint; 90% of dislocations occur posteriorly.

DIAGNOSTIC WORKUP & INITIAL MANAGEMENT

History and physical examination

- Assess onset, duration, and character of pain
- Carefully examine the hand, wrist, elbow, and shoulder of the affected side
- Evaluate for paresthesias, bony point tenderness, crepitus on palpation, swelling, ecchymosis, limited range of motion, and neurovascular compromise (e.g., coolness, pallor, loss of distal pulses)
- Observe the bones and soft tissues, including color changes and swelling
- Assess range of motion both actively and passively (grinding or popping suggests degenerative joint disease) and muscle strength

Initial diagnostic workup

- Standard radiographs include anteroposterior, lateral, and oblique views
  - The anterior humeral line should intersect with the anterior middle third of the capitellum
  - A radial capitellar line should be present
  - Any visible posterior fat pad or enlarged anterior fat pad is evidence of joint effusion
- Aspiration may be diagnostic as well as therapeutic for bursitis; send for cultures and crystals
- Occasionally, nerve conduction tests are indicated to evaluate nerve entrapment and/or carpal tunnel syndrome
- CT or MRI is rarely necessary; if treatment is not progressing as planned, consider to clarify findings on plain-film radiographs or to evaluate cartilage, nerves, tendons, and ligaments

Initial patient management

- Orthopedic referral may be necessary
- High-risk injuries (e.g., intra-articular fracture, neurovascular compromise, crush injury, difficult anatomic reductions, supracondylar fractures, medial condylar fractures) warrant immediate orthopedic consultation and possible hospital admission
- General principles of fracture management include immobilization, analgesia, NSAIDs, and elevation
- Immediate anatomic reduction is required in cases of neurovascular compromise
- Nondisplaced fractures should be immobilized with the elbow flexed at 90°
- Displaced or intra-articular fractures usually require open reduction with internal fixation
- Joint aspiration may relieve pain if effusion is present
- Epicondylitis is treated with rest, NSAIDs, and physical therapy
- Elbow dislocation requires reduction (place traction–countertraction on arm and forearm, then press downward on the proximal forearm while flexing the elbow); follow with splint immobilization
- Splinting may be beneficial
- Physical therapy referral to improve strength, range of motion, and proprioception

DIFFERENTIAL DIAGNOSIS

Fracture (listed from proximal to distal)
- Humeral shaft (may be associated with radial nerve injury)
- Supracondylar (most common elbow fracture in children)
- Intracondylar (common in the elderly)
- Capitellum (often associated with radial head fracture)
- Epicondylar (may occur in children from repetitive stress)
- Radial head (most common elbow fracture in adults); usually caused by a fall on an outstretched arm and resulting in pain on supination
- Olecranon (may be associated with ulnar nerve injury); results in pain on extension
- Distal humerus (less common)

Dislocation
- Dislocations may be posterior (90%) or anterior
- 20% have an associated ulnar or median nerve injury
- Nursemaid's elbow (subluxation of radial head) occurs in young children who were pulled by an outstretched arm; children will refuse to move the arm
- In adults, dislocations generally occur secondary to falling on an outstretched arm; 80% are associated with an olecranon fracture

Bursitis
- Trauma
- Inflammation
- Infection

Epicondylitis
- Degeneration of the tendinous insertion at the lateral or medial epicondyles
- Lateral epicondylitis ("tennis elbow") is caused by extensor muscle overuse (results in pain on pronation and wrist dorsiflexion)
- Medial epicondylitis ("golfer's elbow") is caused by flexor muscle overuse (results in decreased grip strength and pain on pronation or wrist flexion)

Ulnar nerve entrapment
- Usually in the groove of the posterior aspect of the medial epicondyle
- Occurs acutely after direct trauma or with prolonged pressure or overuse
- Causes acute medial aching with numbness and tingling in 4th and 5th digits

Chronic arthritis
- Osteoarthritis
- Rheumatoid arthritis
- Gouty arthritis

Disorders of biceps or triceps tendons
- Biceps or triceps tendonitis
- Distal biceps or triceps tendon rupture

Pronator syndrome
- Median nerve entrapment distal to the elbow caused by racquet or throwing sports
- Anterior pain on resisted pronation and distal paresthesias

Radial tunnel syndrome
- Compression of the radial nerve as it crosses the head of the radius

Other
- Trauma
- Loose body (e.g., bone fragment)
- Bone tumor or cyst
- Rotator cuff injury
- Adhesive capsulitis
- Infection

Joint Pain and Swelling, Knee

INTRODUCTION

The knee is a critical weight-bearing joint and is subject to many forms of injury. Recognizing the anatomy of the knee can be helpful in determining the cause of knee pain. The ACL provides anterior stability and is commonly injured by the pivoting required in a number of sports (e.g., skiing, football, soccer). The PCL provides posterior stability and may be injured by strong anterior forces on a flexed knee (e.g., "dashboard injury"). The MCL and LCL may be injured by lateral or medial forces to the knee. Patellofemoral pain syndrome may result from processes that affect the patellofemoral joint; in some cases, this may be associated with degeneration of the patella, known as chondromalacia patellae.

DIAGNOSTIC WORKUP & INITIAL MANAGEMENT

History and physical examination (often diagnostic)

- Note onset, duration, and description of pain; evaluate the mechanism of injury (best predictor of injury type)
- Assess the knee, ankle, lower leg, hip, and related bones and soft tissues
- Assess symmetry between the knees; note swelling, deformity, erythema, and atrophy
- Assess range of motion both actively and passively (grinding or popping suggests degenerative joint disease) and muscle strength
- Assess ability to walk and bear weight; if the patient can, inspect gait for limitations of motion or other abnormalities
- Evaluate neurovascular status, including pulses, color, and capillary refill; a high risk of neurovascular injury (popliteal artery and nerve) exists following posterior knee dislocations
- If an effusion is not immediately present, one can "milk the joint" by compressing the suprapatellar bursa to force fluid into the joint space
- The drawer test is used to detect a rupture in the cruciate ligament; with the patient lying supine and knee flexed to 90°, attempt to pull the tibia forward (anterior drawer) and push backward (posterior drawer)
- Other tests to consider: Lachman maneuver (more sensitive than anterior drawer for detecting ACL rupture); valgus and varus stress on the lateral aspects of the knee (to assess integrity of MCL and LCL); and McMurray test (to detect torn meniscus)

Initial diagnostic workup

- Plain-film radiography of the joint is usually indicated
  - Anteroposterior, lateral, and sunrise views (patella) of both knees
  - When possible, also obtain weight-bearing anteroposterior films
  - Merchant and sunrise radiographs of the patella evaluate patellar alignment and injury
  - Tunnel views of the knee may rarely be useful (e.g., to diagnose osteochondritis dissecans)
- Joint aspiration may be indicated in patients with joint effusions; fluid analysis includes cell count with differential, crystals, Gram's stain, and culture
- CT or MRI may further evaluate an injury; MRI may help to confirm specific injuries and plan surgery (e.g., PCL tear, meniscus tear, osteochondritis dissecans)
- In some cases, blood work may include CBC, ESR, CRP, alkaline phosphatase, or uric acid

Initial patient management

- General injury management includes rest, ice, compression dressing, elevation of the leg, and pain control with NSAIDs and/or narcotics
- Ligamentous and meniscal injuries generally require only conservative therapy and orthopedic follow-up; splinting or bracing may be indicated
- Consider angiography to evaluate vascular structures in dislocations, PCL tears, or decreased peripheral pulses
- Physical therapy is often indicated to improve strength, range of motion, and proprioception

DIFFERENTIAL DIAGNOSIS

Degenerative joint disease (osteoarthritis)
- Knee osteoarthritis is extremely common with increasing age

Ligamentous injury (strain, tear)
- ACL: Positive Lachman (more sensitive) and anterior drawer tests
- PCL: Positive posterior drawer test
- MCL: Pain and/or increased laxity with valgus stress
- LCL: Pain and/or increased laxity with varus stress

Meniscus tear
- Patient may complain of pain and locking
- Positive McMurray test (not sensitive; negative test does not exclude a meniscal tear)

Patellofemoral syndrome (chondromalacia patellae)
- Pain at superior aspect of knee, especially during activities involing knee extension (e.g., climbing stairs)
- May be apparent on radiography performed while the knee is fully flexed ("sunrise view")

Iliotibial band syndrome
- Pain along the lateral aspect of the knee accompanied by a palpable or audible snapping
- Occurs almost exclusively in runners

Bursitis
- Prepatellar bursitis (housemaid's knee)
- Infrapatellar bursitis
- Baker's (popliteal) cyst
- Pes anserine bursitis: Patients complain of pain along the medial aspect of the knee (at pes anserinus insertion); caused by repetitive movement that creates an inflammatory response

Joint effusion
- May occur secondary to osteoarthritis, inflammatory arthritis, ligament injury, gout, pseudogout, or infection

Joint infection (septic joint)
- *Staphylococcus aureus* is most common
- *Neisseria gonorrhoeae* is common in adolescents and young adults
- *Salmonella* is common in sickle cell patients
- *Haemophilus influenzae* is common in children

Fracture
- Fractures may occur at the patella, femur, or tibial plateau

Dislocation
- Knee (tibiofemoral) dislocation
- Patellar dislocation

Malignancy
- Primary osteosarcoma
- Metastatic adenocarcinoma

Osteochondritis dissecans
- Results in osteonecrosis of subchondral bone; most common at the knee

Pediatric injuries
- Osgood-Schlatter disease
- Physeal injury
- Discoid meniscus

Other
- Compartment syndrome
- Hip or foot/ankle disease with referred pain to the knee

Joint Pain and Swelling, Shoulder

INTRODUCTION

The shoulder is held in place by the rotator cuff, an arrangement of 10 muscles that act on the scapula, clavicle, and humerus. Rotator cuff tears may occur in the setting of trauma, particularly with activities that require forceful overhead motions. Shoulder impingement syndrome results from inflammation of the rotator cuff and may occur in the setting of repetitive use. The shoulder includes three articulations—acromioclavicular, glenohumeral, and sternoclavicular—each of which may be subject to injury. The glenohumeral joint is the most frequently dislocated joint in the body, and 95% of cases involve anterior dislocation.

DIAGNOSTIC WORKUP & INITIAL MANAGEMENT

History and physical examination

- Note history of present illness, including onset, duration, characteristics of pain, and associated symptoms
- Note weakness, disuse atrophy, palpable crepitus, range of motion, and pain with active or passive motion
- Inspect for asymmetry, dislocation, or muscle atrophy
- Perform a complete neurovascular exam

Initial diagnostic workup

- Plain-film shoulder radiographs (anteroposterior, axillary, and scapular Y views); cervical spine and chest radiographs may also be useful
- Radiography or CT may identify chronic degenerative arthritis
- Shoulder MRI evaluates the anatomy of the rotator cuff and associated soft tissue; may differentiate partial from complete tears
- EMG can help discern nerve entrapments, cervical disk disease, or brachial plexus injury
- Diffuse shoulder or acromioclavicular pain may require workup for the presence of systemic illness

Initial patient management

- In acute trauma, reduction, ice, sling immobilization, and pain control may be necessary; severe trauma (e.g., sternoclavicular dislocation, acromioclavicular injury, humeral head fracture) should be referred to an orthopedic specialist
- Conservative therapy (rest, ice, NSAIDs) is beneficial for most cases of shoulder pain
- Slings may be used for comfort, but early range of motion (24–48 hours) is advised to prevent adhesive capsulitis
- Subacromial cortisone injection may be helpful if other anti-inflammatory methods fail; however, multiple injections are discouraged because of development of tissue atrophy
- Physical therapy is generally the mainstay of treatment for most shoulder injuries
- In some cases, surgical repair may be necessary (e.g., full-thickness rotator cuff tear, comminuted fractures, displaced distal clavicle fractures)
- Adhesive capsulitis may require surgical lysis of adhesions

DIFFERENTIAL DIAGNOSIS

Trauma and sports-related injuries
- Acromioclavicular dislocation ("separated shoulder")
- Sternoclavicular dislocation
- Glenohumeral dislocation
- Proximal humeral fractures

"Impingement syndrome"
- Progressive degeneration and inflammation of the subacromial contents (rotator cuff and subacromial bursa), which results in part from compression between the acromion and the head of the humerus
- May ultimately result in a rotator cuff tear

Rotator cuff strain, tear, or rupture
- May occur acutely (secondary to significant trauma) or, more commonly, from a relatively mild (e.g., reaching overhead) insult to a chronically degenerative rotator cuff

Degenerative joint disease
- The shoulder is a relatively infrequent presentation of osteoarthritis

Tendonitis
- Rotator cuff tendonitis
- Bicipital tendonitis

Bursitis
- Subacromion bursitis
- Subcapsular bursitis

Adhesive capsulitis ("frozen shoulder")
- Thickened, scarred joint capsule that occurs secondary to prolonged postinjury or postsurgery immobilization

Calcific tendonitis
- Deposition of calcium crystals in the rotator cuff, with resulting inflammation and severe pain

Other
- Acromioclavicular joint inflammation
- Suprascapular nerve entrapment
- Cervical disk disease and radiculopathy
- Gout
- Pseudogout
- Connective tissue disease (e.g., rheumatoid arthritis, SLE)
- Brachial plexus injury
- Septic arthritis
- Referred pain from acute coronary syndrome, cholecystitis, or splenic injury
- Malignancy (e.g., apical lung tumor)
- Fibromyalgia
- Thoracic outlet syndrome
- Reflex sympathetic dystrophy
- Rib dislocation/rib pain
- Acute axillary vein thrombosis (Paget-Schroetter disease)

Joint Pain and Swelling, Toe/Foot

INTRODUCTION

Toe pain and swelling is commonly caused by trauma and is a common consequence of sports that place stress on the feet (e.g., running or basketball). Metatarsalgia is pain at the ball of the foot (which overlies the metatarsal joints). Especially among women, this may result from wearing ill-fitting shoes and can be associated with hammertoes, bunions, or Morton's neuroma. Arthritis is another common cause of toe and foot pain. Rheumatoid arthritis may present with metatarsalgia before affecting the hands. Podagra, which is severe pain and swelling at the base of the great toe (i.e., the 1st metatarsophalangeal joint), is a classic presentation for gout. Less intense toe and midfoot pain may result from osteoarthritis.

DIAGNOSTIC WORKUP & INITIAL MANAGEMENT

History and physical examination
- Assess the toes, foot, ankle, and lower leg
- Evaluate neurovascular status, including pulses, color, and capillary refill
- Observe the bones and soft tissues, including color changes, ecchymoses, swelling, and tenderness
- Assess range of motion (both actively and passively) and muscle strength

Initial diagnostic workup
- Initial laboratory studies may include CBC, electrolytes, BUN and creatinine, calcium, magnesium, phosphorus, and ESR
  - Blood cultures and Lyme titers may be indicated
  - Iron studies (ferritin, iron, total iron-binding capacity) may be useful if suspect pseudo-gout, because many patients have underlying hemochromatosis
- Aspiration of the affected joint and synovial fluid analysis may be indicated
  - Look for infection, inflammation, blood (hemarthrosis of trauma), and crystals
  - Gram's stain, culture, and polarized light microscopy
  - Fluid cell counts typically reveal <50,000 white blood cells/mL in inflammatory processes and >50,000 white blood cells/mL in infectious arthritis
  - Gout: Needle-shaped, negatively birefringent crystals
  - Pseudogout: Linearly shaped, weakly positively birefringent crystals
- Radiography or CT may reveal fractures, chondrocalcinosis (pseudogout), signs of osteomyelitis (septic arthritis), or erosive distal bone changes (psoriatic arthritis)

Initial patient management
- Gout: NSAIDs, corticosteroids, colchicines for acute attacks; colchicine, urate-lowering agents (e.g., allopurinol, probenecid) for chronic management
- Ingrown toenails: warm soaks, removal of toenail if persistent
- Pseudogout: NSAIDs, corticosteroids, colchicine for acute attacks; NSAIDs and colchicine for chronic management
- Trauma: Most closed toe fractures can be treated with stiff-soled shoes (to unload the metatarsal heads); "buddy-tape" immobilization may help to relieve pain; rest, ice, NSAIDs, and elevation may be helpful
- Reiter's syndrome: Prednisone, indomethacin, sulfasalazine, methotrexate; local injection of steroids
- Septic arthritis: Treatment is based on clinical scenario and initial Gram's stain; ceftriaxone for gram-negative and cefazolin for gram-positive infections; add a fluoroquinolone for pseudomonal infections

DIFFERENTIAL DIAGNOSIS

Gout
- Monosodium urate crystal deposition occurs secondary to hyperuricemia
- Severe pain, redness, and swelling occurring in one joint (80% of cases), usually of the lower extremity and most classically at the metatarsophalangeal joint of the great toe (podagra)
- Tophi (collections of solid urate in connective tissue) may be present

Ingrown toenail
- Causes severe pain in the distal nail folds, with associated erythema, edema, and tenderness

Trauma
- Contusion
- Fracture
- Dislocation
- "Turf toe" (a tear in the capsule of the 1st metatarsophalangeal joint at the metatarsal neck)
- Puncture wound (e.g., stepping on a nail)

Pseudogout
- Calcium pyrophosphate deposition disease
- Can affect the toe, but the knee is the most common site

Seronegative spondyloarthropathy
- Psoriatic arthritis: A spondyloarthropathy involving middle-aged patients at multiple joints and associated with classic skin lesions
- Reiter's syndrome: Presents with arthritis, uveitis, and urethritis

Septic arthritis
- Presents with fever, joint redness, pain with passive and active range of motion
- Most often caused by skin flora (e.g., *Staphylococcus aureus* and various *Streptococci*)
- Often associated with previous penetrating toe trauma

Less common etiologies
- Cholesterol emboli
- Septic emboli secondary to infective endocarditis
- Lyme disease
  - Presents as monoarticular arthritis in 10% of cases
- Paronychia (bacterial infection of the posterior nail folds)
- Plantar fasciitis
- Tarsal tunnel syndrome

Joint Pain and Swelling, Wrist/Hand

INTRODUCTION

The wrist is composed of 8 carpal bones that are held in alignment by a series of ligaments and cartilage. Wrist pain is fairly common in primary care; wrist and hand injuries account for nearly 10% of emergency department visits. Osteoarthritis (degenerative joint disease) commonly affects the hands and wrists and may explain pain experienced by older patients when performing activities that stress these joints (e.g., opening jars, turning door knobs, weeding). Pain at the base of the thumb (i.e., at the carpometacarpal joint) is an especially common complaint among patients with osteoarthritis. Repetitive motion injuries (e.g., carpal tunnel syndrome, De Quervain's tenosynovitis) are common causes of hand and wrist complaints as well.

DIAGNOSTIC WORKUP & INITIAL MANAGEMENT

History and physical examination

- Assess the hand, wrist, fingers, elbow, and shoulder
- Assess onset, duration, and character of the pain; evaluate for paresthesias, bony point tenderness, crepitus on palpation, swelling, ecchymosis, limited range of motion, and neurovascular compromise (e.g., coolness, pallor, loss of distal pulses)
- Test the fingers for tendon involvement:
  - Weakness to resisted flexion/extension or inability to fully flex/extend the finger
  - Weak or absent thumb adduction, abduction, or opposition
- Tinel's sign and Phalen's sign may indicate carpal tunnel syndrome:
  - Tinel's sign is positive if pain is elicited by tapping the anterior wrist
  - Phalen's sign is positive if wrist flexion for at least 30 seconds elicits pain or numbness

Initial diagnostic workup

- Labs are usually unnecessary but may include RF, ANA, ESR, CBC, uric acid, TSH, and pregnancy testing (carpal tunnel disease is more common during pregnancy)
- Standard radiographs include posteroanterior, lateral, and oblique views
- Suspicion of a carpal fracture may require additional radiographs (e.g., scaphoid view)
- EMG and nerve conduction studies may be indicated if suspect carpal tunnel syndrome or other neuropathy
- Arthrocentesis with crystal analysis may be indicated if warmth and redness are noted in the wrist and MCP joints
- Bone scan may be necessary to assess avascular necrosis, occult fracture, or infection
- Rarely, CT or MRI is indicated
- Shoulder or chest CT may be indicated to evaluate for masses resulting in nerve entrapment or vascular compromise

Initial patient management

- Orthopedic referral may be necessary; significant long-term morbidity can be associated with missed or improperly treated fractures
- Hospital admission is generally required for open fractures, neurovascular injury, compartment syndrome, and open reduction with internal fixation (ORIF)
- General principles of fracture management include immobilization, analgesia, NSAIDs, and elevation; use of cock-up splints applied during activities and while sleeping reduces strain from repetitive use and reduces symptoms
- Immediate anatomic reduction is required in cases of neurovascular compromise
- Displaced or intra-articular fractures usually require ORIF
- Physical and occupational therapy, biofeedback, and relaxation therapy may be beneficial
- Corticosteroid injection for carpal tunnel syndrome improves symptoms in most patients; surgery may be warranted to release the transverse ligament and decompress the nerve entrapment

DIFFERENTIAL DIAGNOSIS

Carpal tunnel syndrome
- The most common cause of significant wrist discomfort and morbidity
- Associated with repetitive use activities (e.g., typing)
- Pain and numbness result from entrapment of the median nerve under the transverse ligament

Overuse injury
- Sports
- Occupational

Osteoarthritis
- The most commonly involved joints include the carpometacarpal, proximal interphalangeal, and distal interphalangeal joints

Rheumatoid arthritis
- The most commonly involved joints include the metacarpophalangeal and wrist joints

Tenosynovitis (De Quervain's) of the radial wrist
- Results from inflammation of tendon sheaths of the extensor pollicis brevis and abductor pollicis longus
- Presents with wrist pain extending to the thumb

Ganglion cysts
- Common growths of tendons and ligaments in the wrist area, occurring on both the dorsal and ventral surfaces
- Cysts are compressible, round, often tender, and mobile

Trauma and fracture
- The most common mechanism of injury is a fall on an outstretched hand
- The most commonly fractured carpal bone is the scaphoid
- Other mechanisms include direct blows, crush injuries, fall on an angulated wrist, and severe twisting motions
- Distal radius fractures include Colles' fracture (dorsal displacement and angulation with "dinner fork" deformity), Smith's fracture (volar displacement and angulation), Barton's fracture (intra-articular fracture with carpal dislocation), and Chauffeur's fracture (intra-articular radial styloid fracture)
- Galeazzi's fracture of the distal radial shaft along with radioulnar dislocation
- Monteggia's fracture of the proximal ulna along with radial head dislocation
- Fracture of a finger or volar plate

Dislocation
- Radioulnar dislocation: Ligament tear associated with a distal radius fracture
- Perilunate dislocation: Capitate displaced posteriorly to the lunate
- Lunate dislocation: Lunate displaced volarly off the radius ("spilled teacup" sign)

Other
- Ligament sprain
- Compartment syndrome
- Fibromyalgia
- Chest or shoulder masses, resulting in compression of lymphatic or venous systems
- Venous thrombosis of the subclavian or distal veins
- Flaccid paralysis following a stroke
- Rheumatologic disease
- Peripheral neuropathy
- Insect or animal bite/sting
- Infection (e.g., *Staphylococcus aureus*, streptococci)
- Contusion

Jugular Venous Distension

INTRODUCTION

Examination of the jugular venous pulse for abnormalities of the waveform or for estimation of central venous pressure is a critical component of the cardiovascular exam. It can aid in the assessment of volume status and the diagnosis of certain cardiac and noncardiac diseases.

DIAGNOSTIC WORKUP & INITIAL MANAGEMENT

History and physical examination

- The right internal jugular vein is easiest to evaluate and is seen best in tangential light from the foot of the bed with the patient at 30° of head elevation
- Distinguish venous pulsations from arterial pulsations (venous, but not arterial, pulsations can be obliterated by compression)
- The right atrium lies 5 cm below the sternal angle of Louis and is used as a reference point
- Normal central venous pressure is measured at <8–9 cm above the sternal angle of Louis
- The hepatojugular reflex is a helpful adjunct in patients suspected of having right heart failure
- Kussmaul's sign (the presence of an inspiratory increase in jugular venous distension) may be a sign of cardiac tamponade
- "Cannon" A waves may be a sign of AV dissociation and complete heart block
- Prominent V waves can be seen with severe tricuspid regurgitation
- A prominent x descent may be seen with cardiac tamponade, right ventricular overload, or atrial septal defect
- A steep y descent may be seen with constrictive pericarditis (Friedreich's sign)

Initial diagnostic workup and patient management

- ECG may be normal or reveal atrial fibrillation, ventricular tachycardia, right ventricular infarction, heart block, or other pathology
- Chest radiography may reveal signs of congestive heart failure or cardiomegaly
- Echocardiography is helpful to evaluate for valvular disease, ventricular function, and pericardial disease
- Additional diagnostic testing depends on the suspected pathology

DIFFERENTIAL DIAGNOSIS

- Congestive heart failure
- Constrictive pericarditis
- Restrictive cardiomyopathy
- Cardiac tamponade
- Superior vena cava syndrome
- Tricuspid regurgitation
- Complete heart block
- Atrial fibrillation
- Right ventricular infarction and/or failure
- Tricuspid stenosis
- Pulmonic valve stenosis
- Hypervolemia
- Ventricular tachycardia

Low Back Pain

INTRODUCTION

Low back pain is the second most common cause of doctor visits in the United States and the most common cause of disability. Up to 90% of the population will experience back pain at some point during their lives. At any given time, up to 20% of the population is experiencing some form of low back pain. The specific anatomic cause is often impossible to determine. Most cases result from mild muscle injury; however, all patients should be evaluated for the presence of neurologic deficits or other "red flags" that might signal a more serious problem.

DIAGNOSTIC WORKUP & INITIAL MANAGEMENT

History and physical examination

- Assess history of present illness, including onset, duration, severity, radiation, exacerbating and alleviating factors, functional disability, and associated symptoms (e.g., night pain, constitutional symptoms, morning stiffness, numbness, weakness, bowel/bladder dysfunction)
- Evaluate range of motion, sensation, strength, straight-leg raise test, reflexes, and neurovascular status
- Evaluate for "red flags" that may indicate serious conditions; if present, further workup is necessary (e.g., radiography, CBC, ESR, alkaline phosphatase, bone scan, metastatic workup)
  - Red flags suggesting fracture: Trauma, strenuous lifting in an older or osteoporotic patient
  - Red flags suggesting tumor or infection: Age (>50 or <20 years), history of cancer, presence of constitutional symptoms, IV drug use, immunosuppression, worsening pain at night
  - Red flags suggesting cauda equina syndrome: Saddle anesthesia, recent onset of incontinence, severe or progressive neurological deficit in leg

Initial diagnostic workup

- Plain-film radiography is rarely useful in the initial evaluation of back pain
- MRI and CT demonstrate abnormalities in asymptomatic patients; thus, positive findings in patients with back pain are frequently of questionable clinical significance; consider these studies in patients with worsening neurologic deficits or a suspected systemic cause of back pain (e.g., infection, neoplasm)
- If red flags are absent, no imaging is necessary; if pain persists, MRI is the most useful study
- MRI or CT myelography is indicated in patients with evidence of cord compression, red flag symptoms, or suspicion of epidural abscess or osteomyelitis
  - MRI depicts soft tissue and the spinal canal; can rule out malignancy, epidural abscess, osteomyelitis, nerve root and cord compression, cauda equina syndrome, and disk herniation
  - CT will only depict bone (CT myelography may be used to depict spinal cord/canal in patients unable to undergo MRI)
- Consider CBC, ESR (elevated ESR is very sensitive for vertebral osteomyelitis, epidural abscess, and metastases), and other testing as indicated by the clinical evaluation

Initial patient management

- In the absence of red flags, return to activity as soon as possible; rest is not beneficial
- Acetaminophen, NSAIDs, opioids, and/or muscle relaxants for pain; epidural corticosteroid injections may be indicated for resistant pain
- Patient education (weight loss, exercise, proper back biomechanics and ergonomics)
- Physical therapy, including pain-relief modalities (ice, heat, ultrasound), stretching, strengthening, aerobic conditioning, and relaxation therapy
- Surgery may be indicated for refractory disease, large neurologic deficits, unbearable pain, or significant limitations

DIFFERENTIAL DIAGNOSIS

Arthritic pain
- Osteoarthritis/degenerative joint (or disk) disease
- Rheumatoid arthritis
- Spondyloarthropathies

Mechanical pain
- Disk or facet disease
- Lumbar disk herniation
  - May have unilateral radiation down the leg
  - Increased pain with sitting
- Spondylolisthesis
- Vertebral fracture
  - Often associated with trauma or osteoporosis

Postural pain
- Osteoporosis
- Poor posture
  - Excessive demands of back musculature to support weight causes lactic acid buildup and pain

Myofascial pain
- Muscle or ligament strain
  - Lumbosacral muscle strain is the most common etiology of low back pain and the most common cause of temporary disability in adults
- Fascial tension
- Fibromyalgia
- Sacroiliac joint dysfunction
  - Often presents as unilateral upper buttock pain that is relieved by movement

Secondary gain
- Drug seeking
- Disability or liability issue

Other serious etiologies
- Spinal stenosis ("pseudoclaudication")
  - Back and bilateral buttocks and thigh pain that is relieved by rest
  - Increased pain with standing
- Cauda equina syndrome
- Infection (e.g., osteomyelitis, epidural abscess)
- Malignancy (especially prostate, breast, or lung metastases; multiple myeloma)
- Paget's disease
- Inflammation (e.g., ankylosing spondylitis)
- Referred pain (e.g., AAA, peptic ulcer disease, kidney stones, endocarditis, pancreatitis, others)
- Congenital spine malformations (e.g., occult spina bifida, spondylolisthesis)

Lymphadenopathy

INTRODUCTION

The lymphatic system is comprised of lymph vessels, nodes, and lymphoid tissues distributed throughout the body. It functions to drain interstitial fluids, ultimately returning fluid via the thoracic duct and right lymphatic duct to the thoracic venous system. It also serves as an organ of the immune system; pathogens are brought through the lymphatics to regional nodes, where cell-mediated immune functions respond to infections.

Lymphadenopathy refers to enlargement of the lymph nodes. Localized lymphadenopathy involves one lymph region; generalized lymphadenopathy involves more than one region. The majority of cases result from nonspecific causes or upper respiratory illnesses. Underlying malignancy must be ruled out, but <1% of cases are associated with malignancy.

DIAGNOSTIC WORKUP & INITIAL MANAGEMENT

History and physical examination

- Characterize the affected lymphatics: Regional vs. generalized, acute vs. subacute vs. chronic, number, size, texture (hard nodes may suggest malignancy; rubbery nodes may suggest lymphoma; fluctuant nodes suggest a suppurative etiology; fixed nodes may suggest malignancy or other inflammatory process), tenderness (suggests infection), and associated symptoms (lymph node pain results from expansion of the node capsule and is *not* a predictor of malignancy)
- Note signs of inflammation, skin lesions, petechiae, splenomegaly, and hepatomegaly
  - There may be an associated rash, as in the case of Lyme disease
  - A history of arthropod (flea, tick) exposure may be present
  - Travel history is important: Many parasitic diseases are Third World (e.g., trypanosomiasis) or tropical (e.g., filariasis) diseases
  - Immune status is also important because of the prevalence of toxoplasmosis as an AIDS-associated disease
- Thorough head and neck exam in adult patients with cervical adenopathy and/or history of tobacco use to evaluate for lesions suggestive of squamous cell carcinoma
- Supraclavicular and epitrochlear lymphadenopathy carry a high risk of malignancy or other abnormality and are rarely normal or reactive
- Lymph nodes > 1 cm (particularly > 2 cm) are likely to be pathologic

Initial diagnostic workup

- Initial labs may include CBC with peripheral smear, ESR, CRP, liver function tests, uric acid, and blood cultures
  - Leukocytosis often indicates infection
  - Atypical lymphocytes suggest a viral illness
  - Immature leukocytes/blasts may suggest leukemia
- Biopsy of affected lymph nodes may aid the diagnosis
  - Strongly consider biopsy if node is >2.0 cm, associated with abnormal chest radiograph, and/or patient is >40 years
  - Biopsy should be performed on the largest, most abnormal node, if possible (in descending order of preference of location: supraclavicular, cervical, axillary, inguinal)
- Consider HIV testing and skin testing for tuberculosis
- Immune globulin titers for EBV or cytomegalovirus
- Ultrasound of regional lymphatics, chest radiography, and chest CT may be indicated
- Bone marrow aspiration may infrequently be necessary to rule out underlying malignancy

Initial patient management

- If the node itself is infected, incision and drainage may be indicated
- Diagnosed malignancies must be staged and treated as appropriate

DIFFERENTIAL DIAGNOSIS

Generalized lymphadenopathy (e.g., cervical, supraclavicular, axillary, inguinal lymphadenopathy; hepatomegaly; splenomegaly)

Infection
- Viral (e.g., EBV, cytomegalovirus)
- Bacterial (e.g., *Staphylococcus, Streptococcus*, tuberculosis)
- Secondary syphilis
- Mononucleosis
- HIV/AIDS
- Kawasaki's syndrome
- Typhoid fever
- Parasites (e.g., toxoplasmosis)
- Fungi

Hypersensitivity reaction
- Serum sickness
- Drug reaction (e.g., hydantoin, phenytoin, hydralazine, allopurinol, primidone, penicillin, cephalosporins, sulfonamides, atenolol, captopril, quinidine)

Malignancy
- Lymphoma
- Leukemia
- Lymphoproliferative disorders
- Metastatic cancer is especially common in cases of left supraclavicular lymphadenopathy (Virchow's node), which may be associated with abdominal malignancies (e.g., stomach, pancreas, gallbladder, testis, ovary, kidney, prostate cancers)

Other
- Connective tissue disorders (e.g., SLE, rheumatoid arthritis)
- Chronic granulomatous disease
- Sarcoidosis
- Amyloidosis
- Churg-Strauss vasculitis
- Endocrine disorders (e.g., hyperthyroidism, hypothyroidism, hypoadrenalism, Addison's disease)
- Castleman's syndrome (angiofollicular lymph node hyperplasia)
- Kikuchi's disease

Localized lymphadenopathy

Reactive hyperplasia, local inflammation
- Dermatitis
- Recent vaccination
- Trauma

Infection
- Viral: mononucleosis, cytomegalovirus, HIV, rubella, mumps
- Bacterial: *Streptococcus,* tuberculosis, salmonella, cat-scratch disease (*Bartonella henselae*), gonorrhea, chlamydia, other STDs
- Parasitic: Malaria, toxoplasmosis
- Fungal: Histoplasmosis, coccidioidomycosis

Malignancy
- Lymphoma
- Metastatic disease (e.g., head and neck squamous cell cancer leads to cervical lymphadenopathy)

Myalgias

INTRODUCTION

Myalgia, or muscle pain, is a common complaint. When evaluating a patient with myalgia, it is important to determine if objective evidence exists for muscle breakdown (e.g., elevated levels of aldolase, creatinine phosphokinase, or aspartate aminotransferase), which may indicate the presence of rhabdomyolysis (can occur in the setting of trauma, seizure, metabolic disorders, or cocaine use) or myositis (inflammation of the muscle, which may be the result of infection or autoimmune disease). Myalgia in the absence of muscle breakdown may be associated with a number of unrelated conditions and should prompt a broad investigation for the underlying cause.

DIAGNOSTIC WORKUP & INITIAL MANAGEMENT

History and physical examination

- History should focus on the temporal events surrounding the occurrence of myalgias (e.g., postexercise, trauma, new vocational or avocational activities, onset of pain coinciding with initiation of new medications, recent illness)
- Distinguish focal versus generalized muscle pain
- Review of systems and associated symptoms (e.g., myoglobinuria causes tea-colored urine in cases of rhabdomyolysis)
- Physical exam should be directed at determining whether muscular weakness and features of systemic illness are present

Initial diagnostic workup

- Labs may include electrolytes, BUN and creatinine, glucose, creatine phosphokinase, aldolase, creatinine, urinalysis, myoglobin, thyroid function tests, ESR, and CBC
- EMG may be helpful to rule out nerve-related disorders
- MRI of the involved area can rule out masses or mechanical impingement, localized muscle edema (usually seen in injury or localized myositis), or generalized muscle edema (usually seen in inflammatory myositis)
- Muscle biopsy may be useful for evaluation of suspected inflammatory myopathies, muscular dystrophies, or metabolic myopathies
- Consider malignancy workup, particularly in older individuals

Initial patient management

- Address obvious, reversible causes (e.g., remove offending drugs or identified toxins, correct electrolyte imbalances, address endocrine disorders, treat infectious etiologies)
- Overuse injury is generally treated by rest, followed by gradual conditioning exercises
- Inflammatory myopathies may require steroids or other immunosuppressive therapies
- Severe muscle trauma may require surgical treatment

DIFFERENTIAL DIAGNOSIS

Inflammatory etiologies
- Autoimmune disorders
  - Dermatomyositis
  - Polymyositis
  - SLE
  - Scleroderma
  - Other connective tissue diseases
- Paraneoplastic myositis
- Intramuscular injections
- Systemic febrile illness (e.g., influenza)
- Infectious muscle disease (e.g., viral, bacterial, parasitic)

Metabolic etiologies
- Genetic enzymatic disorders of glycolysis and glycogen/lipid synthesis
- Endocrinopathies
  - Hypothyroidism or hyperthyroidism
  - Parathyroid disease
  - Adrenal disease
  - Diabetes mellitus (muscle infarcts)
- Drug-induced (e.g., alcohol, statins, zidovudine, corticosteroids, cocaine)
- Inherited myopathies (e.g., mitochondrial myopathy)

Mechanical etiologies
- Chronic myofascial pain syndrome
- Fibromyalgia
- Posttraumatic (e.g., "whiplash")
- Sleep deprivation
- Osteoarthritis with nerve compression
- Localized muscle injury
- Chronic overuse syndromes (frequently related to occupational or vocational activities)
- Acute muscle overuse/excessive physical exertion

Other
- Trauma
- Muscle ischemia (e.g., claudication in patients with peripheral vascular disease)
- Electrolyte disturbances, especially of potassium, calcium, or magnesium
- Rhabdomyolysis
- Dystrophies (e.g., mitochondrial myopathies)
- Polymyalgia rheumatica
- Psychogenic
- Distinguish muscle pain from pain of associated or nearby structures (e.g., tendons, ligaments, bone, connective tissue)

Nail Disorders

INTRODUCTION

Nail disorders are common and range from onychomycosis (fungal infection of the nail) to onycholysis (separation of the distal nail from the underlying nail plate, usually with nail thickening and subungual debris) to nail pitting to paronychia (an infection next to the nail plate that can be exquisitely painful). Various focal, skin, and systemic disorders must be considered in the differential diagnosis.

DIAGNOSTIC WORKUP & INITIAL MANAGEMENT

History and physical examination

- Assess onset, duration, characteristics, associated symptoms, history (e.g., psoriasis), family history, exposures, occupation and hobbies, and medications
- Physical exam should include complete skin assessment
- Evaluate the nail for shape (i.e., clubbing), pits, yellowish oil spots, pallor, ridges, and notching

Initial diagnostic workup

- Onychomycosis (nail fungus) is diagnosed by clipping the affected nail and curetting subungual debris for PAS (fungal stain) and/or culture
  - PAS stain is less expensive, quicker, and more sensitive than culture
  - Cultures are more helpful when a patient is refractory to systemic therapy; certain non-dermatophytes (e.g., *Aspergillus*, *Fusarium*) can act as nail pathogens and are difficult to eradicate with some antifungal drugs
- Acute paronychia requires incision and drainage for fungal and bacterial cultures to determine appropriate topical or systemic treatment and to relieve pain
- Chronic paronychia often results from *Candida* and should be treated with oral or topical antifungals and avoidance of excessive moisture to the nails
- Pigmented streaks in the nails often require nail matrix biopsy to rule out melanoma
- Lesions under the nail plate often require nail bed biopsy for definitive diagnosis
- Ingrown nails are sources of pain and infection and can be easily treated surgically
- Dermatology referral is indicated in unusual, recalcitrant, or potentially malignant cases

Initial patient management

- Nail fungus can be treated with systemic antifungals (e.g., terbenafine, itraconazole)
  - Fingernail fungus often requires 6 weeks of systemic therapy; toenail fungus requires 12 weeks of treatment to achieve a 70%–80% cure rate
  - Treat diabetics appropriately; nail fungus can compromise integrity of the nail bed, allowing bacterial pathogens to enter, and may lead to extremity cellulitis
  - Topical ciclopirox has low success rate (20%)
  - Educate the patient that risk of recurrence is quite high; modify lifestyle to prevent reinfection (e.g., use antifungal powders on feet/shoes)
- Intralesional steroids into the nail matrix are very painful but may offer long-term improvement in nail dystrophy because of lichen planus, psoriasis, and atopic eczema
- Nail psoriasis may be treated topically with limited success; systemic antipsoriatic therapies (e.g., cyclosporine, methotrexate, TNFα inhibitors, efaluzimab) are also used

DIFFERENTIAL DIAGNOSIS

Onychomycosis
- A very common cause of nail thickening, yellowing, and subungual debris; may also result in white, superficial flaking on the nail plate
- Caused by a dermatophyte infection
- May affect one or all fingernails and toenails
- Patients often have coexisting tinea pedis or tinea manum

Psoriasis
- More than half of patients with psoriasis have associated nail changes, including pits, "oil spots," and onycholysis
- Distinguishing nail fungus from psoriasis can be difficult on clinical exam
- Most patients with nail disease have other skin manifestations (e.g., plaques of thick, silvery white, adherent scalp scale that overlies well-demarcated patches of erythema)

Paronychia
- Tenderness, erythema, and peeling around the nail following minor cuticular trauma
- Very common and exquisitely painful
- Often exacerbated by "wet-work" (e.g., dishwashing)
- May have bacterial and/or yeast (*Candida*) component
- Can cause nail dystrophy without treatment

Nail trauma
- Very common (especially the great toenails and thumbnails)
- Easily misdiagnosed as fungal disease
- Can cause separation of the nail from the nail plate

Malignancy
- Subungual melanoma and squamous cell carcinoma
- Require biopsy and immediate surgical intervention

Endocrine disease (e.g., hyper- and hypothyroidism)
- May cause nail splitting, drying, and other nail changes

Lichen planus and atopic eczema
- Various nail dystrophies can be seen in atopic dermatitis

Alopecia areata
- A disorder of patchy autoimmune hair loss
- Can be associated with nail pits as well, often in a scotch plaid pattern

Other
- Several congenital disorders (e.g., ectodermal dysplasia) can cause nail dystrophy in association with other skin and systemic disorders
- Koilonychia: Spoon-shaped nails may indicate iron deficiency
- Terry's nails (white nails): Associated with liver disease, diabetes, CHF, malnutrition
- Lindsay's nails (half-and-half nails): Associated with renal failure
- Clubbing: Associated with lung disease, inflammatory bowel disease, cirrhosis, congenital heart diseases
- Yellow nails: Associated with bronchiectasis, lymphedema, immunodeficiencies
- Distal notching with red and white stripes: Associated with Darier's disease (a congenital disorder of abnormal keratinization)
- Muehrcke's lines: Associated with hypoalbuminemia
- Mee's lines: Associated with arsenic poisoning

Nasal Congestion

INTRODUCTION

Nasal congestion is a common complaint in primary care. Although usually a sequela of an upper respiratory infection, it can also be a sign of acute or chronic illness and may result in sleep disorders, emotional problems, and impaired functioning and learning in both children and adults. Regardless of the cause, successful management of nasal congestion often significantly improves the patient's quality of life.

DIAGNOSTIC WORKUP & INITIAL MANAGEMENT

History and physical examination (with attention to the head and neck)

- Note onset, duration, recurrence pattern, associated symptoms (e.g., cough, sneezing, fever, itchy palate or eyes, postnasal drip, rhinorrhea), medication and illicit drug use, family history, occupational history, exposures (e.g., home environment, presence of mold, triggers, resolution of symptoms during vacation), and seasonal variability of symptoms
- Patients may also have loss of smell, inability to taste, snoring, frequent throat clearing, functional decline, and daytime fatigue
- Examine the eyes, ears, sinuses, nares, oral mucosa, tongue, pharynx, neck, and chest
- Allergic "shiners" (dark circles under the eyes) may occur due to venous congestion
- Many children develop a nasal crease caused by chronic rubbing of the nose
- Turbinate edema and nasal passage occlusion can be visualized on exam
  - Nonallergic rhinitis may cause mucosal erythema
  - Allergic rhinitis causes pale or blue mucosa or turbinates
- Shiny polyps may be visualized; consider cystic fibrosis in children with polyps

Initial diagnostic workup

- Allergy (skin prick) testing for common inhaled antigens will be positive in patients with perennial and seasonal allergic rhinitis (perform only if chronic or recurrent)
- Nasal lavage with identification of cell type
  - Increased eosinophils occur in NARES and perennial and seasonal allergic rhinitis
  - Increased PMNs in infectious etiologies
- Rhinoscopic exam/flexible nasopharyngolaryngoscopy may reveal polyps, deformity, mucosal inflammation, or discharge draining from sinus meatus
- CT of the sinuses is usually reserved for patients who are resistant to medical therapy for 6–8 weeks
  - May see opacification and air-fluid levels in cases of sinusitis
- Other tests, such as nasal cultures, blood eosinophil counts, and total IgE levels, are less sensitive and specific and have little clinical value

Initial patient management

- Avoid allergens (e.g., mattress and pillow casings for dust mite allergy)
- Nasal saline lavage can reduce symptoms significantly; if not, intranasal steroids are safe and effective and improve quality of life, including daytime somnolence
- Systemic antihistamines are useful in cases of allergic rhinitis; newer, second-generation medications (e.g., cetirizine, fexofenadine, loratadine) have more favorable side effect profiles
- Topical nasal antihistamines (e.g., azelastine) may be effective for both types of rhinitis
- Treat bacterial infections (e.g., sinusitis) with appropriate antibiotics (e.g., amoxicillin, doxycycline, trimethoprim-sulfamethoxazole)
- Immunotherapy for persistent symptoms in patients with allergic rhinitis can reduce medication needs and significantly improve quality of life

DIFFERENTIAL DIAGNOSIS

Upper respiratory infection
- The most common cause of nasal congestion
- Usually of viral origin (e.g., adenovirus, rhinovirus)

Perennial allergic rhinitis
- Usually associated with a family history of allergy and atopy
- Associated with persistent, watery nasal discharge
- No variation with season

Seasonal allergic rhinitis
- Associated with itchy, teary eyes; sneezing; and watery nasal discharge
- Varies with season
- May be associated with exposure to allergens (e.g., dust, mold, pollen)

Perennial nonallergic rhinitis
- No variation with season
- The nasal obstruction may alternate nares
- Swollen nasal mucosa on exam

Sinusitis (acute or chronic)
- Patients often have a history of sinusitis
- Associated with craniofacial discomfort (especially on leaning forward), sinus headaches, pain with percussion of the sinuses or teeth, retro-orbital pain on coughing or sneezing in cases of ethmoid sinusitis, and mucopurulent nasal drainage

Rhinitis medicamentosa (rebound rhinitis)
- Results from prolonged use of intranasal decongestants

Inflammatory rhinitis
- Wegener's granulomatosis
- Sarcoidosis

Structural
- Foreign body in nose
- Deviated nasal septum
- Perforated nasal septum (may result from cocaine use)
- Tumor
- Adenoid hypertrophy
- Nasal polyps

Medication side effects
- Aspirin
- β-Blockers
- NSAIDs
- Oral contraceptives
- Reserpine
- Thioridazine

Less common etiologies
- Non-allergic rhinitis with nasal eosinophilia syndrome (NARES)
- Vasomotor rhinitis
- Environmental exposures (e.g., smoke, odors, temperature)
- Cystic fibrosis
- Folliculitis of a nasal hair
- Congenital abnormality
- Ciliary dyskinesis
- Postural changes

Nausea

INTRODUCTION

Nausea is a feeling of sickness in the stomach characterized by an urge to vomit. It can occur as a manifestation of a large group of disorders within and outside the gut, as well as a side effect of various drugs and circulating toxins. The chemoreceptor trigger zone, contained in the area postrema on the floor of the 4th ventricle, is particularly sensitive to chemical stimuli and is readily accessible to emetic substances because the blood-brain barrier is poorly developed in this area. Medical complications resulting from persistent nausea include weight loss, electrolyte imbalance and dehydration, delayed oral therapy, and anxiety or depression leading to delayed treatment.

DIAGNOSTIC WORKUP & INITIAL MANAGEMENT

History and physical examination

- Evaluate for fever, weight loss, jaundice, dehydration, abdominal pain, and distension
- Acute onset suggests infection, ingestion of toxins or new medication, pregnancy, head trauma, or acute bowel obstruction; chronic onset suggests partial obstruction, motility disturbance, metabolic, brain tumor, or psychogenic origin
- Note timing and relation to meals: Early morning (before meals) suggests morning sickness of pregnancy, alcoholism, uremia, postnasal drip, or increased intracranial pressure; during meals suggests psychogenic or peptic ulcer disease
- Perform a complete history, including review of systems, medical and surgical history, medications, recent illness, and social history
- Perform a complete physical exam, including head and neck (with ophthalmic exam for nystagmus), cardiac, pulmonary, abdominal (include stool guaiac), and neurologic exams

Initial diagnostic workup

- Initial laboratory testing may include CBC, electrolytes (may reveal hypokalemia, hypochloremia, metabolic acidosis), liver function tests, amylase, lipase, urinalysis, calcium, magnesium, salicylate level, hepatitis serologies, and toxicology screen
- Consider ECG and cardiac enzymes to evaluate for cardiac ischemia
- Upper GI radiography and endoscopy may be helpful when the history and physical exam suggest peptic ulcer disease or gastric outlet obstruction
- Abdominal radiography or CT may be indicated if abdominal pathology is possible
- In patients with chronic nausea and vomiting but normal findings on upper GI series and endoscopy, consider radionuclide solid-phase gastric emptying study
- Consider head CT with and without contrast if suspect CNS lesion
- Consider lumbar puncture with CSF analysis
- Abdominal or pelvic ultrasound is especially helpful in cases of lower abdominal pain in female patients or suspected gallbladder disease

Initial patient management

- Management involves restoration of normal fluid and electrolyte balance, specific treatment of identified underlying disorders, and antiemetic agents
- Neuroleptic agents (e.g., prochlorperazine, chlorpromazine) are effective in treating nausea and vomiting caused by drugs, radiation, or gastroenteritis
- D_2-receptor antagonists (metoclopramide, domperidone) are useful for nausea caused by chemotherapy, gastroparesis, or pseudo-obstruction
- Selective serotonin (5-HT_3) receptor antagonists (e.g., ondansetron) are very effective in controlling chemotherapy-induced nausea refractory to conventional agents
- Patients with refractory nausea may pose significant treatment challenges; newer therapies include somatostatin analogues, pyloric injections of botulinum toxin, implantation of gastric electrical pacemakers and neurotransmitters, and surgical resection of the stomach

DIFFERENTIAL DIAGNOSIS

Gastrointestinal disease
- Gastroenteritis
- Hepatobiliary disease (e.g., cholecystitis)
- Pancreatic disease (e.g., pancreatitis)
- Gastritis and peptic ulcers
- Peritonitis (e.g., ruptured appendix, ascites caused by liver disease, peritoneal dialysis)
- Bowel obstruction
- GI motility disorders (e.g., diabetes, achalasia, scleroderma, amyloidosis)
- Fatty liver
- Other causes of infection or inflammation
- Radiation treatment

Central nervous system disorders
- Increased intracranial pressure, hydrocephalus
- CNS lesion (e.g., tumor)
- Migraine
- Pseudotumor cerebri
- Vestibular disease (e.g., vestibular neuritis)
- Middle ear disease (e.g., Ménière's disease, labyrinthitis, benign positional vertigo)
- Meningitis
- Head trauma
- Subarachnoid or intracerebral hemorrhage
- Conversion disorder

Endocrine disorders or electrolyte disturbance
- Hypothyroidism or hyperthyroidism
- Parathyroid disease
- Hypokalemia
- Hypercalcemia
- Metabolic alkalosis
- Diabetic ketoacidosis
- Uremia
- Adrenal disease

Toxic ingestions
- Chemotherapy agents
- Alcohol
- Salicylates
- Iron
- Arsenic

Other etiologies
- Pregnancy (hyperemesis gravidarum)
- Pyelonephritis
- Testicular torsion
- Ovarian torsion
- Carbon monoxide poisoning
- Food poisoning
- Post-tussive (especially in children)
- Motion sickness
- Acute MI (especially inferior wall MI)
- Drug withdrawal
- Malingering

Neck Masses

INTRODUCTION

Nearly all neck masses are benign, but any mass occurring in a patient older than 30 years must be considered malignant until proven otherwise. In children and young adults, inflammatory and congenital masses are far more common than neoplasms. In adults, neoplasms are more common than inflammatory or congenital masses. Smoking, alcohol use, and history of head/neck radiation increase the likelihood of a malignant neoplasm.

DIAGNOSTIC WORKUP & INITIAL MANAGEMENT

History and physical examination

- Note size and location of the mass, character of the mass (e.g., firm, soft, blottable, pulsatile), and recent growth (malignant lesions are fast-growing); assess for associated symptoms (pain, dysphasia, hoarseness), radiation exposure (risk of thyroid cancer), social history (tobacco, alcohol), and family history (thyroid cancer)
- Location of the neck mass is often helpful in narrowing the differential: Congenital cysts occur predictably based on type (e.g., thyroglossal cysts occur at the midline); the location of upper aerodigestive tract malignant metastases is often predictable based on the primary site (e.g., tonsillar carcinoma metastases are often located in the high jugular chain)
- Duration of neck mass provides a clue to its etiology: Masses present for only a few days suggest an inflammatory lesion; masses lasting months suggest malignancy; masses lasting years suggest a congenital lesion
- Inflammatory masses often present with typical symptoms of infection (e.g., pain, erythema, tenderness, fluctuance, fever, leukocytosis)
- Congenital masses often present after an upper respiratory illness, with symptoms similar to those of inflammatory masses; may also present as asymptomatic, blottable neck mass
- Neoplastic masses usually present as asymptomatic and painless; may also present with symptoms of malignant disease, including weight loss, dysphagia/odynophagia, otalgia, change in voice, fetid odor, oral pain, and hemoptysis/hematemesis
- Physical exam (including direct laryngoscopy) should evaluate for size, color, location and symmetry, consistency, and tenderness

Initial diagnostic workup

- Initial laboratory testing may include CBC, chemistries, BUN/creatinine, TSH, free T_4, parathyroid hormone, ESR, calcium, phosphorus, LDH, PPD, and monospot test
- Imaging is usually necessary
  - CT or MRI is the most helpful
  - Ultrasound, arteriography, and radionuclide scan are helpful in specific instances
- Fine-needle aspiration will often establish the diagnosis and guide management
- Surgical endoscopy with directed biopsy is used if suspect a primary head or neck cancer
- Open biopsy is a last resort if the above workup does not provide a diagnosis

Initial patient management

- Inflammatory masses require appropriate antibiotics, incision and drainage (e.g., for abscess), and/or excision
- Congenital neck masses may be excised or followed
- Neoplastic neck masses require excision or neck dissection
- Lymphoma requires excisional biopsy when possible
- Indications for resection include suspected cancer, hyperthyroidism unresponsive to therapy, hyperparathyroidism, symptoms of pressure or choking, and cosmetic disfigurement

DIFFERENTIAL DIAGNOSIS

Inflammatory or infectious
- Enlarged lymph nodes are the most common neck mass
- Abscess
- Acute lymphadenitis (bacterial, viral, fungal)
- Tuberculous scrofula
- Atypical mycobacteria
- Mononucleosis
- Cat-scratch disease
- Granulomatous processes (e.g., histoplasmosis, blastomycosis)
- Sarcoidosis
- HIV
- Castleman's disease
- Kimura's disease

Congenital
- Thyroglossal duct cyst
- Branchial cleft cyst
- Laryngocele
- Cystic hygroma
- Hemangioma
- Lymphangioma
- Dermoid

Neoplasm
- Local metastases (from primary upper aerodigestive tract tumor)
- Metastases from a distant site
- Lymphoma
- Other primary neck tumors (e.g., thyroid, carotid body, salivary gland, schwannoma)

Thyroid lesion
- Cancer (papillary, medullary, follicular/Hurthle cell, anaplastic)
- Thyrotoxicosis (Graves' disease, toxic multinodular goiter, toxic thyroid nodule)
- Thyroiditis (Hashimoto's disease, acute thyroiditis, subacute thyroiditis, Riedel's tumor)

Parathyroid lesion
- Hyperplasia
- Adenoma
- Carcinoma

Primary tumors
- Thyroid (see above)
- Parathyroid (see above)
- Salivary gland (parotid tumor is most common)
- Soft-tissue tumor (lipoma, sebaceous cyst, inclusion cyst, carbuncle)
- Carotid body tumor
- Neurofibroma
- Schwannoma
- Angioma
- Laryngeal tumor (chondroma)
- Sarcoma
- Skin cancer
- Lymphoma
- Upper aerodigestive tract tumor

Neck Stiffness or Pain

INTRODUCTION

Neck pain or stiffness may be caused by trauma, inflammation, or mechanical disorder. Following trauma, the neck should be immobilized until imaging tests can be performed to evaluate for the presence of fracture. Nuchal rigidity is characterized by an inability to touch the chin to the chest. It is associated with the presence of meningeal inflammation; however, the absence of nuchal rigidity does not exclude the possibility of infectious meningitis. Arthritis can also affect the neck; both osteoarthritis and rheumatoid arthritis can lead to cervical spondylopathy, which, in turn, can lead to a myelopathy characterized by neck stiffness and pain.

DIAGNOSTIC WORKUP & INITIAL MANAGEMENT

History and physical examination

- Assess onset, duration, presence and location of pain, associated symptoms (e.g., vomiting, headache, fever, visual changes, seizures), history (e.g., blood clots, aneurysm, immunocompromise), recent infection or dental work, decreased sensation
- Focus on evidence of trauma and infection
- Maintain all patients with possible traumatic injury in a cervical collar and backboard until the diagnostic workup is complete
- Assess vital signs, head and neck, torso, lungs, and heart
- If suspect meningeal irritation, perform Brudzinski and Kernig tests:
  - Positive Brudzinski's sign: Spontaneous hip flexion in response to passive neck flexion
  - Positive Kernig's sign: Inability to extend at the knee when the hip is in flexion

Initial diagnostic workup

- Initial labs may include CBC, electrolytes, BUN and creatinine, calcium, glucose, and ESR
- Blood cultures are indicated if suspect an infectious etiology
- Lumbar puncture with CSF analysis is useful in cases of suspected infection or subarachnoid hemorrhage
- Cervical spine radiography is indicated in trauma or neck infection (may reveal prevertebral soft-tissue swelling)
- Head CT without contrast may show bleeding in cases of subarachnoid hemorrhage (fails to reveal subarachnoid blood in 10% of cases)
- Neck CT may be indicated in suspected soft-tissue disease (e.g., retropharyngeal abscess) or occult vertebral fracture if not adequately visualized on plain-film radiographs
- MRI of the spine may be indicated in suspected epidural abscess or epidural hematoma

Initial patient management

- The vast majority of cases of nontraumatic, noninfectious neck pain are self-limited
- Follow trauma protocols in cases of trauma or acute neck injury
- In cases of trauma, soft-collar immobilization is no longer routinely recommended
  - Cervical spine fractures may be treated with surgical fixation, halo brace immobilization, or careful observation
  - Soft-tissue injuries to the neck and torticollis are treated symptomatically with NSAIDs and muscle relaxants
  - Subarachnoid hemorrhage is often treated surgically
- Bacterial meningitis requires immediate broad-spectrum antibiotics (e.g., ceftriaxone, vancomycin) and, possibly, steroids; viral meningitis is treated supportively (IV fluids, NSAIDs)
- Inflammatory arthropathies typically respond to NSAIDs, steroids, or antirheumatic agents
- Hospital admission is warranted in patients with progressive neurologic symptoms, with possible serious conditions (e.g., MI) and in those who need further workup to rule out severe pathology (e.g., MRI for epidural abscess)

DIFFERENTIAL DIAGNOSIS

Trauma

- Cervical muscle sprain/strain or spasm
- Paraspinal neck stiffness
  - Commonly results from motor vehicle collisions ("whiplash") or abnormal sleep posture
- Cervical spine fracture with spasm of neck muscles
- Subarachnoid hemorrhage
- Epidural hematoma
- Spinal cord injury without radiographic abnormality (SCIWORA)
  - Occurs in pediatric patients with ligamentous laxity and hypermobility of the cervical spine
- Rotary atlantoaxial subluxation
  - Subluxation of the cervical spine at C1-C2, resulting in sternocleidomastoid spasm with tilt of the head toward the affected side and chin pointed toward the ipsilateral side

Infection

- Meningitis
  - Bacterial (e.g., *Neisseria meningitidis, Streptococcus pneumoniae*) [handwritten: -severe, general fever, HA, stiff neck, photophobia, N/V, altered mentation]
  - Viral (e.g., HIV, EBV, enterovirus, HSV)
  - Other (e.g., fungal, parasitic, chemical)
- Parameningeal infection
- Encephalitis
- Cervical lymphadenitis
- Tonsillopharyngitis
- Epiglottitis
- Retropharyngeal abscess
- Epidural abscess
- Discitis
- Osteomyelitis
- Tetanus
- Dental abscess
- Chagas' disease
- Poliomyelitis
- Trichinosis
- After upper respiratory infection

Inflammatory disorders

- Rheumatoid arthritis
- Spondyloarthropathy
- Ankylosing spondylitis
- Psoriatic arthritis

Other

- Torticollis
- Mechanical disorders (e.g., degenerative joint disease, herniated disk, spondylosis)
- Spinal stenosis
- Tumors (e.g., leptomeningeal metastases, apical lung tumor, posterior fossa tumor)
- Myocardial ischemia or acute coronary syndrome
- Carotid dissection
- Brachial plexus injury
- Thoracic outlet syndrome
- Headache syndrome
- GERD or hiatal hernia may manifest as neck torsion
- Spasm of the pharynx or larynx
- Thyroiditis
- Dystonic reaction, often to psychiatric medications (e.g., haloperidol, prochlorperazine)
- Toxins (e.g., strychnine, lead poisoning, methanol poisoning, hypervitaminosis A)

Night Sweats

INTRODUCTION

Night sweats are a fairly common complaint in primary care medicine. Authors define night sweats variably, but the term generally pertains to drenching sweats that occur at night and are not caused by excessive room temperature or clothing/covering. There are both serious and benign causes for night sweats. A thorough history is the most important tool in determining the cause and directing the workup.

DIAGNOSTIC WORKUP & INITIAL MANAGEMENT

History and physical examination

- Complete history, including onset, associated symptoms (e.g., unintentional weight loss, fatigue, pruritis, flushing, diarrhea, pain, headaches, palpitations)
- Review medical history, social history, and systems for risk factors of HIV and tuberculosis; ask about foreign travel and IV drug use
- Review all medications, including over-the-counter and herbal remedies
- Complete physical exam, including blood pressure, heart rate, temperature, and weight, with a focus on endocrine (thyroid nodules, lid lag, reflexes), lymphatic (spleen and complete lymph node exam), and dermatologic systems

Initial workup and management

- Laboratory testing depends on the presumed etiology; a reasonable initial workup includes CBC with differential, eosinophil count, electrolytes, BUN and creatinine, calcium, magnesium, TSH, urinalysis and urine culture, and ESR
- Further testing may include FSH in perimenopausal women, PPD, chest radiography, HIV viral load/antibody, blood cultures, monospot or Epstein-Barr virus IgM, 3 AM glucose level to assess for nocturnal hypoglycemia, sleep study, free T_4, 24-hour urinary catecholamines, 5-hydroxyindoleacetic acid, echocardiography, and/or CT of the chest, abdomen, and pelvis
- Treatment depends on the etiology, although identifying the correct diagnosis is usually the most difficult aspect of patient management

DIFFERENTIAL DIAGNOSIS

Infection
- HIV
- Tuberculosis
- Infectious mononucleosis
- Fungal (e.g., histoplasmosis, coccidioidomycosis)
- Lung or other abscess
- Endocarditis
- Osteomyelitis
- Chronic eosinophilic pneumonia

Neoplasm
- Leukemia
- Hodgkin's disease and other forms of lymphoma
- Solid tumors (e.g., prostate, adrenal, renal, testicular)
- Endocrine tumors (e.g., pheochromocytoma, carcinoid)

Endocrinopathy
- Menopause/premature ovarian failure
- Hyperthyroidism
- Diabetes mellitus (nocturnal hypoglycemia)

Behavioral and psychiatric
- Anxiety
- Chronic fatigue syndrome
- Substance abuse (including alcohol)

Drugs
- Antipyretics (most common)
- Antihypertensives
- Phenothiazines
- Antiretroviral agents
- Antidepressants

Other
- Pregnancy
- GERD
- Obstructive sleep apnea
- Orchiectomy
- Prinzmetal's angina
- Temporal arteritis
- Takayasu's arteritis

Nystagmus

INTRODUCTION

Nystagmus is an involuntary, rhythmic, biphasic oscillation of the eyes. It is characterized as horizontal, vertical, rotary, or some combination; fast or slow; symmetric or asymmetric; and pendular (equal speed in either direction) or jerking (slow in one direction, followed by fast in the opposite direction). It is usually bilateral, and the abnormal movements occur identically in both eyes. By convention, nystagmus is named in the direction of the fast phase. Nystagmus usually results from a defect in the slow eye movement system (visual fixation, vestibular system, smooth pursuit, vergence, optokinetic, and neural integrator pathways). It may be normal or pathologic, congenital or acquired. Most cases are attributable to brainstem disorders, cranial nerve (especially cranial nerve VIII) disease, or cerebellar disease.

DIAGNOSTIC WORKUP & INITIAL MANAGEMENT

History and physical examination

- Note age of onset, characteristics, medications, and drug use
- Associated symptoms may include oscillopsia (a sense that the surroundings are oscillating), vertigo, diplopia, disequilibrium, tinnitus, facial numbness, nausea and vomiting, dysarthria, dysphagia, and ataxia
- Perform a complete ocular exam, including eye movements in primary gaze and all positions of gaze, iris transillumination (albinism), dilated fundus exam, careful refraction, and vestibulo-ocular reflex
- Perform the Dix-Hallpike maneuver to assess for benign paroxysmal positional vertigo
  - The patient is brought from a sitting to a supine position, and the head is turned 45° to one side and slightly extended; the eyes are then observed for 30 seconds; if no nystagmus is noted, the patient is brought back to a sitting position for 30 seconds, and the test is repeated on the other side
- Consider caloric stimulation
- Perform a complete neurologic exam

Initial diagnostic workup

- Consider drug, toxin, and dietary screen of the urine and serum
- Brain MRI may reveal tumors, demyelinating disease, vascular disease, and congenital malformations
- Consider eye movement recording or ENG, visual-evoked responses, and ERG
- In children with opsoclonus, abdominal CT to rule out neuroblastoma
- In adults, rule out paraneoplastic syndromes via anti-Ri antibodies and malignancy workup
- Workup for myasthenia gravis may be indicated
- Consider neurology and/or ophthalmology consultation

Initial patient management

- Most acquired cases will resolve when the underlying etiology is treated
- Remove offending medications and toxins
- Nystagmus medications (e.g., meclizine for positional vertigo) have varying success rates
- Otolith repositioning maneuvers (Epley, Semont) may be effective for positional vertigo
- Botulinum toxin injection to the extraocular muscles may help in severe, disabling nystagmus
- In cases of congenital nystagmus, maximize vision by refractive lenses, treat amblyopia ("lazy eye") if indicated, and consider eye muscle surgery
- In cases of vestibular nystagmus, a vestibular suppressant (e.g., meclizine, diazepam) and vestibular adaptation exercises may be effective
- Consider baclofen for periodic alternating nystagmus and congenital nystagmus
- Clonazepam may be indicated for downbeat nystagmus

DIFFERENTIAL DIAGNOSIS

Horizontal nystagmus
- May be normal in the extremes of lateral gaze or when tracking an object or a row of objects horizontally; otherwise, most often caused by drug intoxication (e.g., anticonvulsants, sedatives, barbiturates, benzodiazepines, alcohol) or intramedullary brainstem disease

Vertical upbeat nystagmus
- May occur in intrinsic brainstem disease (e.g., multiple sclerosis, stroke)
- May rarely occur in drug intoxications

Vertical downbeat nystagmus
- Commonly occurs with lesions in the region of the foramen magnum (e.g., Arnold-Chiari malformation)

Rotatory nystagmus
- May occur in central or peripheral vestibular disease

Vestibular nystagmus
- Peripheral (horizontal rotary nystagmus, slow phase toward hypoactive side, latency, fatigability, and accompanied by vertigo, tinnitus, or deafness): Etiologies include labyrinthitis, vestibular neuronitis, Meniere's disease, migraine, or benign positional vertigo
- Central (asymmetric, rotary nystagmus that changes direction in different gazes; no latency; not fatigable): Etiologies include lesions of the cerebellum, pons, or cerebellopontine angle

Gaze-evoked nystagmus
- May occur physiologically while fixing on objects with the eyes when the head is turned (e.g., in ballerinas)
- Pathologic (asymmetric) etiologies include toxic-metabolic lesions, cerebellar lesions, or pontine lesions

Dissociated nystagmus (i.e., different nystagmus between eyes)
- Etiologies include internuclear ophthalmoplegia of multiple sclerosis or cerebral disease

Periodic alternating nystagmus
- Disorders of the cervicomedullary junction

Downbeat nystagmus
- Disorders of the cervicomedullary junction
- May be a characteristic of syringobulbia

Upbeat nystagmus
- Brainstem or cerebellum disease when present in primary gaze
- Drug effect if only present in upgaze

Monocular visual loss
- Ipsilateral, slow, vertical oscillation

Head nodding, head turn
- Caused by motor or sensory deficits
- Latent nystagmus (occurs when only one eye is viewing; associated with strabismus)
- Nystagmus blockage syndrome (convergence, esotropia, and head turn)
- Spasmus nutans (resolves by age 5 years)

Myasthenia gravis
- May cause nystagmus as a result of weakness of extraocular muscles

Nonnystagmus eye oscillations
- Saccadic intrusions (e.g., square-wave jerks seen in cerebellar disease, ocular bobbing seen in brainstem infarcts, ocular dysmetria seen primarily in multiple sclerosis, opsoclonus/myoclonus seen in paraneoplastic syndromes)
- "Searching" eye movements (particularly in blind patients)

Oral Ulcers

INTRODUCTION

Recurrent oral erosions are most often a result of herpes simplex virus (HSV) or idiopathic aphthous stomatitis. A thorough review of systems and complete skin exam are the best tools to ensure diagnostic accuracy. Note that serious medical conditions may initially manifest as oral lesions. Referral to an oral surgeon, otorhinolaryngologist, or dermatologist is necessary if a definitive diagnosis cannot be determined.

DIAGNOSTIC WORKUP & INITIAL MANAGEMENT

History and physical examination
- Careful history to evaluate for difficulty swallowing or breathing
- Assess onset, duration, characteristics, and associated symptoms (e.g., fever, prodrome)
- Review the patient's medical history and medication list
- If ulcers occur in the same location with every episode, oral herpes simplex is likely
- In sexually active patients, consider HIV, immunosuppression, or syphilis
- Perform a thorough skin exam to evaluate for rashes or other mucosal lesions (ocular, urethral, vaginal, or perianal)
- Lacy white plaques on the tongue or buccal mucosa may suggest lichen planus
- Ocular or anogenital complaints may suggest Behçet's syndrome, pemphigus, or pemphigoid

Initial diagnostic workup
- Initial evaluation includes a viral swab for culture and/or serum IgG testing for herpes simplex
- Consider RPR for syphilis and CBC for leukopenia
- Consider a punch biopsy of the edge of an ulcer/erosion to determine the presence of viral changes, cytologic atypia, or evidence of an autoimmune bullous disease
- Recurrent aphthous stomatitis is a diagnosis of exclusion but is also the most common diagnosis for recurrent painful oral ulcers after herpes
- Consider fungal culture for oral candidiasis

Initial patient management
- Orabase compounded with high-potency topical steroids (e.g., clobetasol) may offer symptomatic relief and increase speed of healing for autoimmune diseases
- "Magic mouthwash" may be used to swish and spit as necessary for relief (these may contain lidocaine, diphenhydramine, and even liquid tetracycline)
- Aphthous stomatitis will usually resolve spontaneously within 2 weeks; a trial of intralesional triamcinolone may be considered
- Recurrent herpes stomatitis may be treated with 1- to 7-day courses of oral antivirals (e.g., acyclovir) to shorten duration of the episode and speed healing; however, these are effective only if started within 24 hours of onset of the prodrome (tingling or pain at the site of eruption occurring hours before onset)
  - Chronic suppressive therapy with oral antivirals may be indicated if frequent recurrences
- Bullous diseases may be treated with corticosteroids (topical or oral) or other steroid-sparing immunosuppressant agents
- Treat *Candida* with nystatin swish and swallow or oral fluconazole

DIFFERENTIAL DIAGNOSIS

Aphthous stomatitis
- Idiopathic, recurrent, painful oral ulcers that resolve spontaneously

Herpes stomatitis
- Caused by a primary outbreak of HSV
- Severe gingivostomatitis occurs with pain, redness, and erosions around the gum line
- Recurrent oral herpes ("cold sores") often occur at the lip border
- Stress, sun exposure, and many other factors contribute to flare-ups

Self-limited viral disease (e.g., herpangina, hand-foot-mouth disease)
- Most often occurs in children
- Prodrome of malaise and fever, followed by a 5- to 10-day outbreak of oropharyngeal erosions or vesicles

Chemotherapeutic drugs
- 5-Fluorouracil
- Methotrexate

Squamous cell carcinoma
- Always consider in cases of a nonhealing ulcer or oral erosion

Bullous diseases
- Pemphigoid
- Pemphigus
- Lichen planus

Behçet's syndrome
- An uncommon but well-known cause of oral ulcers
- Patients must exhibit other symptoms (e.g., uveitis, CNS problems, GI complaints, genital ulcers) before the diagnosis can be made

Erythema multiforme (Stevens-Johnson syndrome)
- Characterized by oral ulcers, ocular involvement, and simultaneous targetoid, erythematous, or bullous skin lesions
- May be triggered by HSV infection, *Mycoplasma* infection, or drugs (e.g., phenytoin, sulfonamides)

Syphilis
- Primary syphilis is characterized by a painless chancre
- Secondary syphilis manifests with mucous patches

Agranulocytosis or leukopenia
- Presents with nondistinctive oral ulcerations

Histoplasmosis
- Especially common in immunosuppressed patients

Other
- Allergic contact dermatitis to amalgams in dental work may result in buccal tenderness
- Nicotine stomatitis
- Trauma (e.g., burn or cut in the mouth)

Orthopnea

INTRODUCTION

Orthopnea is defined as difficulty breathing (dyspnea) while in the recumbent position. The dyspnea is usually caused by increased venous return to the lungs while recumbent, resulting in increased pulmonary venous and capillary pressures. Elevating the head and chest toward an upright position relieves the dyspnea. Orthopnea implies left-sided heart failure in ~95% of cases.

DIAGNOSTIC WORKUP & INITIAL MANAGEMENT

Initial management
- Attention to airway, breathing, and circulation
- Assess vital signs, including pulse oximetry
- Administer supplemental oxygen as needed
- If an obvious cause is identified, begin treatment as necessary (e.g., inhaled bronchodilators for asthma or COPD, nitroglycerin for ischemic disease)

History and physical examination
- Note onset (sudden or chronic, progressive), timing (persistent or intermittent), associated symptoms (e.g., chest discomfort, syncope), medical history, family history, and medications
- Perform complete cardiovascular and pulmonary exams

Initial workup and management
- Initial laboratory testing includes CBC, electrolytes, thyroid function tests, pulse oximetry (resting, ambulatory, and nocturnal), and chest radiography
- ABG will identify barriers to oxygen diffusion (increased A-a gradient), hypoxemia, and chronic hypercapnia
- ECG may reveal evidence of MI, right ventricular strain (e.g., caused by mitral stenosis), left ventricular hypertrophy (e.g., aortic stenosis), low voltage (e.g., pericardial effusion), and arrhythmias
- If the etiology is uncertain, B-type natriuretic peptide (BNP) may be useful to distinguish congestive heart failure from other causes of dyspnea
- Pulmonary function tests may be indicated to identify restrictive or obstructive lung disease and barriers to diffusion
- Echocardiography may be indicated to establish a diagnosis of structural heart disease, valve disease, or left ventricular dysfunction
- Consider referral to a cardiologist and possible cardiac catheterization to evaluate for coronary artery disease, valve disease, cardiomyopathy, and congenital heart disease

DIFFERENTIAL DIAGNOSIS

Congestive heart failure
- The most common cause of orthopnea (95% of cases)
- Etiologies include uncontrolled hypertension, pulmonary embolism, hyperthyroidism, pericardial disease, endocardial disease (e.g., valvular stenosis, valvular insufficiency, valve rupture, endocarditis), and myocardial disease (e.g., myocardial ischemia or infarction, arrhythmias)

Aortic regurgitation
- Common causes include hypertension, rheumatic fever, and endocarditis

Cardiomyopathies
- Dilated cardiomyopathy is most common
  - Etiologies include coronary artery disease, hypertension, valve disease, toxins (e.g., alcohol, amphetamines, cocaine, doxorubicin), peripartum, infection (e.g., viral, *Trypanosoma cruzi*), tachycardia induced, and metabolic conditions (e.g., deficiencies of selenium, carnitine, phosphorus, calcium, or thiamine)
- Restrictive cardiomyopathy is less common
  - Etiologies include endomyocardial fibrosis, Löffler's endocarditis, infiltrative diseases (e.g., amyloidosis, sarcoidosis, radiation carditis), and storage diseases (e.g., hemochromatosis, glycogen storage disease, Fabry's disease)
- Hypertrophic cardiomyopathy and arrhythmogenic right ventricular cardiomyopathy are relatively rare

Pleural effusion
- Etiologies include congestive heart failure, pneumonia, cancer, pulmonary embolism, connective tissue disease (e.g., SLE, rheumatoid arthritis), pancreatitis, and renal or liver disease

Aortic stenosis
- May be associated with angina, syncope, or congestive heart failure

Mitral stenosis
- Usually occurs 15–40 years after rheumatic fever
- Advanced cases result in pulmonary hypertension and right heart failure
- Dyspnea is the most significant symptom
- May present with the classic triad of a diastolic rumble, opening snap, and loud S_1

Congenital heart disease
- May see failure to thrive, progressive symptoms of congestive heart failure, cyanosis, and/or murmur

Diaphragmatic disorders
- Bilateral diaphragmatic weakness or paralysis may be caused by surgical trauma (e.g., interruption of the phrenic nerves), neuromuscular disease (e.g., Guillain-Barré syndrome, amyotrophic lateral sclerosis), and rheumatologic disease (e.g., polymyositis, shrinking lung syndrome in SLE)

Other
- Severe COPD
- Asthma
- Obstructive sleep apnea
- Panic disorder
- Polycystic liver disease
- GERD

Osler's Nodes

INTRODUCTION

Osler's nodes are small, tender, nodular or papulopustular, violaceous, cutaneous lesions in the pads of the fingers or toes. They are most characteristic of subacute bacterial endocarditis. Infective endocarditis can be diagnosed by the Duke Criteria (e.g., positive blood cultures, evidence of a cardiac vegetation, fever of unknown origin, vascular/immunologic phenomena). Osler's nodes are considered to be a minor criterion in the category of immunologic phenomena, but the exact pathogenesis (septic emboli vs. immune complex formation) is controversial.

DIAGNOSTIC WORKUP & INITIAL MANAGEMENT

History and physical examination

- Note history of present illness, associated symptoms (e.g., chest pain, fever, pruritis), medical history (history of endocarditis, valve surgery, structural heart disease, rheumatic fever, recent procedures including dental work, oncologic disease), family history (e.g., valve or autoimmune disease), social history (including IV drug use), HIV status, and medications
- Endocarditis most commonly presents with nonspecific symptoms, including fever, weight loss, myalgias, arthralgias, night sweats, weakness, abdominal or back pain, and new or changing heart murmur
- Physical exam should focus on cardiac, neurologic, ophthalmologic, dermatologic, and musculoskeletal systems

Initial diagnostic workup

- Echocardiography is necessary to evaluate cardiac valves and identify vegetations
- Initial testing includes blood cultures (2–3 cultures from separate sites before initiating antibiotics), CBC, ESR, ANA, anti-dsDNA and anti-SM antibodies, coagulation studies, urinalysis, chest radiography, and ECG
- Duke Criteria for diagnosis of endocarditis: Probable diagnosis requires 2 major criteria *or* 1 major criterion and 3 minor criteria *or* 5 minor criteria; possible diagnosis requires 1 major criterion and 1 minor criterion *or* 3 minor criteria
  - Major criteria: Typical microorganism from 2 separate blood cultures (e.g., *S. viridans, S. bovis,* HACEK group, community-acquired *S. aureus, Enterococcus*) or persistently positive blood cultures for any microorganism; evidence of endocardial involvement; vegetation on echocardiogram; oscillating intracardiac mass on valve or supporting structures or in path of regurgitant jets; perivalvular abscess; new regurgitation
  - Minor criteria: Predisposing heart condition; IV drug use; fever > 38°C; vascular phenomena (e.g., arterial embolism, septic pulmonary infarcts, mycotic aneurysm, Janeway lesions); immunological phenomena (e.g., Osler's nodes, Roth's spots, glomerulonephritis, RF), echocardiographic findings not meeting major criterion), microbiologic evidence (e.g., positive blood culture but not meeting major criterion)
- Additional testing is directed by the suspected etiology
- Biopsy of skin lesions may or may not reveal causative organisms in endocarditis and may reveal evidence of other etiologies (e.g., areas of necrosis in polyarteritis nodosa)

Initial patient management

- Hospitalization is usually required for initial treatment of endocarditis with IV antibiotics
- Begin organism-specific antibiotics as soon as cultures and sensitivities are available
  - The penicillins or vancomycin, often in combination with an aminoglycoside (e.g., gentamicin), are cornerstones of therapy; may be necessary for 4–6 weeks
- Obtain surveillance blood cultures during the early phase of therapy to ensure eradication
- Valve surgery may be required if infection cannot be controlled or embolization occurs

DIFFERENTIAL DIAGNOSIS

Acute bacterial endocarditis
- Common organisms include *Staphylococcus aureus, Streptococcus pneumoniae, and Streptococcus pyogenes*

Subacute bacterial endocarditis
- The most common organisms include *Streptococcus viridans, Enterococcus, Staphylococcus epidermidis*, and fungi

Sterile valve vegetations
- Libman-Sacks endocarditis
- Marantic endocarditis
- Atrial myxoma

Extracardiac infections
- Meningococcemia
- Rocky Mountain spotted fever
- Secondary syphilis
- Infected intravascular device
- Abscess
- Osteomyelitis
- Typhoid fever
- Enterovirus infection (echovirus or coxsackievirus)

Other
- Systemic lupus erythematosus (SLE)
- Thrombotic thrombocytopenic purpura (TTP)
- Idiopathic thrombocytopenic purpura
- Polyarteritis nodosa
- Cutaneous vasculitis
- Immune complex disease
- Serum sickness
- Drug allergy
- Lymphoma
- Erythema multiforme
- Disseminated intravascular coagulation (DIC)
- Lambl's excrescences ("wear and tear" valvular lesions)

Otorrhea (Ear Discharge)

INTRODUCTION

Otorrhea, or ear discharge, usually arises from the external ear canal. In the setting of a non-intact tympanic membrane, the middle and even inner ear may be sources as well. A thorough cleaning of the ear canal (with suction if possible) will help to visualize the tympanic membrane and may be both therapeutic and diagnostically valuable. Ear lavage should be avoided in the presence of otorrhea because of possible injury to the inner ear if the tympanic membrane is perforated. Cerebrospinal fluid otorrhea must always be considered in patients with recent face or head trauma or surgery.

DIAGNOSTIC WORKUP & INITIAL MANAGEMENT

History and physical examination

- History should focus on onset, duration, associated symptoms (e.g., pain and tenderness in acute otitis externa, aural pruritis in chronic or fungal otitis externa), activity history (e.g., swimming), and medical history (e.g., frequent otitis infections, history of tympanostomy tubes, history of middle ear surgery or neurosurgery, trauma, diabetes, dermatologic disease)
- Assess the appearance and quality of the discharge: Malodorous and purulent (infection) versus bloody (trauma, granulation tissue) versus clear and watery (CSF)
- A thorough cleaning of the ear canal under direct visualization (with magnification) using a curette or suction is necessary to examine the tympanic membrane and determine the source of discharge
  - Unless the ear canal is cleaned with suction, many pathologies will not be identified
  - Assess for the presence or absence of tympanic membrane pathology; absence usually signifies that the source of otorrhea is limited to the external ear canal
  - Ear lavage should be avoided in the presence of otorrhea
- Perform a complete exam of the head and neck
  - Note appearance of the skin of the external canal: In acute diffuse otitis externa, the skin is often red and swollen, and the canal is filled with white-colored debris; in chronic otitis externa, the epithelium of the canal is reddened and scaling
  - Views of the involved skin may be obscured by discharge and debris in the canal

Initial diagnostic workup

- Ear cultures from the canal may be helpful in persistent cases; however, contamination by normal ear canal flora usually decreases their value
- If CSF otorrhea is suspected, an assay for β-transferrin will distinguish CSF from other fluids
- CT of the temporal bones is helpful to evaluate patients with suspected cholesteatoma, mastoiditis, and CSF otorrhea
- Gallium and technetium scans may be helpful in patients with malignant external otitis
- In invasive otitis externa, granulation tissue occurs in the posteroinferior wall of the canal, at the junction of the bony and cartilaginous portions of the canal; biopsy of this tissue should be done to identify the etiology of the infection

DIFFERENTIAL DIAGNOSIS

Cerumen
- Often brownish in color
- Rarely associated with pain or pruritis

Otitis externa (swimmer's ear)
- The most common cause of otorrhea
- Usually associated with water contamination or cotton-swab abuse
- Pain occurs with movement of the pinna or tragus
- Usually secondary to *Pseudomonas* or *Staphylococcus* infection

Malignant otitis externa
- Also known as necrotizing external otitis and skull base osteomyelitis
- Suspect in patients with diabetes or immunosuppression who present with persistent otorrhea, ear pain, and granulation tissue in the ear canal
- Usually caused by *Pseudomonas* infection
- Often requires IV antimicrobials and a prolonged treatment course

Foreign body
- Frequently a retained cotton swab
- Often occurs in toddlers

Otitis media (acute or chronic) with perforated tympanic membrane
- Acute perforation may already have closed by the time the patient is examined

Cholesteatoma
- A skin-lined cyst of the middle ear or mastoid that occurs secondary to chronic otitis media
- Most cases have fullness, bulging, or a white mass of the tympanic membrane (may easily be confused with ear wax)
- A benign condition, but often causes aggressive local erosion
- Requires prompt surgical intervention

Mastoiditis
- A serious condition that presents with tenderness or bogginess over the mastoid

Cerebrospina fluid otorrhea (CSF)
- Clear, colorless discharge through a tympanic membrane perforation or tympanostomy tube
- Patients usually have a history of trauma or surgery, but it may occasionally be spontaneous

Perichondritis
- A serious inflammatory or infectious condition of the cartilage of the pinna and ear canal

Myringitis
- Results from tympanic membrane granulation or de-epithelialization

Primary dermatologic conditions
- Eczema
- Psoriasis

Palpitations

INTRODUCTION

Palpitations are a subjective sensation of the heart beating rapidly, forcefully, or irregularly. It often means that a rapid heart rate is present, but palpitations can be seen even when the heart rate is normal (often in anxious patients). Palpitations are a very common complaint among outpatients, accounting for as many as 16% of ambulatory visits. Although typically benign, a thorough history and physical examination and appropriate diagnostic testing may help to identify potentially serious etiologies.

DIAGNOSTIC WORKUP & INITIAL MANAGEMENT

History and physical examination
- Note onset, duration, frequency, precipitating factors, and associated symptoms (e.g., chest pain, dyspnea, diaphoresis, light-headedness, syncope)
- Heart rhythm may be regular or irregular
- May have family history of prolonged QT syndrome, hypertrophic cardiomyopathy, syncope, arrhythmias, sudden cardiac death, or other heart disease
- The description of the palpitations may be a clue to the etiology:
  ○ "Flip-flopping" in the chest: SVT, premature atrial or ventricular contractions
  ○ "Forceful" contraction after a pause: Premature ventricular contractions
  ○ Rapid "fluttering": Supraventricular or ventricular tachycardia, sinus tachycardia, atrial fibrillation
  ○ "Pounding" in the neck: Atrioventricular dissociation
  ○ "Irregular heartbeat": Atrial fibrillation, heart block, premature ventricular contractions
- Sustained ventricular tachycardia may not necessarily be accompanied by hemodynamic instability

Initial diagnostic workup
- ECG in all patients
- If no abnormality is found on ECG, lab studies may be done to rule out organic causes (e.g., anemia, hyperthyroidism), including CBC, electrolytes, glucose, and TSH
- If the diagnosis is still unclear and there are concerning risk factors, ambulatory monitoring (Holter or event monitoring) is indicated
- Echocardiography and/or exercise stress testing may be indicated in some patients
- If there is concern for a malignant arrhythmia, electrophysiologic testing can be performed, particularly in patients with a high pretest probability of a serious arrhythmia (e.g., severe left ventricular dysfunction, long QT syndrome, WPW syndrome)
- Consider toxicology screen

Initial patient management
- Eliminate causative medications, if possible
- If hemodynamic instability is present, urgent cardioversion may be indicated, depending on the cardiac rhythm (atrial fibrillation with rapid ventricular response, ventricular tachycardia)
- Psychiatric causes may require a combination of anxiolytics (e.g., lorazepam, buspirone) and behavioral interventions
- Cardiac arrhythmias may require the guidance of a cardiologist; depending on the etiology, therapy may include medications (e.g., β-blockers, calcium channel blockers, other antiarrhythmics), cardioversion, or invasive therapy (ablation, pacemaker, defibrillator)
  ○ Sinus tachycardia itself is usually benign and often caused by another disease; investigate for the cause (e.g., fever, anxiety, pain, anemia, hypoxia, sepsis)

DIFFERENTIAL DIAGNOSIS

Cardiac etiologies

- Arrhythmias
  - Premature ventricular or atrial contractions
  - Sinus tachycardia
  - Atrial fibrillation
  - Atrial flutter
  - Ventricular tachycardia
  - Prolonged QT syndrome
  - Wolff-Parkinson-White (WPW) syndrome
  - Paroxysmal atrial tachycardia
- Valvular disease
  - Mitral valve prolapse
  - Mitral stenosis
- Myocardial ischemia or infarction
- Heart failure (with exertion)
- Congenital heart disease (e.g., atrial or ventricular septal defect)
- Normal variant (e.g., premature ventricular contractions)

Psychiatric etiologies

- Anxiety/fear
- Panic attack

Catecholamine excess

- Medications (e.g., bronchodilators, theophylline, aminophylline, atropine, epinephrine, MAO inhibitors, amphetamines, pseudoephedrine, ephedrine, steroids)
- Caffeine (e.g., excessive coffee or tea)
- Tobacco
- Cocaine
- Herbs (e.g., ma huang)
- Thyroid extract
- Thyrotoxicosis
- Anemia (with exertion)
- Mastocytosis
- Pheochromocytoma

Other

- Dehydration
- Menopausal syndrome (with hot flashes)
- Severe deconditioning (with exertion)
- Hypoglycemia
- Postural hypotension

Papilledema

INTRODUCTION

Papilledema is swelling or edema (usually bilateral) of the optic discs due to increased intracranial pressure. Clinically, the disc appears elevated and the margins indistinct or blurred, with obscuring of some small and medium vessels. Cotton-wool spots and intraretinal hemorrhages can be seen on exam. Patients may present with transient visual loss (lasting seconds), often precipitated by changes in posture. Papilledema is also commonly associated with headache, double vision, nausea, and vomiting. Rarely, affected patients experience decreased visual acuity. Ocular pain is usually absent.

DIAGNOSTIC WORKUP & INITIAL MANAGEMENT

History and physical examination
- Note medical history, associated symptoms, and current medications
- Complete neurologic and ocular exam, including color vision assessment, slit-lamp exam, posterior vitreous evaluation for white blood cells, and a dilated fundus exam
  - True papilledema presents as bilaterally swollen, hyperemic discs, with blurring of the disc margin that often obscures the blood vessels
  - True papilledema results from increased intracranial pressure; if spontaneous venous pulsations are present, intracranial pressure is probably normal

Initial diagnostic workup
- Noncontrast CT and/or MRI of the head and orbit will identify cerebral tumors, hydrocephalus, and intracranial hemorrhage; always obtain imaging studies before lumbar puncture to avoid risk of herniation
  - Pseudotumor cerebri presents with normal CT and MRI
  - Cerebral tumors appear as space-occupying lesions
  - Hydrocephalus appears as enlarged ventricles
- Lumbar puncture (if CT or MRI is negative) for diagnosis of meningitis or encephalitis
  - Record opening pressure to assess for pseudotumor cerebri if imaging studies are normal
  - Tests include CSF cell counts, Gram's stain, cultures (bacterial, viral, VDRL if suspect neurosyphilis, fungal), cryptococcal antigen, protein, and glucose
  - Note bloody fluid in subarachnoid hemorrhage
- Further laboratory studies may include CBC, thyroid function tests, and blood glucose

Initial patient management
- Aggressive IV blood pressure control in cases of malignant hypertension
- Pseudotumor cerebri may be self-limited; weight loss and discontinuation of offending medications may be effective
- Diuretics (e.g., acetazolamide) may decrease CSF production
- Lumboperitoneal shunting or optic nerve sheath decompression may be indicated in severe cases with progressive optic nerve damage
- Intracranial tumors may require resection
- Hydrocephalus may require surgical correction and/or ventriculoperitoneal shunt
- Intracranial hemorrhage may be treated conservatively or by surgical evacuation, depending on the size and location
  - Acute subdural hematoma: Control elevated intracranial pressure with osmotic and loop diuretics and mild hyperventilation; emergent craniotomy for evacuation of hematomas that result in significant mass effect
  - Epidural hematoma usually does not require surgery; use mild hyperventilation and mannitol to decrease intracranial pressure
- Administer appropriate antibiotic treatment for intracerebral infections

DIFFERENTIAL DIAGNOSIS

Optic disc swelling caused by increased intracranial pressure

Pseudotumor cerebri (idiopathic intracranial hypertension)
- The most common cause of papilledema; most prevalent in obese or pregnant females
- Associated with vitamin A overdose, oral contraceptives, tetracycline, steroid withdrawal

Cerebral tumor
- Primary or metastatic

Hydrocephalus
- Tumor
- Arnold-Chiari malformation
- Aqueductal stenosis
- Postinfectious

Intracranial hemorrhage
- Subdural hematoma
- Subarachnoid hemorrhage
- Hemorrhagic stroke
- Epidural hematoma

Infection
- Brain abscess
- Encephalitis (e.g., herpes)
- Neurosyphilis
- Toxoplasmosis
- Meningitis (e.g., bacterial, viral, tuberculosis)

Malignant hypertension

Preeclampsia

Optic disc swelling *not* caused by increased intracranial pressure

Pseudopapilledema
- The vessels traversing the disc margins are obscured, as in true papilledema
- Etiologies include optic disc drusen or congenitally anomalous disc

Papillitis
- Unilateral, painful, vitreous cells

Papillophlebitis
- Mild visual loss and disc swelling in a young, healthy patient

Central retinal vein occlusion
- Associated with acute, unilateral loss of vision

Diabetic papillopathy
- Disc edema with minimal visual loss, resolves spontaneously

Optic-disc vasculitis/ischemic optic neuropathy
- Giant cell arteritis, temporal arteritis

Graves' ophthalmopathy
- May be associated with lid lag, proptosis, increased intraocular pressure

Uveitis
- Associated with pain, photophobia, and ciliary flush

Orbital optic nerve tumors
- Infiltrative disorders (e.g., lymphoma)
- Mass lesions (e.g., glioma)

Atypical optic neuritis

Paraplegia (Lower Extremity Paralysis)

INTRODUCTION

Paralysis is the total loss of voluntary motor function in an affected area. It usually indicates a serious neurologic problem at the site of distribution in the affected area. Paraplegia refers to paralysis of both legs, whereas quadriplegia refers to paralysis of all four extremities. The key to correct diagnosis of paralytic syndromes is knowledge of the neurologic pathways and dermatomes so that the site of the problem can be defined anatomically, after which a focused imaging examination can define the specific etiology.

DIAGNOSTIC WORKUP & INITIAL MANAGEMENT

History and physical examination

- Determine whether the weakness is more likely secondary to an upper or a lower motor neuron disorder:
  - Symmetric lower extremity weakness with hyperreflexia, positive Babinski sign, and a dermatomal area of sensory loss suggests a brain or, more commonly, a spinal cord lesion
  - Symmetric lower extremity weakness with areflexia and flexor plantar responses suggests a peripheral neuropathy
  - Difficulty with bowel and/or bladder control suggests a myelopathy or cauda equina syndrome

Initial diagnostic workup

- MRI of the spinal cord is the usually the best imaging modality
- EMG and nerve conduction studies to evaluate for possible neuropathy, polyradiculopathy, or myopathy
- CSF examination may show signs of infection, elevated protein in Guillain-Barré syndrome, or findings consistent with multiple sclerosis (oligoclonal bands)
- Laboratory testing may include CBC, electrolytes, calcium, glucose, ESR, vitamin B_{12}, and ANA
- DNA testing is available for many of the inherited ataxias
- Genetic testing may be possible

Initial patient management

- Identify and treat the underlying cause
  - In cases of compressive lesions of the spinal cord, cauda equina, or nerve roots, surgical therapy is usually required
  - Traumatic spinal cord injury frequently requires surgical stabilization; additionally, acute, high-dose steroid treatment is also effective in improving the outcome of traumatic myelopathy
- Treat infectious myelopathies with appropriate antimicrobials
- Physical therapy, assistive devices, orthotics, and wheelchairs may all be beneficial in improving the functional abilities of patients with paraplegia/paresis

DIFFERENTIAL DIAGNOSIS

Myelopathy
- Compressive (e.g., spondylytic, spinal epidural abscess or hematoma)
- Traumatic
- Metabolic (e.g., vitamin B_{12} deficiency)
- Infectious (e.g., HIV or other viral myelitis, botulism)
- Inflammatory (e.g., multiple sclerosis, SLE, vasculitis, transverse myelitis)
- Vascular (spinal cord or cerebral infarct)
- Neoplastic

Congenital
- Dysraphism (spina bifida, tethered cord)
- Cerebral palsy

Cauda equina syndrome
- Caused by compression of the cauda equina, often by a central disk herniation
- Variable presentation, with lower extremity weakness, sensory loss, pain, lower motor neuron findings on exam, and bowel/bladder disturbances

Peripheral neuropathy
- Usually results in chronic or insidious onset of lower extremity weakness (except for Guillain-Barré syndrome, which may result in weakness over hours to days)
- Guillain-Barré syndrome (also results in upper extremity weakness)
- Myasthenia gravis
- Eaton-Lambert syndrome
- Amyotrophic lateral sclerosis

Other
- Syringomyelia
- Polyradiculopathy
- HTLV-1–associated myelopathy
- Hereditary spastic paraparesis
- Spinocerebellar or Friedreich's ataxia
- Myopathies (e.g., muscular dystrophy) may result in paraparesis, but usually also result in upper extremity weakness
- Parafalcine meningioma may result in bilateral lower extremity weakness by compressive effects on the medial frontal lobe bilaterally
- Bilateral anterior cerebral artery infarction
- Medications (e.g., pancuronium)
- Periodic paralysis (secondary to hyper- or hypokalemia)
- Tick paralysis
- Lyme disease
- Psychogenic (e.g., conversion disorder)

Paresthesias

INTRODUCTION

Paresthesias are abnormal sensations, such as numbness or tingling, in the extremities in the absence of stimuli. They may occur secondary to lesions anywhere in the nervous system. The sensations arise spontaneously and may or may not be painful. Common paresthesias include numbness, warmth, cold, burning, prickling, tingling or "pins and needles," skin "crawling," or pruritis. They may be accompanied by hypesthesia (decreased sensation), most commonly noticed in response to painful or tactile stimuli. The etiology of paresthesias is usually suggested by the distribution of the finding and the associated symptoms.

DIAGNOSTIC WORKUP & INITIAL MANAGEMENT

History and physical examination

- Assess time course of onset, duration, frequency, and changes with movement
- Note the anatomic distribution (focal, unilateral, bilateral)
- Identify history of trauma, diabetes, alcohol abuse, cancer, collagen vascular disease, and exposure to heavy metals or toxins
- Note associated weakness, cramping, pain, or loss of position or temperature sense
- Assess medications (e.g., chemotherapy, antibiotics)
- Note family history of neuropathies or muscle problems
- Comprehensive neurologic exam, focusing on cervical or lumbosacral nerve patterns, sensory examination (vibratory, pinprick, position sense), and musculoskeletal exam

Initial diagnostic workup

- Initial tests may include CBC, electrolytes, calcium, magnesium, TSH, glucose, BUN and creatinine, Hb_{A1C}, urinalysis, ESR, vitamin B_{12} and folate, and thiamine level
- Additional tests may be indicated based on history (e.g., lead level, serum or urine electrophoresis to rule out paraproteinemia, Lyme titers)
- Consider radiography of the chest and the affected extremity
- EMG and nerve conduction studies may be used to differentiate neuropathic versus myopathic causes of muscle atrophy
- Nerve (usually the sural nerve) or muscle biopsy is reserved for proof of histologic processes that have an impact on management (e.g., amyloidosis)
- Consider CT or MRI of the brain

Initial patient management

- Treat and control underlying diseases (e.g., diabetes, alcoholism, HIV, renal disease, vasculitis, infections, vitamin deficiencies, offending medications, toxic exposures)
- Painful peripheral neuropathies (diabetic, alcoholic) may be relieved by amitriptyline or desipramine, phenytoin or carbamazepine, or topical capsaicin cream
- Lifestyle interventions, physical therapy, and analgesia may be sufficient for compression or entrapment neuropathies; in severe cases, epidural steroids or surgical release of the entrapped nerve or herniated disk may be indicated
- Surgical removal of compressive tumors

DIFFERENTIAL DIAGNOSIS

Nerve compression or entrapment neuropathy (usually unilateral)
- Lumbosacral disk herniation with nerve root compression
- Lateral femoral cutaneous nerve syndrome
- Posterior tibial nerve compression (tarsal tunnel syndrome)
- Peroneal nerve compression (foot drop)
- Cervical spine spondylosis/disk herniation with nerve root compression
- Median nerve compression (carpal tunnel syndrome)
- Ulnar nerve compression
- Long thoracic nerve compression (winged scapula)
- Pressure palsy

Infections
- HIV/AIDS
- Herpes zoster
- Lyme disease

Metabolic (usually bilateral)
- Diabetic neuropathy
- Alcoholic neuropathy (caused by thiamine deficiency and/or direct toxic effect of alcohol)
- Alcohol withdrawal (may have sensation of "crawling bugs")
- Hypothyroidism
- Amyloid neuropathy
- Uremia

CNS etiologies
- Stroke
- Brain tumor
- Head trauma
- Abscess
- Encephalitis
- Lupus cerebritis
- Multiple sclerosis
- Transverse myelitis

Connective tissue disorder
- Rheumatoid arthritis
- SLE
- Sjögren syndrome

Tumors
- Carcinomatous infiltration or direct compression
- Paraneoplastic syndrome (especially lung cancer)

Toxins
- Heavy metal poisoning (e.g., lead, arsenic, mercury)
- Industrial exposure (e.g., heavy metals, pesticides)
- Medications (e.g., chemotherapy, metronidazole, pyridoxine, isoniazid, vincristine, cis-platin, antiretrovirals, hydralazine)

Other
- Vasculitis
- Guillain-Barré syndrome (usually bilateral)
- Hereditary motor or sensory neuropathies
- Porphyria
- Paraproteinemias (e.g., multiple myeloma, monoclonal gammopathy)
- Amyotrophic lateral sclerosis
- Trigeminal neuralgia
- Respiratory alkalosis

Paroxysmal Nocturnal Dyspnea

INTRODUCTION

Paroxysmal nocturnal dyspnea is defined as severe difficulty breathing or air hunger that awakens patients from sleep (usually 1–3 hours after lying down) and forces them to a sitting or standing position. The patient may gasp and proceed to an open window for fresh air. The shortness of breath tends to resolve within 10–30 minutes. This symptom nearly always implies heart failure.

DIAGNOSTIC WORKUP & INITIAL MANAGEMENT

History and physical examination

- Assess the onset, duration, characteristics, associated symptoms, medical history, family history, and medications
- Pay particular attention to the cardiac and respiratory systems

Initial diagnostic workup

- Initial laboratory studies may include pulse oximetry, CBC, electrolytes, BUN and creatinine, glucose, and calcium
- Chest radiography to evaluate for effusion and heart size
- Echocardiography may be used to evaluate heart valves, chamber size, and ventricular function
- ECG is usually indicated
- Cardiac catheterization may be indicated for valvular disease, cardiomyopathies, and congenital heart disease

Initial patient management

- Attention to airway, breathing, and circulation
- Administer supplemental oxygen as necessary
- Many patients feel relief as a result of cold air blowing in the face
- Consider cardiology consultation

DIFFERENTIAL DIAGNOSIS

Congestive heart failure
- Etiologies include uncontrolled hypertension, pulmonary embolism, hyperthyroidism, pericardial disease, endocardial disease (e.g., valvular stenosis, valvular insufficiency, valve rupture, endocarditis), and myocardial disease (e.g., MI, ischemia, arrhythmias)
- The mainstay of therapy is to decrease preload (by venodilation) and afterload (by arteriodilation and volume removal) to improve forward blood flow and decrease symptoms; nitrates (sublingual and IV), loop diuretics, IV morphine, ACE inhibitors, and spironolactone are commonly used medications; treat refractory respiratory distress with mechanical ventilation (CPAP, BiPAP, or intubation)

Mitral stenosis
- Most commonly occurs 15–40 years after rheumatic fever
- Advanced cases result in pulmonary hypertension and right heart failure
- Dyspnea is the most significant symptom
- Presents with the classic triad of diastolic rumble, opening snap, and loud S_1

Aortic regurgitation
- Common causes include hypertension, rheumatic fever, and endocarditis

Aortic stenosis
- Most commonly results from senile valve degeneration, rheumatic disease, bicuspid valve, or congenital aortic stenosis
- Associated with angina, syncope, and congestive heart failure

"Cardiac asthma"
- Compression of small airways occurs secondary to pulmonary congestion and interstitial edema
- Standing usually decreases lung congestion

Other etiologies
- Cardiomyopathies
- Anxiety
- Severe COPD
- Asthma
- Obstructive sleep apnea
- Obesity-hypoventilation syndrome
- Congenital heart disease
- Tropical pulmonary eosinophilia (filariasis)

Pelvic Masses

INTRODUCTION

Pelvic masses are most common in women, but they occur in men as well. Obvious causes (e.g., bladder distension, pregnancy) must be ruled out before a full workup. Malignancy must be considered in all cases, particularly older patients and those with a history of malignant disease.

DIAGNOSTIC WORKUP & INITIAL MANAGEMENT

History and physical examination

- Note whether the mass is painful (constant or intermittent, cyclic or noncyclic, associated with dyspareunia)
- Note associations with menstrual disturbances (dysmenorrhea and menorrhagia are associated with endometriosis and leiomyomas) or other symptoms (e.g., fever, weight loss/gain, nausea, vomiting, dyspepsia, early satiety, abdominal bloating, constipation, diarrhea, change in stool caliber)
- Full abdominal, breast, lymph node, and pelvic/genital exams, including bimanual and rectal exams
  - The sacral promontory can occasionally be confused with a pelvic mass by inexperienced clinicians

Initial workup and management

- Initial labs may include urine pregnancy test, urinalysis, BUN and creatinine, CBC with differential, Pap smear with DNA probe for gonorrhea and chlamydia, cervical cytology, Hemoccult, and liver function tests
- Pelvic ultrasound may be indicated for adnexal or uterine masses to determine the size, location, and composition of the mass
- Pelvic or abdominal CT
- Colonoscopy to rule out colorectal cancer
- Consider bladder catheterization if suspect bladder distension
- Tumor markers may be indicated if ultrasound is abnormal, but these have variable sensitivity and specificity
  - β-hCG (nongestational choriocarcinomas)
  - α-Fetoprotein (endodermal sinus tumors)
  - Lactate dehydrogenase (dysgerminomas)
  - Serum CA-125 (ovarian cancer)
- Gynecologic referral for suspicious masses

DIFFERENTIAL DIAGNOSIS

Postmenarche and premenopause
- Ovarian etiologies
  - Follicular and corpus luteum cysts are the most common causes of pelvic masses
  - Endometrioma
  - Polycystic ovarian syndrome
  - Neoplasms (benign or malignant)
- Fallopian tube etiologies
  - Hydrosalpinx
  - Fallopian tube cancer
- Infectious etiologies
  - Tubo-ovarian abscess secondary to pelvic inflammatory disease
- Pregnancy
  - Uterine pregnancy
  - Ectopic pregnancy
  - Molar pregnancy
- Leiomyoma (fibroids)
- Retroperitoneal tumors
- Constipation

Postmenopause (increased risk of malignant neoplasms)
- Ovarian fibroma
- Ovarian cyst
- Leiomyoma (fibroids)
- Diverticular abscess
- Enlarged bladder
- Hernia (femoral or inguinal)
- Primary ovarian carcinoma
- Metastatic disease, especially from the uterus, breast, or GI tract
- Colorectal cancer

Newborns and children
- Functional ovarian cysts
- Germ cell tumor
  - Dermoid (benign cystic teratoma)
  - Dysgerminoma
- Wilms tumor
- Lymphoma

Less common etiologies
- Ovarian torsion
- Leiomyoma torsion
- Congenital obstructive genital lesion (e.g., imperforate hymen, blind uterine horn)
- Bicornuate uterus
- Pelvic kidney
- Cervical cancer

Males
- Lymphoma
- Colorectal cancer
- Diverticular abscess
- Metastatic disease, especially from colorectal cancer
- Bladder distension, often secondary to benign prostatic hypertrophy
- Hernia (femoral or inguinal)
- Retroperitoneal tumors
- Constipation

Pelvic Pain, Female

INTRODUCTION

Pelvic pain is a common primary care complaint that should be distinguished as acute (lasting <6 months) versus chronic (lasting >6 months) and as cyclic, noncyclic, or pregnancy-related. It is generally defined as pain localized below the umbilicus that interferes with normal function. Gynecologic, urologic, and intestinal etiologies are common, but psychologic, oncologic, and other causes must also be carefully considered.

Chronic pelvic pain affects 15% of women from 18–50 years of age. Of these women, 25% spend a day in bed each month because of the pain. In addition, 35% of laparoscopies are performed for chronic pelvic pain.

DIAGNOSTIC WORKUP & INITIAL MANAGEMENT

History and physical examination

- Obtain a complete menstrual and gynecologic history, history of symptoms, medical history, psychosocial history, and medication and dietary history
- Note the nature, severity, onset, radiation, and duration of pain
- Note the relation of pain to menstrual cycle, intercourse, or other activities
- Note chronic versus acute
- Inquire about the chance of pregnancy
- Note associated symptoms, including fever, nausea, vomiting, dysuria, frequency, vaginal bleeding or discharge, and abdominal or back pain
- Screen for domestic violence and sexual abuse
- Perform complete abdominal and pelvic exams, including speculum, bimanual, and rectal exams
  - Abdominal exam should assess for surgical scars, hernias, masses, tenderness, rigidity, rebound tenderness, or guarding
  - Pelvic exam should evaluate for signs of infection (including vaginal wet mount and testing for chlamydia and gonorrhea if warranted); uterosacral ligament nodularity or tenderness; cervical stenosis, motion tenderness, or lateral displacement of the cervix; and uterine or adnexal tenderness
  - Rectal exam to rule out masses and assess for point tenderness

Initial workup and management

- Consider an empiric trial of NSAIDs, oral contraceptives, or nonpharmacologic therapies
  - Heating pad on the lower abdomen or back
  - Lifestyle changes (e.g., regular exercise, smoking cessation, decrease in alcohol and caffeine consumption, weight reduction)
- Laboratory studies may include CBC, urine pregnancy test, urinalysis, urine Gram's stain and culture, testing for *Chlamydia* and *N. gonorrhea,* and wet mount of a vaginal smear
- Consider ultrasound if suspect ovarian cyst, torsion, or mass, or to evaluate for intrauterine versus ectopic pregnancy
- Diagnostic laparoscopy may be necessary in suspected endometriosis
- True emergencies (e.g., ruptured tubal pregnancy, appendicitis) may be life-threatening if untreated

DIFFERENTIAL DIAGNOSIS

Acute pain (lasting <6 months)

Pregnancy-related
- Ectopic pregnancy
- Threatened abortion
- Incomplete abortion
- Septic abortion
- Ruptured corpus luteal cyst

Gynecologic (noncyclic pain)
- Ovarian cyst
- Pelvic inflammatory disease
- Tubo-ovarian abscess
- Vaginitis/cervicitis
- Ovarian torsion
- Uterine fibroids
- Pelvic (ovarian, uterine, urinary) neoplasm
- Pelvic floor prolapse (cystocele/rectocele)

Gynecologic (cyclic pain)
- Primary dysmenorrhea
- Endometriosis
- Intrauterine device
- Mittelschmerz (midcycle ovulation)

Nongynecologic
- UTI/pyelonephritis
- Nephrolithiasis
- Appendicitis
- Diverticulitis
- Sexual abuse or trauma
- Abdominal aortic aneurysm (AAA)
- Mesenteric ischemia or infarction

Chronic pain (lasting >6 months)
- Difficult to diagnose and treat; the differential diagnosis includes the gynecologic and nongynecologic etiologies listed above as well as the following:
  - Pelvic adhesions
  - Interstitial cystitis
  - Inflammatory bowel disease (IBD)
  - Adenomyosis
  - Leiomyoma (fibroids)
  - Hernia (femoral or inguinal)
  - Depression
  - Irritable bowel syndrome (IBS)
  - Diverticulosis or diverticular abscess
  - Lymphoma
- Less common etiologies include pelvic congestion syndrome, mesenteric adenitis, surgical adhesions, Asherman's syndrome, foreign body (e.g., tampon), abdominal wall nerve entrapment, and porphyria

Penile Discharge

INTRODUCTION

Penile discharge is a common primary care complaint that results from an acute inflammatory process within the urethra. Infection (particularly sexually transmitted infections) is the most common cause. A thorough history, including a complete and accurate sexual history, as well as a focused physical examination and penile cultures are generally indicated. Of note, lack of circumcision may increase the risk of HIV, gonorrhea, and syphilis.

DIAGNOSTIC WORKUP & INITIAL MANAGEMENT

History and physical examination

- Patients with urethral discharge are often otherwise asymptomatic
- Obtain a complete sexual history
- Note previous instrumentation of genitals and urinary tract; inquire about inserting foreign objects into the meatus (especially in children)
- Assess the onset, duration, and character of discharge (thick vs. thin, color, presence of blood or odor) as well as voiding symptoms and presence of hematuria
  ○ Gonorrhea: Profuse, purulent, thick yellow or gray discharge, dysuria, urgency or frequency
  ○ Chlamydia: Thin, scant, and mucoid (watery) discharge
  ○ *Trichomonas vaginalis*: Usually asymptomatic in men, but may present with discharge and dysuria; female partner tends to be symptomatic, with pelvic pain, itching, and discharge
  ○ Carcinoma of the urethra: Bloody discharge
  ○ Foreign body in the urethra: Pain and bloody discharge
  ○ Reiter's syndrome: Triad of urethritis, conjunctivitis, and arthritis
- Physical exam should assess the meatus, phallus, and testes, and include digital rectal exam; examine joints for arthritis and skin for evidence of rash

Initial diagnostic workup

- Urethral cultures are the gold standard for diagnosis of gonorrhea and chlamydia
  ○ To obtain cultures, hold the penis up, carefully insert the tip of the culture swab into the meatus about one-half inch, and twirl; remove and place in culture medium
- Urinalysis and urine culture
- Wet mount to evaluate for trichomonads
  ○ To express penile discharge, have the patient "milk" the penis from the base up to the tip
- Further workup for STDs may include HIV testing, syphilis testing (RPR), hepatitis B studies, and hepatitis C antibody
- Consider blood cultures, CBC, and joint fluid aspiration if suspect disseminated gonorrhea
- If suspect foreign body, obtain plain-film radiographs of the penis and pelvis

Initial patient management

- Penile discharge without dysuria or frequency should be treated as an STD until proven otherwise; begin empiric antibiotic therapy on clinical suspicion
  ○ Gonorrhea: IM ceftriaxone or oral cefixime, ciprofloxacin, levofloxacin, or oflaxacin
  ○ Chlamydia: Single-dose azithromycin or 7 days of doxycycline, ofloxacin, or erythromycin
  ○ *Trichomonas:* Metronidazole (single dose or 7-day course)
- If cultures are positive, treat accordingly, and test for cure 6–8 weeks later
- Encourage patients to inform sexual partners of the disease so that they can be treated
- Inform the health department, if required
- Emergent urology consult is required for foreign bodies or carcinoma of the penis

DIFFERENTIAL DIAGNOSIS

Infection
- *Neisseria gonorrhoeae* (gonococcal urethritis)
  - Untreated primary gonorrhea may progress to disseminated gonococcal infection; the clinical triad includes tenosynovitis (asymmetric, involving small joints), dermatitis (erythematous macules that progress to pustules with a hemorrhagic component), and arthritis
- *Chlamydia trachomatis*
  - The most common cause of nongonococcal urethral discharge
- *Trichomonas vaginalis*
- Nonspecific urethritis
- Prostatitis
- Reiter's syndrome
  - Triad of urethritis, conjunctivitis, and arthritis ("can't see, can't pee, can't climb a tree") is associated with *Chlamydia* infection
  - Skin lesions (keratoderma blennorrhagicum) involve the palms and soles, begin as vesicles, and become hyperkeratotic

Noninfectious etiologies
- Carcinoma of the urethra
  - Presents with bloody penile discharge
- Foreign body in the urethra
  - Presents with pain and bloody discharge
  - An indwelling Foley catheter can cause urethritis and discharge

Pericardial Rub

INTRODUCTION

The pericardium is a double-layer, fibroelastic sac that envelops the heart. It is composed of a fibrous outer layer (parietal pericardium) and a serous inner layer (visceral pericardium), which are normally separated by a thin layer of pericardial fluid. Rapid or large fluid accumulation can result in marked increases in pericardial pressure and cause cardiac tamponade. A pericardial friction rub is a "creaking leathery" or sandpaper-like sound heard best at end expiration when the patient is leaning forward. It classically consists of three phases, corresponding to atrial systole, ventricular systole, and the rapid filling of early ventricular diastole. A rub is often heard best over the left sternal border with the stethoscope diaphragm. The presence of a rub usually implies pericarditis.

DIAGNOSTIC WORKUP & INITIAL MANAGEMENT

History and physical examination

- Assess associated symptoms (e.g., chest pain, fever, dyspnea, dysphagia, cough, syncope, palpitations), medical history, family history, exposures (e.g., HIV, tuberculosis), recent viral or other illness, and recent trauma
  - Chest pain is the most common symptom of pericarditis; it is usually a sharp, stabbing, pleuritic pain that radiates to the scapula, neck, back, and arms (pain at the trapezius muscle ridge is pathognomonic); it is often exacerbated by inspiration, cough, or recumbency and may be relieved by leaning forward
- Perform a complete cardiovascular and pulmonary exam
  - Pulsus paradoxus (>10 mm Hg fall in systolic pressure on inspiration) and Kussmaul's sign (inspiratory increase in jugular venous pressure) suggest cardiac tamponade
  - Pulsus paradoxus is also seen in marked obesity, severe CHF, asthma, and emphysema
  - A rub would be inaudible in the presence of significant pericardial fluid

Initial diagnostic workup

- Initial evaluation includes ECG, chest radiography, cardiac enzymes, CBC, and ESR
- In cases of pericarditis, the ECG evolves through 4 stages:
  - Diffuse, upward concave ST elevation with reciprocal ST depression in leads aVR and V_1; elevation of PR in aVR; depression of PR in other limb leads and left chest leads, especially V_5 and V_6 (occurs over hours to days)
  - Followed by normalization of ST and PR segments (occurs over several days)
  - Followed by diffuse T wave inversion
  - ECG may then become normal, or T inversions may persist indefinitely
- Chest radiograph is often normal, but cardiomegaly can be seen in patients with substantial pericardial effusion (>250 mL is needed to enlarge the heart silhouette)
- Echocardiography evaluates the presence and size of a pericardial effusion, cardiac chamber compression, and characteristic filling abnormalities (use transesophageal view if transthoracic is suboptimal, particularly in postoperative cardiac surgery patients)
- CT and MRI may be used to visualize the pericardium
- Further testing may include ANA, PPD, HIV serology, and blood cultures

Initial patient management

- Administer oxygen and ensure hemodynamic stability (volume resuscitation, pressors)
- Treat the underlying cause
- Emergent pericardiocentesis may be needed to drain large pericardial effusions with evidence of tamponade and may help in determining the etiology (e.g., malignancy, infection)
- If the effusion is related to aortic dissection or cardiac rupture, remove just enough fluid to improve the hemodynamics and stabilize the patient for emergent surgery
- Pericarditis is treated with NSAIDs; avoid steroids unless the patient is in critical condition
- Surgical pericardial window and/or pericardial biopsy may be needed in some cases

DIFFERENTIAL DIAGNOSIS

Pericarditis (most common cause of pericardial rubs)
- Malignancy is a common cause
- Respiratory viruses (e.g., coxsackievirus, echovirus) are common causes
- Bacterial pericarditis is usually a complication of contiguous pulmonary infections (e.g., pneumonia, empyema); organisms include *S. pneumoniae*, *M. tuberculosis*, *S. aureus*, *H. influenzae*, *K. pneumoniae*, *Legionella*
- Disseminated fungal infection (e.g., *Histoplasma, Coccidioides*) may cause septic pericarditis
- Drugs (e.g., procainamide, hydralazine, isoniazid, phenytoin), metabolic disorders (e.g., myxedema, uremia, dialysis-related), and vasculitis or connective tissue diseases (e.g., SLE, rheumatoid arthritis, sarcoidosis, scleroderma, Reiter's syndrome) may also result in pericarditis
- Postoperative pericarditis following cardiac surgery is very common
- Idiopathic in 30% of cases

Nonpericardial etiologies
- MI
- Myocarditis
- HIV
- Toxoplasmosis
- Trauma
- Mediastinal radiation
- Neoplasm
- Leukemic infiltration
- Sarcoidosis
- Amyloidosis
- Familial Mediterranean fever
- Parasitic (amebic) infection
- Pulmonary embolism
- Means-Lehrman scratch (thyrotoxicosis)
- Mediastinal emphysema ("crunching" noise that may be heard with systole after open cardiac surgery)
- Pleuropericardial rub (rub occurs between inflamed pleura and the parietal pericardium)
- Sail sound of Ebstein's anomaly
- Movement of balloon catheter or transvenous pacing catheter across tricuspid valve

Sounds that may mimic a pericardial rub
- Ventricular septal defect
- Mitral regurgitation
- Tricuspid regurgitation
- Diaphragm or intercostal muscle twitch during artificial pacing (scratchy sound unrelated to cardiac cycle)
- Mill wheel murmur (air in right ventricle, with a "slushing" sound during systole and diastole)
- Combined aortic regurgitation and stenosis
- Patent ductus arteriosus
- Ostium primum atrial septal defect

Photophobia

INTRODUCTION

Photophobia is ocular pain or discomfort on exposure to light. It may be a symptom of a primary ocular disorder or an underlying CNS disorder. It should always be thoroughly evaluated unless a known etiology (e.g., migraine headache) is present.

DIAGNOSTIC WORKUP & INITIAL MANAGEMENT

History and physical examination
- Focused history for exposure to foreign bodies (e.g., woodworking or other flying debris), allergens, exposure to others with upper respiratory infection or conjunctivitis, associated systemic symptoms (e.g., arthritis, rash, fever), and medical history
- Physical exam should include a detailed neurologic exam, ocular exam (including dilated funduscopic and slit-lamp exam, if possible), eyelid eversion to rule out foreign bodies, fluorescein staining of the cornea to rule out abrasion, and intraocular pressure measurement
- Conjunctivitis usually causes hyperemia, which is more intense peripherally and less prominent near the limbus, with mucoid or purulent discharge

Initial diagnostic workup
- Head CT without contrast if suspect subarachnoid hemorrhage
- Lumbar puncture if suspect meningitis or subarachnoid hemorrhage
- CBC and/or blood cultures if suspect meningitis
- If suspect anterior uveitis, targeted testing may include CBC, ESR, ANA, ACE level (sarcoidosis), RPR (syphilis), PPD, chest radiography (sarcoidosis, tuberculosis), Lyme titer, *Chlamydia* cultures (Reiter's syndrome), HLA-B27 assay, sacroiliac spine films (ankylosing spondylitis), and colonoscopy (inflammatory bowel disease)
- If optic neuritis is diagnosed, MRI of the brain and orbits is indicated to evaluate for multiple sclerosis

Initial patient management
- Corneal abrasion: Topical antibiotics with or without cycloplegic agents, NSAIDs, and possibly, eye patching
- Bacterial conjunctivitis: Topical antibiotics
- Allergic conjunctivitis: Topical antihistamines and mast cell stabilizers
  - Avoid topical steroids except in severe cases
- Chemical conjunctivitis: Copious irrigation, topical cycloplegics, and topical antibiotics
- Anterior uveitis: Cycloplegic agents, topical steroids
  - Treat secondary glaucoma and any underlying infections as necessary
- Migraine: Abortive therapy (triptan medications), oral pain medication, and antiemetics
- Meningitis: IV antibiotics
- Episcleritis: Topical steroids in moderate to severe cases
- Subarachnoid hemorrhage: Emergent neurosurgery consult

DIFFERENTIAL DIAGNOSIS

Corneal abrasion
- Usually secondary to trauma or foreign body

Conjunctivitis
- Viral etiologies include adenovirus, enterovirus, coxsackievirus, vaccinia virus, molluscum contagiosum, HSV-1 and -2, varicella zoster virus, EBV, human papillomavirus, congenital rubella, influenza viruses, and measles
- Bacterial etiologies are common, including *S. aureus, S. pneumoniae, H. influenzae, N. gonorrhoeae, C. trachomatis,* and *N. meningitidis*
- Toxic conjunctivitis may result from neomycin, aminoglycosides, atropine, and other topical medications as well as from cosmetics and preservatives
- Seasonal allergic conjunctivitis (hay fever) is common, usually caused by exposure to airborne allergens; allergic conjunctivitis may also result from rubbing the eyes with allergen (e.g., cat dander)
- Immunogenic conjunctivitis is associated with systemic immune disorders (e.g., Graves' disease, rheumatoid arthritis, Sjögren's syndrome, SLE, Wegener's granulomatosis, relapsing polychondritis, polyarteritis nodosa)

Migraine headache
- Normal eye and neurologic exam
- Often associated with headache, nausea and vomiting, and phonophobia

Idiopathic anterior uveitis or iritis
- Often associated with a triad of pain, photophobia, and blurred vision
- Because of midbrain connections that cause pupillary constriction of both eyes even if only one eye receives light, unilateral uveitis will still cause eye pain even if that eye is closed
- Ankylosing spondylitis
- Reiter's syndrome
- Inflammatory bowel disease (IBD)
- Psoriatic arthritis
- Sarcoidosis
- Infections (e.g., Lyme disease, herpes simplex, herpes zoster, tuberculosis, syphilis)
- Postoperative reactions

Other
- Meningitis
- Encephalitis
- Subarachnoid hemorrhage
- Influenza
- Lightly pigmented eye
- Mydriatic use
- Keratoconjunctivitis sicca (dry eye syndrome)

Less common etiologies
- Albinism
- Total color blindness
- Vitamin A deficiency
- Measles
- Posterior uveitis
- Congenital glaucoma
- Sinusitis
- Mononucleosis
- Colorado tick fever
- Babesiosis
- Botulism
- Acute viral hepatitis

Pleural Rub

INTRODUCTION

A pleural friction rub is a "creaking leathery" or grating lung sound caused by inflamed visceral and parietal pleural linings that rub over each other during respiration. It usually occurs during both inspiration and expiration and is heard best with the stethoscope diaphragm. The sound tends to be localized and does not change with deep breaths or coughing. A pleural rub is pathognomonic for pleurisy (pleuritis) and tends to be associated with an exudative pleural effusion and sharp chest pain on breathing.

DIAGNOSTIC WORKUP & INITIAL MANAGEMENT

History and physical examination

- Assess onset, characteristics, associated symptoms, medical history, family history, and medications
- May present with localized pain over the affected area that worsens with deep breathing or coughing and is relieved by pressure on the chest wall or abdomen
- Respirations tend to be fast and shallow, with decreased breath sounds and decreased motion on the affected side
- Distinguish a pleural rub from a pericardial rub, which varies with the cardiac cycle and does not vary with respiration

Initial diagnostic workup

- Initial laboratory testing includes CBC with differential, electrolytes, BUN and creatinine, glucose, calcium, and pulse oximetry
- Chest radiography may show pleural effusion and reveal evidence of the underlying etiology (e.g., pneumonia, tuberculosis, tumor)
- Consider blood and sputum cultures if suspect pneumonia or tuberculosis
- Spiral CT, V/Q scan, pulmonary angiography, ABG, and/or D-dimer assay if suspect pulmonary embolus
- Diagnostic thoracentesis of a pleural effusion may be indicated:
  - Elevated WBC count suggests parapneumonic effusion, empyema, tuberculosis, malignancy, or pancreatitis
  - Red blood cell count > 100,000/mm^3 suggests malignancy, pulmonary infarction, or trauma
  - Glucose level < 50% of serum glucose suggests bacterial infection or rheumatoid pleurisy
  - LDH and total protein levels distinguish transudative from exudative effusions
  - Fluid pH <7.2 may necessitate chest tube insertion
  - Gram's stain and culture to assess for infection
  - Cytology to assess for malignant cells

Initial patient management

- Immediately stabilize the airway, and consider intubation if there are signs of airway distress (e.g., cyanosis)
- Administer supplemental oxygen as necessary
- NSAIDs, narcotics, and/or chest wraps may be used for pain
- Respiratory isolation is necessary if suspect tuberculosis or influenza
- Identify and treat the underlying cause

DIFFERENTIAL DIAGNOSIS

- Viral pleurisy (e.g., coxsackievirus B, influenza)
  - Associated with upper respiratory tract symptoms (e.g., runny nose, earache, low-grade fever)
- Pneumonia
  - "Typical" pneumonia (e.g., *S. pneumoniae, H. influenzae*) is characterized by acute or subacute onset of fever, dyspnea, fatigue, pleuritic chest pain, and productive cough
  - "Atypical" pneumonia (e.g., *Mycoplasma, Legionella, C. pneumoniae*, influenza and parainfluenza viruses) is characterized by more gradual onset, dry cough, headache, fatigue, and minimal lung signs
- Pulmonary infarction secondary to a pulmonary embolus
  - Risk factors (Virchow's triad) include venous stasis (e.g., immobility, pedal edema), hypercoagulability (e.g., malignancy, hypercoagulable states, obesity, pregnancy, estrogen replacement therapy, oral contraceptives), and endothelial damage (e.g., recent trauma or surgery, burns, indwelling catheters)
- Tuberculosis
- Rheumatic pleural effusion
- Trauma (e.g., rib fracture, electrical burn, thoracic surgery)
- Connective tissue disease (e.g., SLE, rheumatoid arthritis)
- Pancreatic pleurisy (caused by leakage of pancreatic enzymes into pleural space)
- Hemothorax
- Drug-induced pleural disease (e.g., amiodarone, nitrofurantoin, bromocriptine)
- Uremia
- Radiation therapy
- Pulmonary metastases
- Subphrenic or intra-abdominal abscess
- Less common etiologies
  - Meigs' syndrome
  - Mesothelioma
  - Asbestos-related pleural disease
  - Amebic empyema
  - Chylothorax
  - Esophageal rupture
  - Lymphoma
  - Sarcoidosis

Polyuria

INTRODUCTION

Polyuria is defined as urine output exceeding 3 L/day. Polyuria may result from the primary intake of excessive quantities of fluid, or it may be secondary to one of a variety of disease processes. In primary polydipsia, volume expansion and lowering of the serum osmolality lead to an increase in water excretion. When due to an underlying disease, the output of a large volume of dilute urine leads to volume contraction, which stimulates thirst mechanisms to increase fluid intake.

DIAGNOSTIC WORKUP & INITIAL MANAGEMENT

History and physical examination

- Assess thirst, dry mouth, volume of daily fluid consumption, urinary frequency and volume, difficulty with urination (pain, hesitancy), nocturia, and orthostatic symptoms
- Assess for uncontrolled diabetes mellitus, underlying psychiatric disease, head trauma, abdominal or back pain, constipation, weakness, signs/symptoms consistent with systemic diseases (e.g., sarcoidosis), and medications (e.g., lithium, surreptitious diuretic use)
- Physical exam for evidence of volume depletion (dry mucous membranes, tachycardia, hypotension, poor skin turgor), neurologic deficits (including visual field evaluation), or organ system dysfunction consistent with a systemic illness

Initial diagnostic workup

- Initial laboratory studies include serum glucose, electrolytes (including calcium), osmolality, BUN and creatinine, urinalysis, and urine osmolality
- If necessary, water deprivation test to assess for diabetes insipidus (DI)
  - Give no fluids for 12–18 hours, and measure body weight, plasma and urine osmolality, serum sodium concentration, and blood pressure every 2 hours
  - Stop the test if severe dehydration, significant drop in blood pressure, or hypernatremia occurs (indicates DI is likely)
  - A normal response is a drop in urine output to 0.5 mL/min, with urine osmolality exceeding plasma osmolality
  - In contrast, maintenance of dilute urine with urine osmolality of ~300 mOsm/kg or less indicates DI (central or nephrogenic)
  - Continue the test until a plateau phase occurs (hourly increase of urine osmolality <30 mOsm/kg for 3 consecutive hours), then give 5 units of aqueous vasopressin (antidiuretic hormone, ADH) subcutaneously and measure urine osmolality 1 hour later
- Measure ADH and osmolality during the water deprivation test
  - In nephrogenic DI, ADH is normal or slightly increased; urine osmolality increases <50% after ADH is administered
  - In central DI, ADH level is decreased and urine osmolality increases significantly after administration of ADH
  - In primary polydipsia, serum and urine osmolality are decreased before the test and increase during the test

Initial patient management

- Eliminate causative medications and treat underlying illnesses, if possible
- Treat central DI with intranasal or oral desmopressin acetate, a synthetic analogue of ADH; measure serum osmolality and sodium levels regularly
- Treat nephrogenic DI by addressing the underlying cause and maintaining adequate fluid intake; hydrochlorothiazide may be useful
- Treat primary polydipsia with fluid restriction

DIFFERENTIAL DIAGNOSIS

Diuretic use
- Consider surreptitious diuretic usage

Uncontrolled diabetes mellitus
- Patients have polydipsia and subsequent polyuria secondary to glucose-induced osmotic diuresis

Primary polydipsia
- May occur as part of a psychiatric illness caused by increased water intake (e.g., psychogenic polydipsia, dry mouth because of antipsychotic medications)
- May result from hypothalamic lesions in the thirst centers (e.g., sarcoidosis)

Central DI
Caused by decreased pituitary production of ADH
- Autoimmune
- Head trauma
- Infiltrative diseases (e.g., sarcoidosis, tuberculosis, Langerhans cell histiocytosis)
- Pituitary tumors
- Ischemic brain injury
- Familial
- Idiopathic

Nephrogenic DI
Caused by decreased response of the kidneys to ADH
- Drugs (e.g., lithium, desmopressin, colchicine, fluoride)
- Chronic renal disease
- Hypercalcemia
- Hypokalemia
- Sickle cell disease
- Familial
- Idiopathic

Prolonged Erection (Priapism)

INTRODUCTION

Priapism is an undesired, sustained, and usually painful erection of the penis that may last hours to days. Low-flow (ischemic) priapism is caused by venous occlusion or obstruction of corpora cavernosa outflow, resulting in persistent venous engorgement, decreased blood flow, and penile ischemia (after 6 hours). High-flow (nonischemic) priapism is caused by increased arterial inflow to the corpora cavernosa that exceeds venous outflow and is usually caused by trauma that results in an arterial fistula in the penis. Priapism is a urologic emergency; consultation should be sought immediately. Impotence is the most feared complication, and the risk increases with duration of priapism (especially if >24 hours). Up to 50% of low-flow and 20% of high-flow cases result in impotence.

DIAGNOSTIC WORKUP & INITIAL MANAGEMENT

History and physical examination

- History and physical exam are usually sufficient to establish the diagnosis
- Usually presents as persistent tumescence in the absence of sexual stimulation, predisposing conditions, or drug use
- History should focus on time of onset (usually hours to days), medications (e.g., antidepressants, antipsychotics, sildenafil), medical history (e.g., sickle cell disease, anticoagulation therapy, diabetes mellitus, leukemia, genitourinary malignancies, schizophrenia, depression), previous erectile dysfunction for which treatment has been sought, and activity with onset of erection (e.g., following oral or injection treatment for impotence, with sexual activity, trauma, illicit drug use)
- Physical exam should include abdomen, back, genitalia (palpate the penis for areas of tenderness or induration), digital rectal exam, and neurologic exam
- Assess the penis; note pain, which segments of the penis are involved, and any signs of trauma, injection, or neoplasm
- Assess the testicles and scrotum for masses or evidence of trauma
- Palpate the prostate for signs of neoplasm
- Distinguish low-flow from high-flow priapism:
  ○ Low-flow priapism usually presents with an extremely painful, erect or semierect penis and soft glans penis; the erection may last for hours to days
  ○ High-flow priapism usually presents with a lesser degree of pain and tumescence, the glans is usually firm, the corpora cavernosa are soft, and a penile bruit may be present; a significant delay may occur between the traumatic incident and onset of erection
- Spinal cord injury must be ruled out in any trauma victim with priapism

Initial diagnostic workup

- Laboratory evaluation should include CBC (to rule out sickle cell disease and leukemia), coagulation profile, and urinalysis (to rule out infection)
- Corporeal blood gas analysis distinguishes high-flow from low-flow priapism: Dark blood with pH <7.25, $P_{O_2} < 30$, and $P_{CO_2} > 60$ indicates a low-flow, ischemic state
- Penile Doppler ultrasound may also distinguish high-flow from low-flow priapism
- In high-flow disease, angiography may be necessary to localize the fistula
- Consider urine toxicology screening

Initial patient management

- Priapism, particularly low-flow, is a urologic emergency because of persistently elevated pressure in the corpora cavernosa; seek consultation immediately
- Initial medical therapies (Foley catheterization, perineal ice packs, subcutaneous phenylephrine, corpora cavernosa aspiration) can be attempted; if these are ineffective, emergency surgical intervention is necessary within 36 hours of onset to preserve potency and prevent corporal fibrosis

DIFFERENTIAL DIAGNOSIS

Low-flow (ischemic) priapism
- Intracorporeal injection for impotence (e.g., papaverine, prostaglandin E_1, phentolamine, phenoxybenzamine) is the most common cause in adults
- Sickle cell disease is the most common cause in children
- Leukemia
- Penile infiltration with solid tumors (e.g., bladder cancer, prostate cancer)
- Prescription drugs (e.g., trazodone, chlorpromazine, sildenafil, antihypertensives, phenothiazines, anticoagulants)
- Illicit drugs (e.g., marijuana, crack cocaine, MDMA)
- Alcohol
- Penile or perineal trauma
- Total parenteral nutrition (lipid infusion)
- Dialysis
- Vasculitis
- Idiopathic

High-flow (nonischemic) priapism
- Groin or straddle injury
- Cocaine

Less common etiologies
- Spinal cord trauma or injury to the medulla (clinically similar to high-flow priapism)
- Polycythemia
- Thalassemia
- Amyloidosis
- Fabry's disease
- Snake or scorpion bite
- Rarely, may also occur in the clitoris in females

Proptosis/Exophthalmos

INTRODUCTION

Proptosis, or exophthalmos, may be caused by inflammatory, infectious, neoplastic, traumatic, or vascular etiologies. It usually signals significant pathology. Thyroid-associated orbitopathy is by far the most common cause. Some cases may have a benign course, but others follow a fulminant course that threatens sight and/or life and require urgent diagnosis and intervention. Imaging studies are essential in almost all cases.

DIAGNOSTIC WORKUP & INITIAL MANAGEMENT

History and physical examination
- History should include age, tempo of onset, duration, progression, pain, fever, laterality, other ocular symptoms (e.g., vision loss, diplopia), and associated symptoms (e.g., fever, fatigue, rash, tremors, palpitations)
- Note history of thyroid disease, sinusitis, trauma, diabetes, immunosuppression, or cancer
- Note maneuvers or conditions that worsen the proptosis (proptosis caused by lymphangioma may worsen during upper respiratory infections)
- Physical exam should include ophthalmologic, head and neck, and focal neurologic exams
- Measure proptosis with exophthalmometer

Initial diagnostic workup
- Initial laboratory evaluation may include thyroid function tests, antithyroid antibodies, ESR, CRP, LDH, and CBC
- Consider ANCA if suspect Wegener's granulomatosis and blood cultures if suspect orbital cellulitis
- CT and/or MRI of orbits
- Consider ultrasound with color Doppler to evaluate orbital blood flow and arteriovenous malformation
- Consider biopsy if the diagnosis is uncertain

Initial patient management
- Consider ophthalmology, neurosurgery, and/or endocrinology consultation
- Daily vision testing and optic nerve function evaluation
- Prevent eye injury and discomfort with artificial tears and sunglasses; consider eye patch while sleeping
- Treat the underlying cause; however, treatment of Graves' disease does not always improve ophthalmopathy, and radioactive iodine may make it worse
- Surgical decompression may be indicated in cases of thyroid-associated orbitopathy and retrobulbar hemorrhage resulting in acute optic neuropathy
- Treat infectious etiologies with antibiotics and/or surgical debridement
- Treat noninfectious inflammation with systemic steroids or immunomodulating therapy, particularly if there is acute optic neuropathy
- Incisional or excisional biopsy of orbital tumors

DIFFERENTIAL DIAGNOSIS

Thyroid-associated orbitopathy (associated with Graves' disease)
- Usually results in bilateral, although often asymmetric, proptosis
- More commonly occurs in women, smokers, and patients treated with radioactive iodine

Orbital cellulitis
- Most cases result from contiguous spread from sinusitis, particularly ethmoid sinusitis

Mucormycosis
- Occurs primarily in diabetic and immunocompromised patients

Orbital tumors (adult)
- Metastatic breast, lung, or prostate cancer
- Cavernous hemangioma
- Mucocele
- Lymphoid tumors
- Optic nerve sheath meningioma
- Neurofibroma
- Neurilemoma (schwannoma)
- Fibrous histiocytoma
- Hemangiopericytoma

Orbital tumors (children)
- Capillary hemangioma (most common benign pediatric orbital tumor)
- Rhabdomyosarcoma (most common primary pediatric orbital malignancy)
- Lymphangioma
- Dermoid cyst
- Optic nerve glioma
- Acute leukemia (chloroma or granulocytic sarcoma)
- Metastatic neuroblastoma
- Plexiform neurofibromatosis type 1
- Teratoma

Trauma
- Intraorbital foreign body
- Retrobulbar hemorrhage
- Fracture of orbital bones, with hemorrhage into the orbital space

Orbital vasculitis
- Wegener's granulomatosis
- Polyarteritis nodosa

Arteriovenous malformation
- Carotid-cavernous fistula

Cavernous sinus thrombosis
- Presents with signs of orbital cellulitis plus cranial neuropathies (cranial nerves III, IV, V, and/or VI) and mental status changes
- Usually bilateral and rapidly progressive

Neurofibromatosis type 1
- May present with optic gliomas and orbital/periorbital plexiform neurofibromas

Pseudoproptosis
- Enlarged globe (myopia, buphthalmos)
- Enophthalmos of the fellow eye

Craniosynostosis
- A birth defect characterized by premature closure of one or more fibrous joints between the bones of the skull (cranial sutures) before brain growth is complete
- May be genetic or caused by metabolic diseases (e.g., rickets or hypothyroidism)

Pruritis with Rash

INTRODUCTION

Pruritis, or itching, is the most common dermatologic complaint. Mediators of itch include histamine, serotonin, acetylcholine, leukotrienes, prostaglandins, cytokines, and opioids. Pruritis is not itself serious, but it may be a clinical manifestation of an underlying dermatologic or systemic disease (e.g., urticaria, uremia, liver disease). Identifying the underlying etiology may be difficult, however, and symptomatic treatment may be all that can be offered initially. Pruritis can occur with or without a rash. When pruritis occurs with cutaneous findings, the clinician must carefully analyze the dermatologic findings to identify the underlying cause. Severe pruritis may lead to lifestyle disturbances by causing anxiety, depression, and loss of sleep.

DIAGNOSTIC WORKUP & INITIAL MANAGEMENT

History and physical examination

- Note the presence of skin lesions that preceded the itching, timing (new vs. recurrent, acute vs. chronic), associated systemic symptoms (e.g., fever, malaise, weight loss, night sweats), evidence of systemic disease (e.g., uremia, liver disease), and pregnancy
- Note medical and family history (e.g., asthma, psoriasis) and exposure history (e.g., poison ivy, poison oak, poison sumac); assess exposure to others with similar complaints
- Complete review of systems may identify underlying disease (e.g., change in bowel habits with colon cancer, cold intolerance with hypothyroidism, abdominal pain with liver disease)
- Detailed medication history
- Complete skin examination to determine presence or absence of primary skin disease and to define the type and distribution of rash or specific abnormalities; evaluate especially for rashes on the extensor or flexor surfaces of skin folds and interdigital spaces
- Note morphology (e.g., macule, papule, pustule, plaque, crust, vesicle, bulla, wheal) and configuration (e.g., linear, grouped, annular, geographic) of the lesion

Initial diagnostic workup

- Lab testing if pruritis lasts >2 weeks may include CBC with differential, liver function tests, renal function tests, and thyroid function tests; other testing may be indicated based on clinical suspicions
- Scrape lesions and perform KOH test if suspect fungal infection
- Scrape possible burrow site to identify a mite in cases of scabies
- Patch testing may be done if suspect allergic contact dermatitis
- Punch biopsy may be done to establish a histologic diagnosis
- Consider referral to a dermatologist if the diagnosis remains unclear

Initial patient management

- Symptomatic treatment is often sufficient
  - Avoid hot baths/showers and harsh soaps; bathe with lukewarm water and bath oil; limit use of soap as much as possible
  - Apply an emollient immediately after bathing: Emollients with menthol will provide a cooling sensation; emollients with phenol or camphor will provide an anesthetic effect
  - Oral antihistamines (e.g., hydroxyzine, diphenhydramine) may be used but are sedating (nonsedating antihistamines are less effective in reducing pruritis)
- Oral steroids are a last resort to interrupt the inflammatory cascade; however, a thorough evaluation for a secondary cause (e.g., infection) should be pursued initially
- Infection may result from excessive scratching and excoriation requiring antibiotics
- Treat underlying etiologies as appropriate (e.g., antimicrobials for infections; permethrin cream or lindane lotion for scabies; topical steroids for eczematous dermatitis and lichen planus; topical steroids, tars, retinoids, UV light, and/or immune modulators for psoriasis)

DIFFERENTIAL DIAGNOSIS

Infection

Fungal infection
- Dermatophyte infections (tinea)
- Candidiasis (beefy-red color with satellite papules)
- Seborrheic dermatitis caused by *Pityrosporum* (common in hair-bearing areas)

Bacterial infection
- Erythrasma caused by *Corynebacterium* (frequently in axilla)
- Cutaneous staphylococcal or streptococcal infections

Viral infection
- Chickenpox (varicella)

Insect vectors
- Scabies (areas of papules and excoriated lesions, particularly in digital web spaces, antecubital, and inguinal regions)
- Pediculosis (lice) on trunk, head, or pubic area; the louse or eggs (nits) appear on hair shaft
- Flea bites (typically on legs)

Mixed infections
- Intertrigo (present at skin folds or areas of friction)

Dermatologic disease

Contact dermatitis
- Lesions may be macular or papular and are often erythematous

Atopic dermatitis
- Erythematous rash in the flexural areas
- Patients often have seasonal allergies and/or asthma

Eczematous dermatitis
- Stasis dermatitis (hyperpigmented legs of patients with vascular disease)
- Lichen simplex chronicus (anxious patient who chronically scratches)
- Dyshidrotic eczema (on hands/feet, with scaling, erythema, vesicles, and painful fissures)
- Nummular eczema (round, scaly lesions on dry skin; common in the winter)

Pityriasis rosea
- Mostly on trunk in "Christmas tree" pattern; begins as single, larger "herald" patch

Lichen planus
- Purple, polygonal, pruritic papules
- Koebner's reaction (lesions occur with trauma, such as linear lesions caused by scratching)

Psoriasis
- Pink, silvery, scaling plaques on extensor surfaces and nail pits
- Koebner's reaction (lesions occur with trauma, such as linear lesions caused by scratching)

Urticaria (hives)
- Erythematous, raised wheals with central pallor that appear on the face or extremities
- May present with angioedema (swelling of the face, tongue, larynx, or GI tract)

Mycoses fungoides
- Referred to as Sézary's syndrome when it presents with lymphadenopathy, erythroderma, and atypical circulating white blood cells

Other
- Drug reaction (e.g., aspirin, alcohol, morphine, codeine)
- Psychogenic (e.g., emotional stress)
- Miliaria (heat rash)
- Dermatitis herpetiformis (caused by gluten allergy)

Pruritis without Rash

INTRODUCTION

Pruritis, or itching, is the most common dermatologic complaint. Mediators of itch include histamine, serotonin, acetylcholine, leukotrienes, prostaglandins, cytokines, and opioids. Pruritis is not itself serious, but it may be a clinical manifestation of an underlying dermatologic or systemic disease (e.g., urticaria, uremia, liver disease). Identifying the underlying etiology may be difficult, however, and symptomatic treatment may be all that can be offered initially. Pruritis can occur with or without a rash. When pruritis occurs without cutaneous findings, a thorough history, physical examination, and laboratory tests must be obtained to rule out systemic disease as a cause. The prevalence of an underlying systemic disease in a pruritic patient is as high as 50% in some patient populations.

DIAGNOSTIC WORKUP & INITIAL MANAGEMENT

History and physical examination

- Note the presence of skin lesions that preceded the itching, timing (new vs. recurrent, acute vs. chronic), associated systemic symptoms (e.g., fever, malaise, weight loss, night sweats), evidence of systemic disease (e.g., uremia, liver disease), and pregnancy
- Note medical and family history (e.g., asthma, psoriasis), exposure history, social history, and sexual history
- Complete review of systems may identify underlying disease (e.g., change in bowel habits with colon cancer, cold intolerance with hypothyroidism, abdominal pain with liver disease)
- Detailed medication history
- Complete skin exam to confirm the absence of rashes and assess for other primary skin disease or other abnormalities; stool exam for occult blood, Pap smear, and pelvic exam

Initial diagnostic workup

- Lab testing if pruritis lasts >2 weeks may include CBC with differential, liver function tests, renal function tests, and thyroid function tests; other testing may be indicated based on clinical suspicions
- Rule out internal malignancies (e.g., chest radiography, mammogram)
- Other labs to consider include HIV test, hepatitis B and C panel, serum iron and ferritin, serum and urine protein electrophoresis, stool for ova and parasites, and blind skin biopsy with or without immunofluorescence
- Consider referral to a dermatologist if diagnosis remains unclear

Initial patient management

- Symptomatic treatment is often sufficient
  - Avoid hot baths/showers and harsh soaps; bathe with lukewarm water and bath oil; limit use of soap as much as possible
  - Apply an emollient immediately after bathing: Emollients with menthol will provide a cooling sensation; emollients with phenol or camphor will provide an anesthetic effect
  - Oral antihistamines (e.g., hydroxyzine, diphenhydramine) may be used but are sedating (nonsedating antihistamines are less effective in reducing pruritis); benzodiazepines may be used adjunctively if antihistamines are ineffective
  - Low-dose topical corticosteroids may be used for short durations
  - UV light therapy may be helpful in some cases
- Oral steroids are a last resort to interrupt the inflammatory cascade; however, a thorough evaluation for a secondary cause (e.g., infection) should be pursued initially
- Infection may result from excessive scratching and excoriation, and require antibiotics
- The ultimate treatment is aimed at the underlying etiology

DIFFERENTIAL DIAGNOSIS

Hepatobiliary disorder
- Cholestasis of pregnancy (pruritus is most severe during the third trimester and ceases after delivery)
- Primary biliary cirrhosis
- Biliary obstruction

Endocrine disorder
- Hypothyroidism
- Hyperthyroidism
- Diabetes mellitus (perianal pruritus)

Hematopoietic disorder
- Polycythemia vera (pruritus classically occurs after emerging from a bath and is described as severe and prickling)
- Hodgkin's lymphoma (pruritus may present years before the diagnosis and portends a poor prognosis)
- Iron deficiency anemia
- Multiple myeloma
- Waldenström's macroglobulinemia

Chronic renal failure
- Dialysis (pruritis often begins 6 months after the start of dialysis; affects up to 75% of patients during or immediately after dialysis)
- Uremia

Malignancy
- Adenocarcinoma
- Squamous cell carcinomas
- Carcinoid syndrome

HIV
- Increasing frequency of pruritis occurs with disease progression

Psychogenic state
- May have underlying personality disorder (e.g., obsessive-compulsive disorder)
- Emotional stress
- Psychogenic pruritis or delusions of parasitosis

Senescence
- Elderly pruritis is very common

Drug reaction
- Aspirin
- Alcohol
- Morphine
- Codeine

Other
- Isolated pruritis
- Parasitic infection (e.g., hookworm, onchocerciasis, ascariasis, trichinosis)
- Hepatitis B or C

Ptosis

INTRODUCTION

Ptosis, or drooping of the upper eyelid, is a fairly common condition that results in decreased vision by direct visual obstruction or by inducing corneal astigmatism. Many cases are congenital. Some cases occur after ocular surgery. All cases of acquired ptosis require careful evaluation, because it may be a harbinger of a more serious underlying medical condition (e.g., myasthenia gravis, 3rd nerve palsy secondary to brain aneurysm, Horner's syndrome secondary to tumor).

DIAGNOSTIC WORKUP & INITIAL MANAGEMENT

History and physical examination

- History should include age of onset, medical history, previous surgeries or trauma, variability of ptosis, diplopia, associated symptoms (e.g., dysphagia), medications, and an attempt to observe old pictures of the patient for comparison, if possible
- Exam should include a complete ophthalmologic examination and focused neurologic, head and neck, and chest exams
  - Assess visual acuity and visual fields; perform a dilated fundus exam
  - Assess the visual fields with and without the eyelids taped up to document a superior visual field defect
  - Evaluate for localized lesions of the eyelid, including hordeola, chalazia, and lid cellulitis
  - In children, rule out amblyopia ("lazy eye") from induced astigmatism or occlusion
  - Note levator function, palpebral fissure width, pupils, anisocoria (pupil difference), extraocular motility (especially supraduction), corneal sensation, corneal surface, and Bell's phenomenon (eyes roll up on lid closure)
  - Use Shirmer's strips to quantify basal secretion of tears

Initial diagnostic workup

- Lab testing may include CBC with differential if suspect Horner's syndrome
- Ophthalmologic consultation is often warranted
- Diagnostic testing is based on the suspected etiology:
  - Tensilon test or ice test to rule out myasthenia gravis
  - Topical cocaine and hydroxyamphetamine drops to rule out Horner's syndrome
  - Consider CT or MRI for possible tumors, aneurysm, orbital disease, or scarring
  - Chest radiography to rule out pulmonary lesion if suspect Horner's syndrome
  - MRA in cases of painful ptosis to rule out carotid dissection

Initial patient management

- Treat underlying medical condition when possible (e.g., hot compresses and antibiotics for hordeola, excision of chalazia, antibiotics for lid cellulitis)
- Eyelid crutches attached to glasses may be used as temporizing measures but may limit blinking and result in dry eyes
- Eyelid surgery may be necessary
- In children $<$ 10 years, perform surgical correction as soon as possible if amblyopia is present

DIFFERENTIAL DIAGNOSIS

Acquired ptosis

Aponeurotic or senile ptosis
- Most common type of ptosis
- Caused by disinsertion or dehiscence of the levator aponeurosis
- Normal levator function, high lid crease
- May be exacerbated by any ocular surgery

Mechanical
- Caused by mass effect of tumor or edema or by tethering by scar (cicatricial)

Myogenic
- Poor levator or Miller's muscle function
- Myasthenia gravis
- Chronic progressive external ophthalmoplegia (CPEO)
- Myotonic or oculopharyngeal dystrophy

Neurogenic
- 3rd nerve palsy
  - Has associated supraduction deficit; may have adduction or infraduction deficit (eye may be down and out)
  - May be caused by hypertension, diabetes, aneurysm, or mass lesions
  - Pupil-sparing 3rd nerve palsy is usually caused by ischemia (most commonly diabetes) and often resolves spontaneously over several weeks to months
  - Mass lesions (e.g., posterior communicating artery aneurysm) usually cause mydriasis as well as 3rd nerve palsy and constitute a medical emergency
- Horner's syndrome
  - A sympathetic lesion causing miosis (pupil 1–2 mm), "reverse ptosis" (lower eyelid is abnormally raised), and often anhidrosis
  - May be caused by numerous etiologies, including Pancoast's tumor of the lung, neuroblastoma, aneurysms, inflammatory processes, chest surgery, and trauma

Other
- Migraine
- Botulism
- Poisoning (e.g., lead, arsenic, carbon monoxide)
- Nutritional deficiency (e.g., thiamine, carnitine, vitamin E)

Congenital ptosis
- Simple congenital (myopathic) ptosis resulting in poor levator function
- Blepharophimosis syndrome
- Congenital Horner's syndrome
- Marcus Gunn's (jaw-winking) syndrome
  - Unilateral ptosis occurs at rest; the ptotic lid raises up when chewing or opening mouth
- Mitochondrial myopathies
- Chromosomal disorders (e.g., Turner's syndrome, trisomy 18)
- Fetal drug exposure (e.g., alcohol, hydantoin, trimethadione)
- Inherited syndromes (e.g., Noonan's, Smith-Lemli-Opitz, Aarskog)

Other disorders that may mimic ptosis
- Physical alteration of the eyelid caused by hordeola, chalazia, lid cellulitis, or tumors
- Eyelid edema (e.g., posttrauma)
- Lid retraction caused by chemical stimulation (e.g., phenylephrine) or thyroid disease
- Pseudoptosis/dermatochalasis (excess skin of the upper eyelids)
- Enophthalmos (narrowed palpebral fissure)
- Hypotropia
- Contralateral eyelid retraction, causing asymmetry
- Small eye (phthisis bulbi, microphthalmia, anophthalmia)

Pupillary Constriction (Miosis)

INTRODUCTION

Pupillary size represents an interplay between the sympathetic and parasympathetic nervous systems. Pupillary constriction (miosis) is effected by the action of the iris sphincter muscle, which is under parasympathetic control (cranial nerve III). It may be caused by cholinergic or parasympathomimetic drugs. If parasympathetic action is unopposed by sympathetic action (e.g., Horner's syndrome), anisocoria (unequal pupils) results and is more pronounced in the dark. Pupils also tend to become smaller with advanced years.

DIAGNOSTIC WORKUP & INITIAL MANAGEMENT

History and physical examination

- Complete medical and surgical history, with specific attention to neurologic, ophthalmologic, and head and neck region
- Physical exam should include measurement of pupil size in the light and dark, pupil response to light and convergence, and lid position (especially with upgaze)
- Pupil should be checked for response to light and convergence
  - Normally, a bright light will constrict the pupils, directly and consensually
  - Normal alteration in sympathetic and parasympathetic tone, with pupils becoming dilated and constricted alternately with sustained light stimulation (hippus)
  - Argyll Robertson pupils are bilaterally constricted but often asymmetric; they accommodate but do not react to light

Initial diagnostic workup

- If tertiary syphilis is possible, workup includes RPR or VDRL and FTA-ABS; also perform a lumbar puncture to evaluate CSF for VDRL
- If Horner's syndrome is found, consider chest CT to rule out apical lung mass (Pancoast's tumor), MRI or MRA of the head and neck, carotid Doppler ultrasound, and/or carotid angiography
- Consider ophthalmology and/or neurology consultation

Initial patient management

- Treat underlying disorder, if possible
- Remove offending medications
- Syphilis is treated with high-dose IV penicillin

DIFFERENTIAL DIAGNOSIS

Argyll Robertson pupils
- Tertiary syphilis
- Light-near dissociation
- Diabetes mellitus

Coma
- Pontine lesions result in pinpoint pupils
- Metabolic lesions and hypothalamic lesions result in small, reactive pupils

Pharmacologic
- Systemic opioids (e.g., heroin, morphine, codeine, methadone)
- Systemic cholinergics (e.g., organophosphate and carbamate insecticides, nerve agents, edrophonium)
- Topical cholinergics or miotics (e.g., pilocarpine) or indirect cholinergics (e.g., physostigmine, echothiophate)
- Others (e.g., phencyclidine, clonidine, phenothiazines, phytostigmine)

Horner's syndrome (triad of ptosis, miosis, and anhidrosis)
- Internal carotid artery dissection
- Headache syndromes
- Raeder's paratrigeminal syndrome
- Herpes zoster
- Otitis media
- Cavernous sinus lesions
- Tolosa-Hunt syndrome
- Cervical lymphadenopathy
- Orbit or neck trauma
- Brainstem or cerebral stroke
- Tumor (head, neck, apical lung)
- Basal meningitis
- Cervical cord lesion
- High thoracic or low cervical lesions (e.g., trauma, traction on brachial plexus, surgery, internal jugular vein catheterization)

Iritis
- Presents with eye pain, redness, and anterior chamber reaction

Mechanical
- Posterior iris synechiae (pupil is nonreactive or irregular)

Long-standing Adie's pupil
- Refer to the *Pupillary Dilation* entry

Hippus
- Pupils become alternately dilated and constricted on sustained light stimulation

Anisocoria (unequal pupil sizes)
- Mild anisocoria (<0.5 mm) may be normal (often called "simple anisocoria")
- Pathologic anisocoria may be caused by Wernicke-Korsakoff syndrome, deformities of the iris or eyeball, defects of the efferent papillary pathways, or drugs (e.g., tropicamide scopolamine)

Pupillary Dilation

INTRODUCTION

Pupillary size represents an interplay between the sympathetic and parasympathetic nervous systems. Pupillary dilation (mydriasis) is often caused by relatively unopposed action of the iris dilator muscle, which is under the control of the sympathetic nervous system, versus the iris sphincter muscle, which is under parasympathetic control. A unilaterally dilated pupil may be caused by mydriatic eye drops (e.g., atropine, scopolamine), postganglionic mydriasis (Adie's pupil), or preganglionic mydriasis (cranial nerve III palsy). Bilaterally dilated pupils may be attributable to glutethimide intoxication and/or anoxia. Third nerve palsy involving the pupil must be worked up for an intracranial aneurysm. Posterior synechiae (iris-lens adhesions) may cause mydriasis if the adhesions form while the pupil is dilated.

DIAGNOSTIC WORKUP & INITIAL MANAGEMENT

History and physical examination

- Determine which eye is abnormal
- Obtain a complete medical and surgical history, with specific attention to neurology, ophthalmology, and head and neck region
- Comparison with old photographs may be useful to determine chronicity; mild degrees of anisocoria (unequal pupil sizes) may be congenital and benign
- Patients will complain of light intolerance because of impaired pupillary constriction
- Unilateral pupillary dilation in an otherwise asymptomatic patient is usually the result of mydriatic eye drops (atropine or scopolamine)
- Physical exam should include measurement of pupil size in the light and dark, pupil response to light and convergence, and lid position (especially with upgaze)
- Pupil should be checked for response to light and convergence
  - Normally, a bright light will constrict the pupils, directly and consensually
  - Normal alteration in sympathetic and parasympathetic tone, with pupils becoming alternately dilated and constricted with sustained light stimulation (hippus)

Initial diagnostic workup

- In cases of cranial nerve III palsy involving the pupil, MRI or MRA of the head is indicated to rule out aneurysm
- If Horner's syndrome is found, consider chest CT to rule out apical lung mass (Pancoast's tumor), MRI or MRA of head and neck, carotid Doppler ultrasound, and/or carotid angiography
- Place dilute pilocarpine drops (0.125%) to diagnose Adie's pupil
- Consider ophthalmology or neurology consultation

Initial patient management

- Treat underlying disorder, if possible
- Remove offending medications, if possible
- Recommend eye protection (e.g., sunglasses) if photophobia occurs
- Adie's pupil is treated with pilocarpine drops for cosmesis and to aid in accommodation; it is usually permanent
- Neurosurgical evaluation of compressive lesions, structural lesions, tumors, masses, and aneurysms
- Narcotic overdose may be treated with naloxone

DIFFERENTIAL DIAGNOSIS

Pharmacologic
- Systemic anticholinergics (e.g., atropine, antihistamines, muscle relaxants, tricyclic antidepressants, scopolamine)
- Adrenergic agents (e.g., caffeine, cocaine, amphetamines, methylphenidate)
- Hallucinogens (e.g., LSD, amphetamines)
- Other (e.g., MAO inhibitors)
- Nicotine
- Topical anticholinergics and adrenergic eye drops
- Serotonin syndrome
- Drug withdrawal

Acute closed-angle glaucoma
- Middilated pupil

Trauma/surgery
- Iris sphincter tear or surgical changes
- Iron mydriasis (intraocular iron foreign body)
- Head trauma

Anisocoria greater in light
- The abnormal pupil is larger

Adie's tonic pupil
- Irregular pupil with segmental palsy and vermiform constriction
- Minimal reaction to light; slow/tonic near response (constriction and redilation)
- Supersensitive to weak cholinergics (pilocarpine 0.125%)
- Absent deep tendon reflexes (Adie's syndrome)

Third nerve palsy
- Associated with ptosis and extraocular muscle palsies
- Will not constrict in response to weak cholinergics but will constrict in response to pilocarpine (1%)

Migraine
- Benign episodic mydriasis

Coma/anoxic encephalopathy
- Midbrain: Pupil is midposition and fixed
- Early brain death: Pupil is midposition or dilated and unreactive to light
- Uncal herniation may result in 3rd nerve palsy because of compression at the skull base
- Many other causes

Hippus
- Pupils become alternately dilated and constricted on sustained light stimulation

Other
- Seizures
- Congenital mydriasis

Purpura

INTRODUCTION

Purpura are dark-purple, nonblanching skin lesions that occur secondary to vascular injury and hemorrhage underneath the skin. Small lesions are called petechiae; large lesions are called purpura. Ecchymoses are bruises. Because the differential diagnosis of purpura is large, begin by determining whether the purpura is palpable or nonpalpable. Subsequent workup is dictated by the history, physical, and review of systems to determine appropriate diagnostic tests. If, after careful evaluation, the cause of purpura cannot be determined, refer the patient to an appropriate consultant, usually a hematologist, unless a collagen vascular disorder is likely, in which case a rheumatologist is an appropriate choice.

DIAGNOSTIC WORKUP & INITIAL MANAGEMENT

History and physical examination

- Assess onset, duration, characteristics (e.g., palpable vs. nonpalpable, blanching vs. nonblanching), associated symptoms (e.g., arthralgias, myalgias, fever), medical history, illness exposure, medication history, and complete review of systems
- Note characteristic spread patterns (e.g., Rocky Mountain spotted fever usually starts peripherally and spreads centrifugally onto the trunk) and CNS symptoms (may suggest SLE or meningococcemia)
- Focused physical exam with complete skin exam

Initial diagnostic workup

- Initial labs include CBC with differential, coagulation profile (PT, PTT, INR) to rule out coagulopathy, urinalysis to evaluate for hematuria in Henoch-Schönlein purpura), liver function tests to evaluate for hepatitis, ESR or CRP to assess for characteristic inflammation that occurs in collagen vascular diseases, and BUN and creatinine to evaluate for renal insufficiency that may occur in polyarteritis nodosa, Henoch-Schönlein purpura, SLE, and many other palpable purpura–inducing diseases
- Consider blood cultures and skin cultures by a punch biopsy if the patient is febrile
- ANA, RF, and viral hepatitis serologies may be indicated
- Age-appropriate malignancy screening as necessary
- Urinalysis showing red blood cells is helpful to diagnose Henoch-Schönlein purpura
- Punch biopsy is diagnostic for leukocytoclastic vasculitis

Initial patient management

- Discontinue causative medications
- Correct coagulopathies as necessary
- Treat malignancy as necessary
- Sun protection and avoidance of trauma will prevent actinic and age-related purpura
- Stasis-associated lower extremity purpura can be treated with compression stockings, elevation, and diuretics if edema is present
- Prompt antimicrobial treatment for infections
- High-dose corticosteroids followed by steroid-sparing medications (e.g., methotrexate, cyclosporine, azathioprine, mycophenolate mofetil) for long-term treatment of autoimmune disorders
- Idiopathic pigmented purpuras are most common on the lower legs of men and may resolve spontaneously or persist indefinitely; topical steroids and oral vitamin C sometimes hasten their resolution

DIFFERENTIAL DIAGNOSIS

Palpable purpura (red/purple papules or nodules that do not blanch with pressure)

Leukocytoclastic vasculitis
- A necrotizing vasculitis of small vessels that presents with fever, malaise, fatigue, and arthralgias
- Inciting factors include drugs (e.g., NSAIDs, thaizides, phenothiazines, antibiotics), infection (e.g., *Streptococcus*, Rocky Mountain spotted fever, meningococcemia, viral hepatitis), and blood abnormalities (e.g., cryoglobulinemia, cryofibrinogenemia)
- Vasculitic injury to the kidneys, brain, lung, heart, and GI tract may occur

Other vasculitis disorders
- Henoch-Schönlein purpura
- Granulomatous vasculitis (e.g., Wegener's granulomatosis, Churg-Strauss syndrome)
- Polyarteritis nodosa

Collagen vascular diseases
- SLE
- Sjögren's syndrome
- Rheumatoid arthritis

Internal malignancies
- Multiple myeloma
- Lymphoma
- Leukemia

Drugs
- Aspirin
- NSAIDs
- Warfarin
- Heparin

Nonpalpable purpura (flat macules, patches, or petechiae that do not blanch with pressure)

Coagulopathies (affecting platelet number or function)
- Thrombotic thrombocytopenic purpura (TTP) (pentad of fever, microangiopathic hemolytic anemia, thrombocytopenia, renal insufficiency, and neurologic signs)
- Idiopathic thrombocytopenic purpura
- Disseminated intravascular coagulation (DIC)
- Drug-induced thrombocytopenia
- Bacteremia and many viral diseases

Other
- Trauma
- Advancing age (senile purpura)
- Actinic changes
- Chronic stasis
- Scurvy (vitamin C deficiency)
- TORCH infection can cause congenital purpura ("blueberry muffin baby")
- Many systemic diseases (e.g., Cushing's and diabetes mellitus) have associated nonpalpable purpura
- Anticoagulant therapy

Rales (Crackles)

INTRODUCTION

Rales, also known as crackles, are caused by the opening of collapsed airways. They are discontinuous, nonmusical breath sounds that may be fine (soft, 5–10 milliseconds in duration, high-pitched) or coarse (slightly louder, 20–30 milliseconds in duration, lower in pitch). Distinguish rales from rhonchi, which are caused by air flowing through airway secretions and are continuous (>250 milliseconds), musical sounds of low pitch.

DIAGNOSTIC WORKUP & INITIAL MANAGEMENT

History and physical examination

- Percussion may reveal dullness
- Egophony ("E" to "A" changes) may be present in cases of lobar pneumonia, atelectasis, and postinfectious bronchiolitis

Initial diagnostic workup

- Initial laboratory studies may include pulse oximetry, CBC, electrolytes, BUN and creatinine, glucose, and calcium
- Chest radiography is generally the initial test
  - CHF: Interstitial and alveolar edema, especially in dependent regions; cephalization; Kerley B lines (if chronic); cardiomegaly; may see pleural effusion
  - Interstitial disease: Reticulonodular or interstitial pattern (diffuse lines and/or small nodules)
  - Atelectasis: Decreased lung volume (retracted ribs, deviation of heart and trachea to the affected side, overinflation of contralateral lung), triangular shadow with apex pointing to hilum, and opacification
  - Bronchiolitis: Patchy infiltrate
  - Bronchiectasis: Bronchial dilation, thickened walls ("tram-tracking")
- ABG will evaluate for barriers to oxygen diffusion (increased A-a gradient), hypoxemia, and hypercapnia
- High-resolution chest CT can detect early disease and small lesions that are otherwise unidentifiable on chest radiographs, can distinguish inflammation from fibrosis, and will confirm bronchiectasis ("signet ring" sign)
- Biopsy may be necessary to diagnose interstitial lung disease

DIFFERENTIAL DIAGNOSIS

Pneumonia

- May be community acquired, hospital acquired (i.e., from residence in any health care facility or nursing home in the preceding 10–14 days), or caused by aspiration
- "Typical" pneumonia (e.g., *Streptococcus pneumoniae, Haemophilus influenzae*) is characterized by acute or subacute onset of fever, dyspnea, fatigue, pleuritic chest pain, and productive cough
- "Atypical" pneumonia (e.g., *Mycoplasma, Legionella, Chlamydia*, influenza and parainfluenza viruses) is characterized by more gradual onset, dry cough, headache, fatigue, and minimal lung signs

Pulmonary edema

- Leakage of fluid into the interstitium and alveoli because of elevated capillary pressure (cardiogenic) or abnormal capillary permeability (noncardiogenic)
- Cardiogenic pulmonary edema:
  - CHF (e.g., MI, cardiomyopathy)
  - Valve disease
  - High-output states (e.g., thyrotoxicosis)
  - Volume overload
  - Hypertensive emergency
- Noncardiogenic pulmonary edema:
  - Sepsis
  - Inhalation injury
  - Drugs (e.g., narcotics)
  - Renal failure
  - High altitude
  - Aspiration
  - Pancreatitis
  - Seizure
  - Trauma
  - Emboli (fat, air, or amniotic fluid)
  - CNS injury
  - Airway obstruction (e.g., croup, foreign body)

Atelectasis

- May be acute (e.g., postoperative) or chronic (resulting from obesity, infection, bronchiectasis, lung destruction, or fibrosis)

Interstitial lung disease

- A group of disorders characterized by inflammation and fibrosis of alveolar walls and the interstitium
- Pneumoconiosis
- Hypersensitivity pneumonitis
- Drug-induced: Antibiotics (e.g., penicillin, sulfa drugs), amiodarone, β-blockers, radiation, chemotherapeutics, and antirheumatics (e.g., gold)
- Rheumatologic: Rheumatoid arthritis, SLE, scleroderma, polymyositis-dermatomyositis
- Idiopathic: Sarcoidosis, idiopathic pulmonary fibrosis, interstitial pneumonia, BOOP, pulmonary alveolar proteinosis

Bronchospasm

- Asthma
- Reactive airways disease

Other

- Bronchiectasis
- Congenital heart disease
- Bronchoalveolar cell carcinoma

Rectal Mass

INTRODUCTION

Any mass in the anal canal or rectum should be considered to be cancer until proven otherwise. Colorectal cancer must be considered because it is the second-leading cause of cancer death in the United States, causing more than 40,000 mortalities each year. Early detection and aggressive treatment are the keys to improving survival, and a multidisciplinary approach to anorectal cancer is essential to improve survival.

DIAGNOSTIC WORKUP & INITIAL MANAGEMENT

History and physical examination

- History should include changes in bowel habits or consistency of stool and family history of colorectal cancer
- Bleeding is the most common symptom associated with benign and malignant lesions:
  - Melena suggests upper GI bleeding
  - Blood on toilet paper suggests anal fissure or hemorrhoids
  - Bright-red blood separate from stool suggests hemorrhoids
  - Blood clots in stool suggests a colonic source

Initial diagnostic workup

- Fecal occult blood testing may be used for screening
- Digital rectal exam and anoscopy are used initially to distinguish many anorectal lesions
- Endoscopy (sigmoidoscopy and/or full colonoscopy) with biopsy of all polyps and suspicious lesions
- Barium enema is indicated if colonoscopy is not available
- Endorectal ultrasound is necessary to evaluate for potential rectal cancer, to appropriately stage tumor invasion and lymph node status, and to direct appropriate treatment
- Manometry may be indicated for incontinent patients

Initial patient management

- Rectal and anal cancers are treated by surgical resection (with sphincter preservation), radiation, and/or chemotherapy
- Hemorrhoid treatment is initially conservative: high-fiber diet, appropriate anal hygiene, sitz baths, and topical steroids
  - Surgical options include rubber band ligation of internal hemorrhoids or surgical resection for large refractory hemorrhoids
  - Acute thrombosis of a hemorrhoid may require incision and drainage

DIFFERENTIAL DIAGNOSIS

Common diagnoses
- Hemorrhoids
- Rectal prolapse
- Rectal polyp
- Prostatitis
- Endometriosis
- Rectal intussusception
- Foreign body

Anal cancer (2% of colorectal cancers)

Anal canal tumors (above the anal verge)
- Adenocarcinoma
- Melanoma
- Epidermoid tumors

Anal margin tumors (below the anal verge)
- Squamous cell carcinoma
- Verrucous (from condyloma acuminatum)
- Basal cell carcinoma
- Bowen's disease
- Paget's disease of the anus

Nonanal cancers
- Presacral neurogenic tumor
- Prostate cancer
- Rectal cancer
- Malignant lymphoma
- Teratoma
- Leiomyosarcoma

Less common diagnoses
- Perirectal fistula
- Rectal carcinoid
- Lymphoid hyperplasia
- Lipoma
- Dermoid cyst
- Rectal duplication

Rectal Pain

INTRODUCTION

Rectal complaints are distressing but common. Although most causes of rectal pain and bleeding are benign and treatable, carcinoma must be considered and ruled out in older patients and in those with suggestive findings (e.g., polyps). Many of the rectal pathologies are easily diagnosed; however, non-GI diagnoses (genitourinary or gynecologic) may present with rectal complaints and should be considered.

DIAGNOSTIC WORKUP & INITIAL MANAGEMENT

History and physical examination

- A careful history and physical exam are crucial and often diagnostic for many conditions
  - Acute anal fissure presents as an anal tear (typically posterior) with a tender perineum; no further workup is necessary if the history and exam are classic
  - Chronic anal fissure presents as an open ulcer with drainage and sentinel pile
  - Levator ani symptoms can be elicited by digital rectal exam
  - Proctalgia fugax symptoms cannot be elicited by exam
  - In patients with coccyodynia, palpation of the coccyx reproduces symptoms

Initial diagnostic workup

- In cases of perianal abscess, rule out anal fistula and inflammatory bowel disease (IBD)
- Colonoscopy may be indicated to rule out IBD
- If an underlying disease process is suspected, consider stool cultures, viral titers, serologies, and/or biopsy

Initial patient management

- Acute anal fissure: 90% heal within 3–4 weeks with conservative management (increased fiber and water intake, stool softeners, sitz bath, topical corticosteroids)
- Chronic anal fissure: Only 40% heal with conservative treatment; sphincterotomy is the treatment of choice, but this carries a risk of permanent incontinence
- Perianal abscess: Requires incision and drainage, followed by packing and sitz baths until healed
- Levator ani syndrome: Decrease anal canal pressure via digital massage (3–4 per week), sitz baths, muscle relaxants
- Proctalgia fugax: Self-limited, infrequent, brief attacks; primary treatment is reassurance; treat any underlying psychologic disorders
- Coccyodynia: Warm sitz baths, analgesics, and corticosteroid injections; coccygectomy may be indicated in rare cases
- Thrombosed hemorrhoid: incision and drainage or surgical excision

DIFFERENTIAL DIAGNOSIS

- Anal fissure
  - Acute fissure presents with pain and bleeding (noticed on toilet paper) immediately following defecation
  - Chronic fissure presents with long-standing itching and mild pain, with or without bleeding
- Perirectal abscess (with or without associated fistula formation)
- Thrombosed hemorrhoid
- Levator ani syndrome
- Proctalgia fugax (rectal muscle spasm)
- Coccyodynia/coccygodynia
- Fecal impaction
- Neoplasm (rectal, pelvic, or cauda equina)
- Inflammatory bowel disease (IBD) (ulcerative proctitis, Crohn's disease)
- Solitary rectal ulcer syndrome
  - A misnomer: May be multiple, not restricted to the rectum, and polypoid
  - Neoplasm is a concern
- Pruritus ani
- Trauma
- Anal sex
- Constipation
- Diarrhea
- Idiopathic

Less common causes

- Familial rectal pain
- Endometriosis
- Pelvic inflammatory disease
- Prostatitis
- Myopathies
- Foreign body
- Compression or inflammation of a sacral nerve

Red Eye

INTRODUCTION

Red eye is a diagnostic sign of ocular inflammation. It is a common presenting complaint with numerous causes, most of which are benign and can be managed effectively by a primary care physician. Misdiagnosis of emergent conditions, however, can result in loss of vision. Red eye refers to hyperemia or injection of the superficial vessels of the conjunctiva, episclera, or sclera, and it may be caused by disorders of these structures in addition to disorders of the cornea, iris, ciliary body, or ocular adnexa. Common etiologies include infections, inflammation, trauma, and glaucoma. A careful history, visual acuity testing, and penlight examination may suggest the diagnosis or reveal "red flag" findings that warrant ophthalmologic referral.

DIAGNOSTIC WORKUP & INITIAL MANAGEMENT

History and physical examination

- Note onset, duration, visual changes, pain, photophobia or fever, history of head or eye trauma, previous eye surgeries, use of contact lenses, and medications (blood thinners)
- Note characteristics of associated discharge (clarity, color, and consistency)
- Note history of comorbid conditions (e.g., autoimmune disorders, hypertension, diabetes) that may have associated ocular symptoms
- Physical exam should include testing for visual acuity, extraocular muscle function, pupil reactivity and size, photophobia, disc assessment, and eyelid inspection with eversion
- "Red flags" that suggest immediate ophthalmology referral include photophobia, deep pain, corneal opacification, acute vision changes, nausea/vomiting, blurred disc margins
  - Severe pain often indicates a more serious condition (e.g., elevated intraocular pressure, scleritis, infectious keratitis, endophthalmitis)
  - "Spontaneous" subconjunctival hemorrhage is usually asymptomatic and often caused by Valsalva maneuver (e.g., sneezing, coughing), especially if taking blood thinners
  - Subconjunctival hemorrhage in a patient with a history of trauma warrants immediate ophthalmologic evaluation to rule out intraocular foreign body or intraocular damage

Initial diagnostic workup

- Slit-lamp exam with or without fluorescein dye may help to locate foreign bodies or corneal pathology; may also show anterior chamber reaction/inflammation caused by uveitis, keratitis, scleritis, corneal ulcer, or gonococcal or bacterial infection
- Labs may include culture and sensitivities for suspected infections, CBC and ESR for suspected inflammatory causes, and ANCA if scleritis is present

Initial patient management

- Consider ophthalmologic referral, particularly for herpes simplex or herpes zoster keratitis or conjunctivitis, acute angle-closure glaucoma, scleritis, episcleritis, corneal ulcer, iritis, penetrating foreign bodies, and chemical injuries
- Avoid treating patients with steroid drops without first consulting an ophthalmologist
- Treat the underlying etiology as necessary
  - Allergic conjunctivitis: Avoid offending agents; use cold compress, NSAIDs, ocular decongestants, antihistamines
  - Viral conjunctivitis: Avoid spread with meticulous hand washing and hygiene; provide symptomatic relief (cool compress, artificial tears, topical antihistamine)
  - Bacterial conjunctivitis: Antibiotic eye drops (avoid neomycin)
  - Subconjunctival hemorrhage: Clears spontaneously in 1–2 weeks; cool compress
  - Dry eye syndrome: Lubricating artificial tears
  - Foreign body: Anesthetize with proparacaine, remove with vigorous irrigation or cotton-tipped applicator using a slit-lamp microscope, and treat with antibiotic drops
  - Corneal abrasion: Topical antibiotic drops or ointment and pressure patch

DIFFERENTIAL DIAGNOSIS

Conjunctivitis
- May be caused by allergies, viruses (e.g., adenovirus, HSV, varicella), or bacteria (e.g., staphylococci, streptococci, *Pseudomonas*)

Keratitis
- Inflammation of the cornea caused by HSV, herpes zoster, bacteria, UV light, contact lenses (infections with *Acanthamoeba* or *Pseudomonas*), or dry eye syndrome

Anterior uveitis (iritis)
- Inflammation of iris and ciliary body; most often idiopathic but may be associated with trauma, infection (e.g., tuberculosis, syphilis, herpes, Lyme disease), sarcoidosis, or connective tissue diseases (e.g., rheumatoid arthritis, SLE, Sjögren's syndrome)

Scleritis
- Inflammation of the sclera and deep layers of the globe
- May be the initial symptom of connective tissue disease or infection

Episcleritis
- A benign, self-limited inflammation superficial to the sclera
- Often idiopathic but may be associated with connective tissue disease or infection

Keratoconjunctivitis sicca
- A common cause of dry, red eyes
- May result from drugs (e.g., antihistamines, anticholinergics), Sjögren's syndrome, rheumatoid arthritis, or sarcoidosis

Subconjunctival hemorrhage
- Benign rupture of small vessels caused by underlying coagulopathy, trauma, coughing, or excessive eye rubbing

Other
- Corneal abrasion, ulceration, or perforation
- Acute angle-closure glaucoma
- Pinguecula
- Pterygium
- Trauma (foreign body, globe injury)
- Chemical burns (e.g., cyanoacrylate injury)
- Orbital cellulitis (especially in children)
- Acute ethmoiditis
- Eyelid abnormalities
- Trichiasis
- Entropion or ectropion
- Molluscum contagiosum
- Kawasaki's disease
- Measles
- UV radiation–induced photokeratitis
- Pseudotumor cerebri
- Blepharitis
- Dacrocystitis
- Endophthalmitis

Restless Legs

INTRODUCTION

Restless legs is one of the most common causes of insomnia. It is a common complaint that cannot simply be diagnosed as "restless legs syndrome" without an appropriate evaluation to assess for other etiologies. A careful sleep and medication history, coupled with a complete neurologic examination, are often all that are needed to establish the correct diagnosis.

DIAGNOSTIC WORKUP & INITIAL MANAGEMENT

History and physical examination
- Inquire about sleep patterns and sleep history from patient and bed partner
- Determine whether pain is relieved by movement
- Include complete medication history (e.g., tricyclic antidepressants are often prescribed for insomnia but tend to worsen restless legs)

Initial diagnostic workup
- Initial laboratory testing may include CBC, iron studies, fasting glucose, BUN and creatinine, electrolytes, calcium, magnesium, TSH, vitamin B_{12}, and pregnancy test
- If anemic, a workup for blood loss is warranted (e.g., colon and upper GI evaluation, urinalysis for hematuria, consider endometrial biopsy in older women)
- Sleep study may be indicated to define sleep pathology

Initial patient management
- Withdraw medications that may cause extrapyramidal side effects (e.g., tricyclic antidepressants, reserpine, propranolol, phenothiazines, metoclopramide, methyldopa, haloperidol, oral contraceptive pills)
- Treat anemia with iron replacement and treatment of underlying pathology (e.g., colon cancer)
- Dopamine agonists (e.g., carbidopa plus levodopa, pergolide, pramipexole, ropinirole) are often useful
- Carbamazepine is useful but may result in cognitive impairment and fatigue
- Gabapentin has been very effective and has fewer side effects (especially useful in patients with concomitant neuropathy)
- Clonidine is useful in patients with hypertension
- Narcotics may be used for short-term relief
- Offer emotional support

DIFFERENTIAL DIAGNOSIS

Normal snoring with periodic limb movements
- Should occur primarily during sleep but not with rest

Nocturnal leg cramps
- Associated with painful, crampy calves

Chronic insomnia
- Sleep-related breathing disorders
- Medical comorbidities (e.g., sleep apnea, congestive heart failure, COPD, asthma, chronic pain syndromes, GERD)
- Psychological disorders (e.g., depression, anxiety)
- Sleep anxiety

Sleep disturbance caused by medication/drugs
- Commonly associated with decongestants, steroids, caffeine, and β-blockers
- May be caused by withdrawal from tobacco, alcohol, or illicit drugs
- Akathisia (e.g., neuroleptics, dopamine antagonists, drug withdrawal)
- Extrapyramidal symptoms caused by medications (e.g., dystonic reaction, pseudoparkinsonism, neuroleptic malignant syndrome from antipsychotics)

Restless legs syndrome
- Feelings of creeping, crawling, burning, pulling, itching, tugging, and discomfort in the legs that are relieved by involuntary leg movement
- Most patients are >50 years
- Often unilateral
- Positive family history in one-third of cases
- Symptoms are exacerbated by pregnancy, end-stage renal failure (dialysis increases restless legs activity; kidney transplant improves symptoms), and some medications (e.g., lithium antidepressants, dopamine antagonists)

Peripheral neuropathy
- Associated with numbness, tingling, and pain
- Leg pain not relieved by movement
- Consider diabetes and vitamin B_{12} deficiency

Other
- Peripheral vascular disease
- Deep venous thrombosis
- Venous stasis
- Delayed deep sleep syndrome
- Hyperthyroidism
- Sleep deprivation
- Spinal cord or vertebral disc disease
- Periodic limb movement disorder

Romberg's Sign

INTRODUCTION

Romberg testing is used to examine proprioception. The test is performed by having the patient stand with feet together and eyes closed, which eliminates the visual cues that help to maintain posture. Patients with diminished proprioception begin to fall or move their feet to maintain balance. Patients with vestibular dysfunction may also exhibit Romberg's sign, although eye closure simply potentiates this form of unsteadiness. With true sensory loss, there is often no unsteadiness until the eyes are closed.

DIAGNOSTIC WORKUP & INITIAL MANAGEMENT

History and physical examination

- Include a comprehensive neurologic exam, including Romberg's sign
- Be sure to include other tests of proprioception, cerebellar function, and strength (e.g., finger-to-nose testing)
- Most patients with a positive Romberg's sign will also exhibit abnormal proprioception and vibratory testing

Initial diagnostic workup

- Laboratory testing may include CBC, electrolytes, glucose, calcium, BUN and creatinine, ESR, vitamin B_{12} and folate levels, RPR, drug screen, and serum and urine protein electrophoresis
- EMG and nerve conduction studies are the best way to document or exclude a large-fiber, sensory neuropathy
- MRI is the most effective imaging option if suspect structural spinal cord or cerebellar disease
- CSF examination may suggest the etiology (e.g., elevated protein in Miller-Fisher variant of Guillain-Barré syndrome, presence of oligoclonal bands or elevated IgG index in multiple sclerosis)

Initial patient management

- Point out that to prevent falls, patients need to exercise caution when standing with eyes closed (e.g., standing under the shower) or in poor lighting (e.g., when going to the restroom at night)
- Assistive devices (e.g., cane, walker) may be useful
- Surgical therapy may be necessary for compressive myelopathy (e.g., spondylotic myelopathy)
- Supplementation as necessary for deficiency states
  - Patients with vitamin B_{12} deficiency require further evaluation to determine the cause of the underlying deficiency and whether parenteral supplementation is necessary
- Eliminate exposure to offending toxic substances
- Infectious causes may be treated with the appropriate anti-infective agent (e.g., penicillin for tabes dorsalis)

DIFFERENTIAL DIAGNOSIS

Myelopathy
- Multiple sclerosis
- Vitamin B_{12} deficiency
- Structural spinal cord disease (e.g., spondylotic myelopathy, tumor)
- Infectious myelopathy (e.g., tabes dorsalis, HIV-related vacuolar myelopathy)

Peripheral neuropathy
- Vitamin B_{12} deficiency
- Chronic idiopathic demyelinating polyneuropathy (CIDP)
- Monoclonal gammopathy of unknown significance (MGUS)
- Inherited demyelinating neuropathies (e.g., Charcot-Marie-Tooth disease)

Cerebellar dysfunction
- Multiple causes (e.g., stroke, brain tumor)
- Most patients with midline cerebellar dysfunction have difficulty standing on a narrow base; this effect will not appreciably worsen with eye closure

Vestibular dysfunction (peripheral)
- Vestibulopathy
- Acoustic schwannoma

Drug intoxication
- Alcohol
- Cisplatin
- Pyridoxine (vitamin B_6) overdose
- Anticonvulsant toxicity (especially phenytoin) may cause difficulty standing on a narrow base, but this may not necessarily worsen with eye closure

Other
- Friedreich's ataxia
- Miller-Fisher variant of Guillain-Barré syndrome
- Paraneoplastic sensory neuropathy
- Vitamin E deficiency

Scalp Rash

INTRODUCTION

Scalp dermatitis or infection is easy to diagnose, but it can be challenging to treat. Topical therapy or topical plus systemic therapy for prolonged periods are often necessary to successfully control these disorders. Seborrheic dermatitis is a chronic condition that can be managed successfully but is rarely "cured," whereas tinea capitis is usually treated successfully and resolves completely. Scalp lesions caused by psoriasis and discoid lupus erythematosus must be treated as aspects of systemic disease.

DIAGNOSTIC WORKUP & INITIAL MANAGEMENT

History and physical examination
- Assess onset, duration, characteristics, associated symptoms (e.g., pruritis, constitutional symptoms, joint pain), medical history, family history, and medications
- If the scalp scale is nonadherent and greasy, yellow, or white, seborrheic dermatitis is the likely diagnosis

Initial diagnostic workup
- Bacterial culture from any intact scalp pustule or suppurating area may be helpful to confirm bacterial folliculitis or dissecting cellulitis
- KOH prep of scalp scale or scalp hair can be assessed under a microscope in the office to confirm presence of fungus in the hair or branching hyphae in the scalp scale
- Fungal cultures can be obtained from the drainage of a kerion or from a scalp scale scraped by a tongue depressor or sterile toothbrush
  - Hairs from the affected area may be sent for fungal culture to rule out tinea capitis; hairs must be plucked so that the root is available
  - Cultures may take several weeks, and sensitivities vary widely based on clinician technique and lab handling
- A punch or shave biopsy is usually unnecessary but can aid in the diagnosis of seborrheic dermatitis
- Some fungi that cause tinea capitis will fluoresce under a Wood's lamp

Initial patient management
- Treat seborrheic dermatitis with zinc pyrithione, ketoconazole, tar, and salicylic acid shampoos
  - If monotherapy fails, addition of a topical steroid solution or ointment (e.g., betamethasone, fluocinonide) during flare-ups may be useful
- Treat tinea capitis and kerion with systemic antifungal therapy (e.g., griseofulvin, diflucan, terbenafine, ketoconazole, itraconazole) for 4–8 weeks
- Treat scalp folliculitis with a short course (2–4 weeks) of first-generation cephalosporin or tetracycline derivative
  - Topical clindamycin or erythromycin solutions may also be used
- Treat discoid lupus erythematosus with intralesional steroid injections and/or systemic treatments aimed at the underlying disease
- Treat psoriasis with combination salicylic acid or tar shampoos and topical steroids; if severe, systemic therapy may be necessary, including methotrexate, biologic therapies, or cyclosporine
- Treat dissecting cellulitis by incision and drainage of suppurative lesions, intralesional steroids, and systemic retinoids or antibiotic therapy

DIFFERENTIAL DIAGNOSIS

Seborrheic dermatitis ("cradle cap," "dandruff")
- An inflammatory condition that causes itching; loose, yellow-white scale on scalp; and occasionally, blepharitis
- The most common scalp condition; occurs across all age ranges
- May be caused by *Pityrosporum ovale*
- May also affect the eyebrows, nasolabial folds, external auditory canals, chin, anterior chest, upper back, and groin
- Does not usually cause hair loss
- The scalp and other affected skin areas may be red, greasy, or oily

Tinea capitis
- Most commonly caused by *Trichophyton tonsurans* or, rarely, *Microsporum canis*
- Presents as patches of scale and/or pruritus with broken hairs and patchy hair loss ("black dot alopecia")
- May progress to a kerion

Kerion
- A boggy, tender, subcutaneous fungal (dermatophyte) infection
- Often has associated drainage and hair loss
- Often requires treatment with both oral antifungals and steroids

Scalp folliculitis
- Presents as recurrent, itchy, crusted papules or pustules
- May be caused by an overgrowth of *Staphylococcus aureus*

Psoriasis
- Usually presents with plaques of thick, silvery, adherent scalp scale that overlies well-demarcated patches of erythema
- Often occurs at the ears and occipital area
- May be limited to the scalp but is often associated with skin disease, nail pitting, or nail dystrophy

Dissecting cellulitis of the scalp
- Chronic, tender, boggy, often suppurative, subcutaneous fluctuant masses
- Often occurs in black patients
- May be associated with acne keloidalis, which can cause a scarring hair loss at the occiput

Discoid lupus erythematosus
- Presents initially as well-demarcated, erythematous plaques of patchy, scarring scalp hair loss, then spreads centrifugally

Scoliosis and Kyphosis

INTRODUCTION

Some degree of curvature of the spine is normal. Looking at the patient from the side, there is an outward (concave) curve to the thoracic spine ("kyphosis") and an inward (convex) curve to the cervical and lumbar spine ("lordosis"). Too much kyphosis leads to a hunched posture; too much lordosis leads to a "swayback" posture. Scoliosis refers to curvature of the spine that is apparent when the patient faces away from you. It is defined as a measured, lateral deviation of the normal vertical orientation of the spine by >10°. Scoliosis is always abnormal. Idiopathic scoliosis accounts for 80% of patients with structural scoliosis and is divided into three groups: infantile, juvenile, and adolescent. Of these, adolescent scoliosis is the most common. School-based screening programs facilitate early diagnosis, but most cases do not require treatment.

DIAGNOSTIC WORKUP & INITIAL MANAGEMENT

Scoliosis

- The Scoliosis Research Society recommends screening children between 10–14 years of age; the American Academy of Pediatrics recommends screening at ages 10, 12, 14, and 16 years
- A measurement of ≥7° trunk rotation should prompt an orthopedic referral
- Evaluate medical history, family history (strong family history; possible autosomal dominant inheritance), pain (although back pain is uncommon, it is a presenting complaint in 20% of patients), and associated symptoms
  - When a patient complains of back pain, a thorough history and physical exam should be performed to rule out a more menacing problem (e.g., tumor, infection)
- Associated signs may include rib rotation deformity, limb-length discrepancy, shoulder slumping, protuberant hip, or waistline asymmetry
- Rotational deformities become exaggerated when the patient flexes forward at the waist
- Perform a thorough neurologic evaluation by assessing limb reflexes, abdominal reflexes, and motor/sensory examination to rule out neural axis pathology

Initial workup and management

- Standing A/P and lateral radiographs of entire spine with extra-long cassette ("scoliosis series"): Measure the curve size by Cobb angle (the angle made by a line drawn along the superior end plate of the uppermost tilted vertebra and a line drawn along the inferior end plate of the lowest vertebra in the curve)
- MRI in patients with neurologic compromise, excessive kyphosis, onset of scoliosis before age 11 years, rapid curve progression, structural abnormalities noted on plain-film radiographs, severe pain, or leftward curves
- Pulmonary function tests are indicated in severe disease to evaluate for pulmonary dysfunction caused by decreased rib cage space
- Observation alone may be sufficient, because many curves do not progress enough to require treatment; no treatment is necessary for curves < 20°
- Treatment options include bracing or surgery
  - 20–40° of deformity may require bracing (preferably worn 23 hours/day) to halt progression
  - >40° of deformity generally requires surgery (posterior spinal fusion with rods)
- Exercise and electrical stimulation have not been shown to alter the natural progression
- Treat the underlying cause if applicable (e.g., tumor)

Kyphosis

- Focused history and physical exam
- Inspect the spine for curve greater than normal (25–45°) in the thoracic spine; assess the patient's ability to extend to correct the curvature
- Rarely, supine hyperextension films are indicated
- Bracing or surgery may be indicated (similar to scoliosis)

DIFFERENTIAL DIAGNOSIS

Scoliosis

Idiopathic scoliosis (75–80% of cases)
- Usually occurs in otherwise healthy patients
- Pain and neurologic deficits are rare
- Right thoracic curve is most common (named by convex side)

Neuromuscular scoliosis
- Common with paralytic disorders (e.g., muscular dystrophy, myotonic myopathy, spinal muscular atrophy, cerebral palsy)
- More severe, almost always progressive
- Pulmonary complications occur with severe curves (>90°)

Congenital scoliosis
- Failure of formation or segmentation of the spinal vertebrae
- Rapid progression and worse prognosis are associated with unilateral unsegmented bar with contralateral hemivertebra

Limb-length discrepancy

Kyphosis

Postural roundback

Scheuermann's disease
- The second most common pediatric spinal deformity
- Cannot voluntarily correct
- Angulation occurs in the mid to low thoracic spine

Congenital kyphosis

Less common etiologies
- Post-thoracotomy
- Marfan's syndrome
- Neurofibromatosis
- Metabolic bone disorders
- Achondroplasia
- Diastrophic dwarfism
- Infection
- Tumor
- Specific neuromuscular disorders (e.g., syringomyelia, poliomyelitis, muscular dystrophy, cord tumor or trauma, cerebral palsy)

Scrotal Masses

INTRODUCTION

Scrotal masses and swelling can involve the contents or wall of the scrotum. Ultrasound should initially be used in evaluating scrotal masses, and most solid masses should be evaluated by surgical exploration. Torsion of the testis should be reduced as quickly as possible; however, surgical intervention will still be needed to prevent future torsion in the affected or contralateral testis. Swelling of the scrotum without a mass is usually associated with an underlying medical condition (e.g., heart failure, anasarca). A painless scrotal mass should be considered as testicular cancer until proven otherwise. Masses that are easily separable from the testicle are much more likely to be benign.

DIAGNOSTIC WORKUP & INITIAL MANAGEMENT

History and physical examination

- Note onset and duration of symptoms, evidence of trauma, medical history (e.g., cryptorchidism, testicular atrophy or dysgenesis), family history of testicular cancer, sexual activity, and history of genitourinary instrumentation
- Note constitutional symptoms (e.g., fever, weight loss)
- Complete review of systems, including head and neck (e.g., parotid glands are enlarged in cases of mumps), breast (e.g., gynecomastia), penis (e.g., ulcers, plaques, induration, urethral discharge), scrotum, and testicles
- Compare size, position, and tenderness of the testicles; transilluminate all masses; palpate spermatic cord and inguinal canals (explore for hernias, hidden testicles, cord tenderness); perform digital rectal exam
- Lift the testicle up over symphysis pubis: Pain is relieved in epididymitis (Prehn's sign), but there is no change in testicular torsion

Initial diagnostic workup

- Initial laboratory testing may include CBC, urinalysis, and urethral Gram's stain and culture
- Scrotal ultrasound is indicated in all patients; include Doppler flow study to assess blood flow and ischemia if suspect torsion

Initial patient management

- Testicular torsion is a surgical emergency
  - If surgery is not available, manual detorsion may be attempted
  - Detorsion maneuver: Infiltrate the spermatic cord with 10–20 mL of 1% lidocaine, then twist the testes toward the outside of the body on the affected side; successful detorsion is indicated by immediate relief of pain
- Intratesticular masses are considered to be cancer until proven otherwise; for a solid mass, consider a full workup, including chest radiography, CT of the abdomen, serum tumor markers (α-fetoprotein, β-hCG), LDH, electrolytes, BUN and creatinine, calcium, coagulation studies (PT/PTT), and urology consult; oncology consult may be necessary
- Incarcerated inguinal hernias and testicular rupture require immediate surgical repair
- Epididymitis and orchitis are treated with antibiotics
  - Patients < 35 years (presumed to be sexually acquired): Treat with ceftriaxone or a fluoroquinolone, plus doxycycline, azithromycin, or tetracycline
  - Patients > 35 years: Trimethoprim-sulfamethoxazole or a fluoroquinolone, unless history reveals that infection is sexually acquired
  - Analgesics and scrotal support may be used

DIFFERENTIAL DIAGNOSIS

Painful masses

Torsion of the spermatic cord
- Presents with sudden pain in one testicle, followed by swelling and erythema of the scrotum
- Testicle rides higher on the affected side
- Usually occurs in patients < 25 years

Epididymitis
- Testicle position is normal; tenderness is felt at the top and posterior of the testicle
- May occur at any age
- In patients < 35 years, usually sexually transmitted (e.g., *Chlamydia*, *N. gonorrhea*) or a postinfectious inflammatory reaction (prepubertal males)
- In patients > 35 years, usually caused by Enterobacteriaceae

Orchitis
- Testicle position is normal
- Usually occurs with epididymitis caused by *E. coli*, *Klebsiella*, or *Pseudomonas* or as part of mumps infection

Strangulated hernia

Trauma

Nonpainful masses

Hernia

Varicocele
- A collection of dilated tortuous veins posterior to and above the testis

Testicular cancer
- Most common in men aged 20–50 years
- 40 times more common in patients with cryptorchidism
- Generally has a gradual onset, though may only be noticed incidentally following trauma

Spermatocele
- A firm, cystic mass containing sperm above and posterior to the testis

Hydrocele
- Caused by a collection of serous fluid between the parietal and visceral layers of the tunica vaginalis
- Covers the anterior surface of the testicle
- Seen in infants, but usually closes before 1 year of age; may reappear in men > 40 years

Scrotal edema
- Caused by cardiac, hepatic, or renal failure

Epididymal cyst
- More common in males with in utero diethylstilbesterol (DES) exposure

Sperm granuloma
- Usually occurs at the site of a previous vasectomy

Less common etiologies
- Torsion of the appendices of the testis and epididymis
- Urinary extravasation
- Lipoma of the spermatic cord
- Pyogenic or granulomatous orchitis
- Chord lipoma
- Chord adenoma

Seizures/Convulsions

INTRODUCTION

Seizures are sudden, brief behavioral changes caused by an abnormal synchronization of cerebral activity. They may or may not be associated with convulsive activity. A seizure is a symptom of an underlying disease; it is not a disease in itself. Seizures are classified as generalized (global onset) or partial (focal onset). Partial seizures are further classified as complex (accompanied by a change in consciousness) or simple (no change in consciousness). During their lifetime, 10% of the population will have a single, unprovoked seizure; 1% of the population is diagnosed with epilepsy (defined as $\geq$2 unprovoked seizures).

DIAGNOSTIC WORKUP & INITIAL MANAGEMENT

History and physical examination

- An observer's account of the seizure can be useful (duration, time of onset, tongue biting, loss of bowel or bladder control); a thorough description of the seizure activity (e.g., focal vs. generalized) is most important
- Note recent illness or change in medications; note risk factors for epilepsy
- Neurologic exam should evaluate focal findings (e.g., weakness, reflex asymmetry, Babinski's sign); evidence of postictal paralysis may suggest the part of the brain involved
- General exam should evaluate for fever, elevated blood pressure, meningismus, and dermatologic abnormalities (e.g., rash, birth marks)

Initial diagnostic workup

- Initial laboratory testing includes screening for metabolic abnormalities (e.g., sodium, calcium, magnesium, glucose) or evidence of infection (e.g., blood cultures, urine cultures)
- Lumbar puncture may be indicated if the patient has fever, meningismus, or HIV
- CT may be indicated to rule out an acute bleed
- Some patients require MRI to look for structural lesions and EEG to characterize seizures; both can be performed as an outpatient once the above workup has been completed
- If in doubt, inpatient monitoring can be performed to observe seizure activity by video EEG
- Prolactin levels may be elevated but may not be specific for seizure
- CSF exam if suspect CNS infection (e.g., meningitis) or subarachnoid hemorrhage
- Consider drug screen and ethanol level

Initial patient management

- Initial treatment includes protecting the patient: Place patients on their side so they do not aspirate, and protect them from injuring themselves on sharp objects or hard surfaces; however, nothing should be placed in their mouths, and they should not be held down
- Administer supplemental oxygen
- It is common to abort the seizure with IV benzodiazepines; however, some neurologists do not recommend benzodiazepine administration immediately in a new-onset seizure patient, because it may interfere with the neurologic exam
- Remove offending intoxicants or medications, and correct metabolic abnormalities
- Treatment after the first seizure is determined by weighing the risks and benefits of medical treatment versus observation; consider withholding treatment in low-risk patients until a second seizure occurs, because most patients have only one lifetime seizure
  - If treatment is initiated, monotherapy is always preferred
  - Older antiepileptic drugs (e.g., carbamazepine, phenobarbital, valproate) are as effective as newer drugs (e.g., gabapentin, lamotrigine, topiramate, oxcarbazine); newer drugs may have fewer side effects and easier dosing and may not require frequent monitoring
  - For most seizures, valproate, carbamazepine, and phenytoin are the initial choices
- Regular sleep patterns may be important, because sleep deprivation can trigger seizures

DIFFERENTIAL DIAGNOSIS

Partial seizure (involves only part of the brain)
- Simple (no altered consciousness)
- Complex (altered consciousness)

Generalized seizure (involves both hemispheres)
- Tonic-clonic
- Atonic
- Tonic
- Myoclonic
- Absence

Epilepsy
- Recurrent, unprovoked seizures of any or multiple types, which may be idiopathic or symptomatic

Secondary seizure
- Metabolic abnormalities (e.g., electrolyte disturbances, hypoglycemia, hyperglycemia, uremia, hypoxia)
- Drug effects (e.g., amphetamines, tricyclic antidepressants, antibiotics, lidocaine), intoxication (e.g., cocaine, alcohol), or withdrawal (e.g., benzodiazepines, alcohol)
- Head injury or trauma
- Febrile seizures in children
- Structural lesions (e.g., tumor, subdural hematoma)
- Cerebrovascular etiologies (e.g., cerebral infarct, intracerebral hemorrhage, subarachnoid hemorrhage, sinus thrombosis, hypertensive encephalopathy, eclampsia)
- Cardiac arrhythmia
- Hypoxic-ischemic encephalopathy
- Infection (e.g., meningitis, encephalitis)
  - Neurocysticercosis is the most common cause of acquired epilepsy worldwide
- Degenerative dementia
- Sleep disorders (especially if seizures are purely nocturnal)

Nonepileptic seizure
- Not associated with abnormal electrical activity in the brain
- Patients with loss of consciousness secondary to cerebral hypoperfusion (fainting, syncope) may occasionally exhibit brief periods of twitching or convulsive movements resembling seizure activity
- Convulsive syncope
- Psychogenic seizures result from stressful psychological conflicts (e.g., major trauma) and almost always occur in patients with a significant underlying psychiatric history
- Conversion disorder ("pseudoseizure")
- Panic attack

Inborn errors of metabolism
- Disorders of amino acid metabolism
- Organic acidemias
- Urea cycle disorders
- Mitochondrial disorders
- Peroxisomal disorders
- Glycogen storage disorders
- Disorders of sugar metabolism

Rasmussen's encephalitis
- Causes seizures and progressive hemispheric dysfunction in infants

Idiopathic
- Cryptogenic
- Hereditary

Skin Lesions, Genital

INTRODUCTION

Skin lesions in the genital area are common, and the etiology can range from simple irritation to STDs to malignancy. The appearance of the lesion, the presence of pain and/or itching, and a description of how the lesion has changed over time can help to narrow the differential diagnosis. Genital herpes, syphilis, and chancroid are the most common causes of genital ulcers in the U.S. The CDC recommends that evaluation of all patients with genital ulcers should include a serologic test for syphilis and a diagnostic test for genital herpes; in areas where chancroid is prevalent, a test for *Haemophilus ducreyi* is also recommended. Genital ulcers are associated with an increased risk for HIV infection.

DIAGNOSTIC WORKUP & INITIAL MANAGEMENT

History and physical examination

- Assess onset, duration, characteristics, associated symptoms (e.g., fever, discharge, lymphadenopathy), medical history, sexual/social history, family history, and medications
- Presentation is often based on whether the lesion is painful and on the characteristics of associated inguinal adenopathy; however, initially painless lesions may become painful because of secondary infection
  - Herpes simplex ulcer is painful and associated with tender, nonfluctuant inguinal adenopathy
  - Chancroid ulcer is painful and has tender, fluctuant inguinal adenopathy
  - Syphilis ulcer is painless, with mildly tender adenopathy
  - Granuloma inguinale ulcer is painless and bleeds easily; firm inguinal adenopathy may mimic lymphogranuloma venereum or be absent
  - Lymphogranuloma venereum ulcer is painless and has tender, unilateral, fluctuant adenopathy; however, the ulcer is usually absent by the time the patient seeks care
  - Behçet's disease is painful, with minimal adenopathy
- Physical exam includes a complete skin and genital exams

Initial diagnostic workup

- Serology and dark-field exam or direct immunofluorescent test for *T. pallidum*; RPR or VDRL tests may also be used, but they only become positive 6–8 weeks after primary infection
- Culture and antigen testing or serology for HSV
- Culture for *H. ducreyi*
- Biopsy for unusual ulcers or ulcers that do not respond to treatment
- Complement fixation titers > 1:64 are diagnostic for lymphogranuloma venereum
- Condyloma acuminatum can be diagnosed by applying acetic acid (will turn white)
- Molluscum contagiosum is diagnosed by appearance
- Wood's lamp may be used to detect erythrasma (looks coral red)
- Shave biopsy is diagnostic for psoriasis, Zoon's balanitis, lichen planus, and neoplasms
- In older patients, lesions that are changing in size, appearance, or texture should always be biopsied to rule out carcinoma
- Patients with suspected STD require full workup for HIV, syphilis, hepatitis B/C, pregnancy

Initial patient management

- Patients should often be treated empirically for the most likely disease based on clinical presentation and epidemiologic circumstances; however, diagnosis based solely on history and physical exam is insensitive because "classic" findings are often not too common
- Treat infections with appropriate antimicrobials
- Condyloma acuminatum lesions can be destroyed with podophyllin, cryotherapy, cantherone, trichloroacetic acid, or laser ablation
- Treat psoriasis, Zoon's balanitis, and seborrheic dermatitis with topical steroids

DIFFERENTIAL DIAGNOSIS

Herpes Simplex Virus (HSV)
- The most common cause of genital lesions in the U.S.
- Presents with prodromal tingling and genital discomfort before lesions
- Lesions are always painful and appear as grouped vesicles on an erythematous base
- Can be severe and resistant to acyclovir in HIV-positive patients

Condyloma acuminatum ("genital warts")
- Caused by human papilloma virus; lesions are usually painless and pearly, with a smooth surface, but may be filiform, fungating, and/or lobulated
- If in perianal area, anal Pap smear is indicated to rule out anal dysplasia

Tinea cruris
- Inguinal erythema, with itch or tenderness and fine scale
- Generally spares the scrotum and penis

Candida intertrigo
- Inguinal erythema, with itch or tenderness; often very red, with satellite lesions
- Frequently involves the labia or scrotum

Syphilis
- Primary stage: Painless solitary ulcer (chancre) on the labia, penis, or oral mucosa that heals in 2–3 weeks
- Secondary stage: Condyloma lata (moist, hypertrophic papules on genital and oral regions)
- Tertiary stage: Cardiac, neurologic, and other systemic effects

Molluscum contagiosum
- Multiple, very small, painless, dome-shaped, skin-colored papules with umbilicated centers

Chancroid
- Painful, solitary, and erythematous lesions caused by *H. ducreyi*
- May present with dyspareunia and/or dysuria

Erythrasma
- A chronic superficial infection (*Corynebacterium minutissimum*) of the intertriginous areas

Lymphogranuloma venereum
- Caused by a strain of *Chlamydia trachomatis*
- May result in inguinal ulcerations, proctocolitis, fistulas, and strictures

Granuloma inguinale (donovanosis)
- Caused by *Calymmatobacterium granulomatis*
- Endemic in India, Papua New Guinea, central Australia, and southern Africa

Behçet's syndrome
- Oral and genital ulcers, retinitis, uveitis

Lichen planus
- Shiny, flat-topped, reddish-purple bumps of unknown etiology
- In the genital area, may present with ulcers, patches, or annular plaques; often itchy

Scabies
- Contagious infestations of the arthropod *Sarcoptes scabiei* that can cause intense pruritis
- Genital, perianal, buttocks, umbilicus, axilla, and web spaces are commonly affected areas

Zoon's plasma cell balanitis
- Inflammation of the glans characterized by subepithelial infiltration of plasma cells

Other
- Inverse psoriasis
- Genital squamous cell carcinoma
- Plaque psoriasis
- Seborrheic dermatitis
- Extramammary Paget's disease
- Fixed drug eruptions

Skin Lesions, Hand & Foot Rashes

INTRODUCTION

Hand and foot rashes are generally nonspecific, but their presence or absence might help in establishing the diagnosis for a wide variety of conditions. The palms and soles are covered with stratum corneum that is thicker than in other parts of the body and also hairless; the innervation is abundant and contains specialized receptors. Edema is likely to be noticeable early because of relative skin excess. Dyshidrotic and irritant eczema are by far the most common etiologies of hand and foot rashes.

DIAGNOSTIC WORKUP & INITIAL MANAGEMENT

History and physical examination

- Assess onset, duration, characteristics, and pattern of the rash, desquamation, edema, involvement of other areas of the body, associated symptoms (e.g., fever, pruritis, oral lesions, arthritis, genital chancre), medical history, family history (e.g., psoriasis, allergy, atopy), recent travel, medications, and social history
- Note chronic exposure to chemicals or potential irritants at work or in hobbies
- Look closely for small, clear, "water blisters" under the skin that may indicate pompholyx
- Examine nails for evidence of coexisting onychomycosis (very common in tinea pedis and manus, and a nidus for frequent reinfection), "oil spots," or nail pitting (may suggest psoriasis)
- Examine joints for arthritis (psoriasis, Reiter's syndrome), eyes (Reiter's syndrome), and genitalia (psoriasis, Reiter's syndrome)

Initial diagnostic workup

- Labs may include CBC, ESR, and various serologies depending on clinical suspicions
- Consider KOH preparation using scale scraped from the palms, soles, or between the toes to determine presence of branching hyphae of tinea or scabies mites
- Culture any intact pustules
- Consider performing a patch test to rule out allergic contact dermatitis
- A punch biopsy is not usually helpful to distinguish psoriasis or pityriasis rubra pilaris from other common eczematous diseases of the hands and feet
- Fungal culture of nail clipping if onycholysis (nail thickening) is present
- Dermatology referral is often indicated in resistant cases

Initial patient management

- Pompholyx, psoriasis, and most noninfectious hand eczemas are treated with topical, high-potency steroid ointments (e.g., temovate, diprolene) for short periods
- Irritant eczema is treated with bland, heavy emollients (e.g., petroleum jelly, mineral oil, various cream formulations with a dimethicone base) to rehydrate the skin and prevent recurrence; avoid wet work, irritants, and harsh soaps
- Tinea manuum and pedis are treated with topical antifungal preparations or a short course of oral fluconazole or terbenafine (2 weeks); if onychomycosis is present (confirmed by nail clipping and PAS stain or culture), treat with oral antifungals for 6–12 weeks
- Topical or systemic phototherapy PUVA can significantly improve palmoplantar eczemas that are refractory to topical monotherapy
- Systemic methotrexate and cyclosporine are also used to treat severe dyshidrotic disease or psoriasis

DIFFERENTIAL DIAGNOSIS

Infection

- Enterovirus infection (e.g., hand-foot-and-mouth disease, other non-polio enteroviruses)
- Kawasaki's disease
- Scabies
- Candidal skin infection
- Rickettsial rash (e.g., Rocky Mountain spotted fever, murine typhus)
- Mononucleosis
- Measles
- Scarlet fever
- Poststreptococcal infection desquamation rash
- Infectious endocarditis (Janeway lesions, Olser's nodes)
- Spirochete infection (e.g., secondary syphilis, Lyme disease)
- Toxoplasmosis
- Rat-bite fever (*Streptobacillus moniliformis, Spirillum minus*)
- Varicella
- Meningococcemia
- Erythema multiforme
- Tinea manus (hand) and tinea pedis (foot)

Immune-mediated

- Urticaria
- Rheumatoid arthritis
- SLE
- Raynaud's phenomenon
- Acute graft-versus-host disease
- Drugs (e.g., ampicillin, especially in patients with infectious mononucleosis)

Skin disorders

- Dyshidrotic eczema (pompholyx)
- Irritant or allergic hand eczema
- Psoriasis
- Reiter's syndrome
- Pityriasis rubra pilaris
- Keratoderma
- Lichen simplex
- Olmstead's syndrome
- Papillon-Lefevre syndrome
- Acrodermatitis enteropathica (zinc deficiency)

Other

- Chronic liver disease
- Metabolic disease (e.g., gangliosidosis)
- Malignancy (e.g., acute leukemia, lymphoma)

Skin Lesions, Janeway Lesions

INTRODUCTION

Janeway lesions are among the stigmata of infective endocarditis. They are irregular, erythematous, flat, painless macules that may appear on the palms, soles, and thenar and hypothenar eminences of the hands, fingertips, and plantar surfaces of the toes. In acute endocarditis, the lesions may be hemorrhagic or purple. Infective endocarditis can be diagnosed by the Duke Criteria (e.g., positive blood cultures, evidence of cardiac vegetation, fever of unknown origin, vascular phenomena). Janeway lesions are considered to be a minor criterion in the category of vascular phenomena.

DIAGNOSTIC WORKUP & INITIAL MANAGEMENT

History and physical examination

- Note history of present illness, associated symptoms, medical history (including history of endocarditis, valve surgery, structural heart disease, rheumatic fever, recent procedures including dental work, oncologic disease), family history (e.g., valve or autoimmune disease), social history (including IV drug use), HIV status, and medications
- Endocarditis most commonly presents with nonspecific symptoms, including fever, weight loss, myalgias, arthralgias, night sweats, weakness, abdominal or back pain, and new or changing heart murmur
- Physical exam should focus on cardiac, neurologic, ophthalmologic, dermatologic, and musculoskeletal systems

Initial diagnostic workup

- Echocardiography is necessary to evaluate cardiac valves and identify vegetations
- Initial testing includes blood cultures (2–3 cultures from separate sites before antibiotics are given), CBC, ESR, coagulation studies, urinalysis, chest radiography, and ECG
- Duke Criteria for diagnosis: Probable diagnosis requires 2 major criteria *or* 1 major criterion and 3 minor criteria *or* 5 minor criteria; possible diagnosis requires 1 major and 1 minor criterion *or* 3 minor criteria
  - Major criteria: Typical microorganism from 2 separate blood cultures (e.g., *S. viridans, S. bovis,* HACEK group, community-acquired *S. aureus, Enterococcus*) or persistently positive blood cultures for any microorganism; evidence of endocardial involvement; vegetation on echocardiogram; oscillating intracardiac mass on valve or supporting structures or in the path of regurgitant jets; perivalvular abscess; new valvular regurgitation
  - Minor criteria: Predisposing heart condition; IV drug use; fever > 38°C; vascular phenomena (e.g., arterial embolism, septic pulmonary infarcts, mycotic aneurysm, Janeway lesions); immunologic phenomena (e.g., Osler's nodes, Roth's spots, glomerulonephritis, rheumatoid factor), echocardiographic findings not meeting major criteria, microbiologic evidence (e.g., positive blood culture but not meeting major criterion above)
- Biopsy of skin lesions may reveal neutrophilic dermal microabscesses; organisms may or may not be found

Initial patient management

- Hospitalization is usually required for initial treatment with IV antibiotics
- Begin organism-specific antibiotics as soon as cultures and sensitivities are available
  - The penicillins or vancomycin, often in combination with an aminoglycoside (e.g., gentamicin), are cornerstones of antibiotic therapy and may be necessary for 4–6 weeks
- Obtain surveillance blood cultures during the early phase of therapy to ensure eradication
- Valve surgery may be required if infection cannot be controlled medically
- Treat other etiologies by established treatment protocols

DIFFERENTIAL DIAGNOSIS

Acute bacterial endocarditis
- Common organisms include *Staphylococcus aureus*, *Streptococcus pneumoniae*, and *Streptococcus pyogenes*

Subacute bacterial endocarditis
- Most common organisms include *Streptococcus viridans*, enterococci, *Staphylococcus epidermidis*, and fungi

Sterile valve vegetations
- Libman-Sacks endocarditis
- Marantic endocarditis
- Atrial myxoma

Extracardiac infections
- Meningococcemia
- Rocky Mountain spotted fever
- Secondary syphilis
- Infected intravascular device
- Abscess
- Osteomyelitis
- Typhoid fever
- Enterovirus infection (echovirus or coxsackievirus)

Other
- Systemic lupus erythematosus (SLE)
- Thrombotic thrombocytopenic purpura (TTP)
- Idiopathic thrombocytopenic purpura
- Polyarteritis nodosa
- Cutaneous vasculitis
- Immune complex disease
- Serum sickness
- Drug allergy
- Lymphoma
- Erythema multiforme
- Disseminated intravascular coagulation (DIC)
- Lambl's excrescences ("wear and tear" valvular lesions)

Skin Lesions, Nodular

INTRODUCTION

A palpable lesion < 1 cm in size is known as a papule. Nodules are often > 1 cm, palpable, and have significant substance to them. Nodules can be on the skin (exophytic), within the skin (intraepidermal or dermal), or beneath the skin (subcutaneous). The differential diagnosis of skin nodules is enormous. The color, rapidity of appearance or growth, associated symptomatology, and underlying medical condition of the patient guide the workup and diagnosis.

DIAGNOSTIC WORKUP & INITIAL MANAGEMENT

History and physical examination

- Assess onset, duration, characteristics, associated symptoms, medical history, family history, and medications
  - Note whether the lesion is changing in appearance or increasing in size
  - Note whether the lesion is tender or symptomatic
  - Note medical history of cutaneous or systemic malignancies and arthritis (e.g., gout, rheumatoid disease)
  - Note immunosuppression, which makes patients more vulnerable to malignant skin nodules
  - Note family history of melanoma and/or lipomas

Initial diagnostic workup

- When in doubt, skin biopsy is indicated
  - Shave biopsy is sufficient for exophytic lesions
  - Punch, excisional, or incisional biopsy may be warranted for intradermal or subcutaneous nodules
  - Excisional, full-thickness biopsy allows full staging when melanoma is considered
- Obtain appropriate cultures from tender or suppurative lesions

Initial patient management

- Treatment depends on the diagnosis and often includes excision for symptomatic and/or cosmetic purposes
- Epidermoid cysts are generally removed
  - Lesions that are actively inflamed must "cool down" before excision can be performed successfully
  - Intralesional steroids and/or oral first-generation cephalosporins will cause the inflammatory reaction to subside more quickly
  - Incision and drainage is indicated for tense and painful, inflamed cysts
  - Once the infection and/or inflammation has resolved, the cyst can be excised
  - The cyst must be marsupialized (the entire cyst contents and its complete lining must be removed) to prevent recurrence

DIFFERENTIAL DIAGNOSIS

Epidermoid or epidermal inclusion cyst
- These may change in size, become intermittently tender and erythematous, or even have a central punctum with extrusion of caseous or "cheesy" material
- Although benign, these lesions may become secondarily infected

Pilar cyst
- Usually occurs on the scalp
- Usually asymptomatic

Dermatofibroma
- Flesh-colored or hyperpigmented, fibrous lesions that dimple when pinched
- May occur after minor trauma
- Common on the lower extremities

Pyogenic granuloma
- Erythematous, papular, friable lesion caused by capillary proliferation
- May occur after minor trauma
- Bleeds easily
- May regress on their own, but can be easily removed surgically

Ganglion cyst
- A somewhat mobile lesion that appears most frequently on the dorsal wrist or over the joints of the hands

Lipoma
- Common; usually nontender, freely mobile, very soft, and pliable

Erythema nodosum
- Tender, erythematous nodules, usually on the shins
- Can be associated with many disorders, including sarcoidosis, inflammatory bowel disease, and infections, or it may be idiopathic
- Treatment is based on the underlying disease

Nodular vasculitis (erythema induratum)
- Seen on the posterior lower legs
- Associated with tuberculosis

Panniculitis
- Generally tender, erythematous nodules or plaques on the legs
- Results from a variety of causes, including vasculitis, pancreatic disease, arterial disease, trauma, and post–steroid injection

Other
- Many benign neoplasms of the skin present as indolent dermal nodules
- Dermal or subcutaneous neoplasms can arise from the hair follicle, sweat glands, blood vessels (hemangiomas), or nerves (neurofibromas)
- Subcutaneous nodules on the extensor surface of joints may be tender, which may indicate gout, calcification of the bursa or calcinosis cutis (seen in renal failure), or rheumatoid nodules
- Nodular melanomas, metastatic tumors, and lymphomas can present as isolated skin nodules that appear suddenly and/or grow rapidly in size
- Hypertrophic scars and keloids can appear as pink, tender skin nodules
- Yellow skin nodules (e.g., xanthomas) may portend an underlying lipid disorder
- Red skin nodules may indicate bacillary angiomatosis or other infection
- Kaposi's sarcoma may present as purplish skin nodules and tumors

Skin Lesions, Papulosquamous

INTRODUCTION

Papulosquamous skin lesions are red, scaly, and often papular in appearance. Papulosquamous rashes are defined as exanthems that have palpable epidermal changes with scale. The potential diagnoses are quite broad and must be considered systematically on the basis of history and physical examination and, occasionally, with a biopsy. The distribution of the lesions is a key characteristic in establishing the diagnosis.

DIAGNOSTIC WORKUP & INITIAL MANAGEMENT

History and physical examination

- Evaluate onset, duration, characteristics, associated symptoms, medical history, family history of psoriasis and other skin diseases, and medications
- Assess fingernails for pitting, subungual debris, distal separation of the nail plate from the nail bed (called onycholysis), and "oil spots" (extravasated proteins under the nail) that are characteristic of psoriasis; always consider psoriasis if the scale is markedly silver and very thick or is adherent to the skin
- Seborrhea of the face and scalp is far more common than psoriasis of these areas, and it has a much thinner and lighter scale (often greasy in appearance)
- Pityriasis rosea presents in healthy, young adults after a viral prodrome; observe carefully for the larger, thicker herald patch to confirm the diagnosis; patients can often pinpoint the first patch, because it appeared several days before the more diffuse eruption
- Consider atopic dermatitis in a young patient with allergic rhinitis or asthma and a very itchy, chronic, or subacute rash that is often symmetric on the flexural skin

Initial diagnostic workup

- A KOH preparation and exam by light microscope can quickly establish the diagnosis of dermatophyte infection
- Patch testing for potential allergens and review of a patient's chemical exposure can help to rule in allergic contact or irritant dermatitis, respectively

Initial patient management

- Psoriasis can be treated with topical calcipotriene (Dovonex), topical steroids, tar and anthralin preparations, intralesional steroids, salicylic acid and UV light therapy, methotrexate, acitretin, cyclosporine, and newer biologic therapies (e.g., TNF-α inhibitors, efaluzimab
  - Avoid using systemic steroids, because they may cause severe flare-ups of the disease on completion of the course of treatment
- Pityriasis rosea is managed symptomatically, with oral antihistamines, topical steroids, topical antipruritics (e.g., sarna, calamine), and in severe cases, oral steroids, erythromycin, or phototherapy
- Atopic dermatitis must be approached as a disease of skin barrier function; it is crucial to repair that function with the use of gentle cleansers and emollient creams and/or oils

DIFFERENTIAL DIAGNOSIS

Allergic and irritant contact reactions
- A common, self-limited cause of papulosquamous lesions

Drug-induced rashes
- Almost any drug can cause a papulosquamous eruption

Psoriasis
- Affects 2% of the U.S. population
- May present acutely as guttate (drop-like), round plaques with minimal scale; this form often occurs after streptococcal infection
- Psoriasis vulgaris is more common; presents as thick plaques of silvery, adherent scale on an erythematous base on the extensor joints

Seborrheic dermatitis
- An inflammatory "dandruff" that manifests as light scale on a greasy and/or erythematous background around the hairline, upper lip, nasolabial creases, chin, external ears, eyebrow areas, and scalp
- Caused by overgrowth of *Pityrosporum ovale*

Pityriasis rosea
- A common exanthem that is self-limited; etiology is unclear
- Presents with initial "herald patch," with subsequent scaly, pink papules/plaques over the trunk in a "Christmas tree" distribution
- May be very itchy and is often confused with guttate psoriasis

Atopic dermatitis
- Common among children with a history of asthma, hay fever, or seasonal allergies
- Manifests as itchy, eczematous plaques on the antecubital and popliteal fossae
- Often becomes secondarily lichenified (thickened with chronic rubbing changes)
- 60% of patients have initial symptoms before 1 year of age
- The disease often lasts 15–20 years

Fungal infections of the skin
- Caused by dermatophytes
- Often present as itchy, scaly, papulosquamous rashes that can mimic nummular eczema

Nummular eczema
- An idiopathic disease that is common in the winter months

Lichen planus
- Presents with flat-topped, polygonal, and purplish papules that may have white streaks or "Wickham's striae"

Eczematous diseases
- Eczema craquele
- Lichen simplex chronicus

Pityriasis rubra pilaris
- A systemic disease with salmon-colored or pinkish erythroderma, with islands of sparing, yellowish desquamation of the palms and soles, nail dystrophy, and scale

Other infections
- Secondary syphilis
- Meningococcemia
- Rocky Mountain spotted fever

Skin Lesions, Pigmented

INTRODUCTION

Pigmented skin lesions are extremely common. The more common lesions are benign, but the physician must accurately rule out a malignant lesion or biopsy the lesion for a definitive diagnosis. Nevi, seborrheic keratoses, and dermatofibromas are common benign lesions that often require evaluation by a physician. In children, certain pigmented lesions may be a sign of a genetic syndrome.

DIAGNOSTIC WORKUP & INITIAL MANAGEMENT

History and physical examination

- Note changes in appearance of the lesion, pruritis, increase in size, or frequent bleeding or irritation
- Note "ABCD" changes to predict malignancy and need for biopsy:
  - Asymmetry
  - Borders (irregular, jagged, streaked, or "faded" edges)
  - Color (>1 color; gray or black pigment or loss of pigment within borders of a lesion)
  - Diameter (consider biopsy for lesions > 6 mm in diameter)
- Moles newly acquired after 40 years of age should be closely examined for dysplasia and malignancy
- Note family history of malignant melanoma and personal history of skin cancer or abnormal moles removed in the past
- Patients with light skin and blue eyes have a higher risk of abnormal moles and malignant melanoma
- Patients with >50 nevi, a history of dysplastic nevi, or a strong history of sun exposure are also at higher risk for melanoma

Initial diagnostic workup

- When in doubt, perform a biopsy
  - Shave biopsy is adequate for suspected actinic keratoses or seborrheic keratoses
  - Punch biopsy of the entire lesion or excisional biopsy to sample the entire depth of the lesion is indicated if suspect a dysplastic nevus or melanoma
- Consider referral to a dermatologist or plastic surgeon if an appropriate differential diagnosis cannot be made or if melanoma is possible

Initial patient management

- All patients should use sunscreen to prevent solar-induced lesions
- Pigmented actinic keratoses and seborrheic keratoses can be successfully removed with topical cryotherapy
- Solar lentigines and freckles are benign; if desired, they can be removed with lasers and intense pulsed light sources
  - Solar lentigines may be lightened by topical hydroquinones and retinoids
- Patients with dysplastic nevi or history of malignant melanoma require (at least) annual full skin exams by a dermatologist and close follow-up of their nevi with body mapping, if possible

DIFFERENTIAL DIAGNOSIS

Benign mole (nevus)
- May be junctional (flat, pigmented), compound (usually raised and pigmented), or dermal (raised, usually not pigmented)

Seborrheic keratosis
- Very common and benign; increase in number with age
- Pink to dark brown; appear as "stuck on" skin; usually waxy and rough

Freckle (ephelides)
- Very common and benign

Solar lentigo ("liver spot" or "sunspot")
- Light- to dark-brown macules up to 2 cm in diameter; very common on the face, hands, and other sun-exposed areas
- If multicolored or abnormal borders, consider a diagnosis of lentigo maligna melanoma, which requires biopsy

Dermatofibroma
- A firm, nodular, asymptomatic or slightly pruritic, often hyperpigmented or violaceous lesion, most often on the lower extremities
- May result from minor trauma (e.g., a scratch or insect bite), but the cause is generally unknown
- Dermatofibromas have a positive "dimple" sign: When squeezed between two fingers, the subcutaneous lesion puckers down into the skin

Dysplastic nevus ("atypical moles")
- May be sporadic or familial; may have "ABCD" changes
- 5–10% risk of malignant melanoma

Blue nevus
- Usually benign; deep dermal pigmentation gives blue color

Malignant melanoma
- May have malignant "ABCD" changes
- The superficial spreading type is most common; other subtypes include acral lentiginous, nodular, and lentigo maligna
- May arise in acquired, dysplastic, or congenital nevi, de novo on normal skin, or extracutaneous (e.g., ocular, leptomeningeal)
- Risk factors are fair skin, >50–100 nevi, multiple dysplastic nevi, excessive sun exposure, xeroderma pigmentosum, immunosuppression, and certain genetic syndromes

Cafe-au-lait macule
- Light brown; present at birth or shortly thereafter in 10% of children
- Consider neurofibromatosis if ≥5 cafe-au-lait spots of >1.5 cm in diameter and axillary freckling are present after puberty
- May also be seen in McCune-Albright syndrome, tuberous sclerosis, and Bloom's syndrome

Other
- Pregnancy
- Oral contraceptive use
- Postinflammatory hyperpigmentation
- Nevus spilus
- Pigmented actinic keratosis
- Pigmented basal cell carcinoma
- Mongolian spots
- Congenital melanocytic nevi
- Other nevi: Becker's, Spitz, halo, blue, Ito's/Ota's, zosteriform, lentiginous
- Tinea versicolor (caused by the fungus *Malassezia furfur*)
- Urticaria pigmentosa (most common form of mastocytosis)
- Incontinentia pigmenti

Skin Lesions, Vesicular and Bullous

INTRODUCTION

A vesicle is a small, discrete, clear fluid–containing bubble on the skin. It is <1 cm, whereas a bulla is >1 cm. Vesicles and bullae can result from a variety of causes, including infection, contact dermatitis (e.g., poison ivy or oak), and autoimmune disorders.

DIAGNOSTIC WORKUP & INITIAL MANAGEMENT

History and physical examination

- Assess onset, duration, characteristics, associated symptoms, exposure history (especially to outdoor weeds), medical history, family history, and medications
- Determine whether the lesions are focal or diffuse
- Include a thorough review of systems
- Physical exam should include a thorough skin exam

Initial diagnostic workup

- Culture from bullous lesions is not usually indicated because most bullous reactions to bacteria are caused by toxin production (thus, bacteria are not commonly found)
- Consider a viral etiology if the patient has low-grade fever, myalgia, pharyngitis, or other systemic symptoms
- If HSV-2 (genital herpes simplex) is the suspected etiology of a vesicular eruption, viral culture is the gold standard for diagnosis; obtain a culture by unroofing an intact vesicle and scraping the floor of the erosion; serum IgM and IgG antibodies can also aid in establishing the diagnosis
- Suspected orolabial HSV-1 infection is diagnosed based on a history of similar recurrent episodes; culture may also be obtained as above
- Tzanck smear may also be done for suspected HSV or varicella infection
- If suspect varicella zoster, direct fluorescent antibody testing yields quick results
- Skin biopsy with direct immunofluorescence if suspect autoimmune blistering disease
- In patients with widespread bullae, consider incipient toxic epidermal necrolysis; skin biopsy may aid in the diagnosis, but because this disease can quickly prove fatal, frozen sections must be examined urgently

Initial patient management

- Topical or systemic steroids may be needed for severe contact dermatitis
- Herpes simplex and zoster can be treated with antiviral medications (e.g., acyclovir, famciclovir); early therapy may decrease the risk of postherpetic neuralgia
- Bullous impetigo can be treated with topical mupirocin or systemic antibiotics (e.g., erythromycin, cephalexin)
- Dyshidrotic eczema can be difficult to treat; it is not curable but can be controlled with high-potency topical steroids ointments and heavy emollients
- Polymorphous light eruption is preventable with sun avoidance and zinc- or titanium-based sunblocks; topical steroids can diminish the pruritus that accompanies an episode
- Stevens-Johnson syndrome and toxic epidermal necrolysis are treated supportively along with discontinuation of the offending drug; patients may require specialized care in a burn center; IVIG is sometimes used
- Systemic immunosuppressants (e.g., prednisone, cyclosporine, azathioprine) are often necessary to control autoimmune bullous diseases (e.g., pemphigus vulgaris)

DIFFERENTIAL DIAGNOSIS

Localized

Allergic contact dermatitis (e.g., rhus)
- Localized vesicular and bullous eruptions

Varicella zoster (shingles)
- Caused by reactivation of latent varicella zoster virus
- Presents as painful vesicles on an erythematous base in a dermatomal distribution, beginning with fever, dysesthesia, and/or malaise

Herpes simplex virus (HSV)
- Herpetic lesions present as painful, recurrent vesicles on an erythematous base
- HSV-1 usually affects the oral mucosa and vermilion border
- Genital HSV (most commonly HSV-2) may manifest as nonspecific symptoms (e.g., dysuria, urethritis)

Bullous impetigo
- Most common in children
- Presents as flaccid vesicles and bullae with honey-colored crust

Burns and friction blisters
- Common causes of bullae, especially on hands

Dyshidrotic eczema (pompholyx)
- Causes itching, scaling, erythema, minute vesicles, and painful fissures

Other
- Insect bite
- Many viral infections of childhood can present with focal vesicles, especially hand-foot-and-mouth disease
- Diabetics can develop bullae on the legs

Diffuse

Polymorphous light eruption
- A common reaction to UV light
- Presents as itchy vesicles or erythematous papules on sun-exposed areas

Varicella ("chickenpox")
- Presents with vesicles in crops and in many stages of evolution

Stevens-Johnson syndrome and toxic epidermal necrolysis
- Serious skin disorders that cause epidermal sloughing and significant mortality
- These are severe forms of erythema multiforme
- Nearly all cases result from drug reactions (e.g., sulfonamides, certain antibiotics, anticonvulsants)
- Following a 1- to 3-day, flu-like prodrome, an erythematous, confluent, morbilliform or bullous eruption occurs that rapidly evolves into exfoliation of the skin at the dermal–epidermal junction, resulting in large sheets of necrotic epidermis and underlying shiny, denuded dermal surface

Blistering diseases (present with coalescing vesicles and bullae)
- Bullous pemphigoid
- Pemphigus vulgaris
- Porphyria cutanea tarda
- Epidermolysis bullosa

Sore Throat

INTRODUCTION

Sore throat is a common symptom. Most cases are caused by infection, and many patients incorrectly believe that antibiotics improve the clinical course. Although the vast majority of sore throats are of viral origin and should be managed conservatively, an appropriate history and physical examination usually identify other causes of sore throat. Use of the clinical criteria listed below to determine the likelihood of streptococcal pharyngitis will assist in making the workup more accurate and cost-effective.

DIAGNOSTIC WORKUP & INITIAL MANAGEMENT

History and physical examination

- History and physical exam is often sufficient to establish the diagnosis
- Assess onset, duration, severity, frequency, and associated symptoms (e.g., odynophagia, dysphagia, fever, malaise, headache)
- Consider age, exposure history, medical history (e.g., immunocompromised states), sick contacts, use of inhaled steroids (e.g., with candidal pharyngitis), immunization history, and allergy history
- Focus on head and neck, lung, and abdominal exams
  - Nasal exam for evidence of rhinosinusitis
  - Oral exam for ulcerations, masses, tonsil size, erythema, and exudates
  - Assess for lymphadenopathy
  - Skin exam for rashes
  - Chest exam for wheezes and asymmetry
- Streptococcal pharyngitis is often a clinical diagnosis
  - Distinguish streptococcal infection from viral infection to determine appropriate treatment
  - The presence of 3 out of the 4 following criteria suggests the diagnosis: Exudative pharyngitis (not just a red throat), tender anterior cervical lymphadenopathy, presence or history of fever, and absence of a cough
  - If none or only 1 of the above criteria exists, group A β-hemolytic streptococci are unlikely

Initial diagnostic workup

- Streptococcal culture is the gold standard for diagnosing streptococcal pharyngitis; it is inexpensive and identifies group A streptococci and others, but it takes 1–2 days for results
- Rapid strep testing is more expensive and identifies only group A streptococci, but it gives immediate results; it is very specific (95%) but less sensitive (60%–70%), so consider culture if negative but clinical suspicion exists
- Monospot testing or CBC showing atypical lymphocytes is diagnostic for mononucleosis
- Radiography (inspiratory and expiratory) may be indicated to diagnose a suspected foreign body; laryngoscopy if unable to verify
- Lateral neck radiography may diagnose epiglottitis and retropharyngeal abscess
- CT may be necessary to assess for complications of an infection (e.g., abscess formation)
- Gonococcal and diphtheria cultures if necessary
- Barium swallow, upper GI radiography series, or EGD to assess for GERD

DIFFERENTIAL DIAGNOSIS

Infectious etiologies
- Viral pharyngitis or laryngitis
  - The most common cause of sore throat
  - Common viruses include rhinovirus, adenovirus, coxsackievirus, and herpesvirus
  - Influenza occasionally causes sore throat with high fever, cough, severe myalgias
  - Acute HIV infection should also be considered
- Mononucleosis
  - Associated with fever, headache, and excessive fatigue
  - May have associated lymphadenopathy, splenomegaly, hepatitis, or encephalitis
- Streptococcal pharyngitis
  - May be associated with scarlatiniform rash, fever, exudative pharyngitis, tender cervical lymphadenopathy, and absence of cough
  - More common during winter months, in those aged 5–10 years, and in those with a history of group A streptococci exposure
- Gonococcal pharyngitis
- Fungal pharyngitis (e.g., *Candida*)
- Sinusitis and postnasal drip
- Deep neck space infection
  - Retropharyngeal abscess
  - Peritonsillar abscess
  - Ludwig's angina
- Epiglottitis or bacterial tracheitis
  - Occurs in children aged 2–7 years and increasingly in adults
- Diphtheria
- Lymphadenitis (cervical)

Noninfectious etiologies
- Allergic pharyngitis
- Rhinosinusitis and postnasal drip
- Foreign body in throat
  - Associated with sudden onset of audible wheezing, stridor, and drooling
- GERD
- Chemical irritation
  - Inhalants (e.g., cigarette smoke, environmental pollutants)
  - Alcohol
  - Hot foods
  - Caustic ingestions
- Pharyngeal drying (e.g., mouth breathing)
- Voice abuse (e.g., excessive screaming)
- Trauma
- Cancer and tumors
  - Leukemia
  - Rhabdomyosarcomas
  - Squamous cell carcinoma secondary to oral ulcerations
  - Tonsillar cancer
  - Tongue cancer
  - Laryngeal cancer
  - Esophageal cancer
- Thyroiditis
- Systemic/rheumatologic disorders
  - Kawasaki's disease
  - Behçet's syndrome
  - Reiter's syndrome
- Angina pectoris or acute coronary syndrome

Splenomegaly

INTRODUCTION

The spleen is the largest lymphatic organ of the body. One of its primary functions is to filter defective and/or foreign cells from the blood. Splenomegaly, or enlargement of the spleen, occurs when the spleen exceeds 12 cm in length, 7 cm in width, or 150 g in mass. Although a normal spleen is not usually palpable, dullness can be percussed between the 9th and 11th ribs (Traube's space) with the patient lying on the right side. Palpation is best performed while the patient is supine with knees flexed. The spleen is best felt as it descends during inspiration; however, physical diagnosis is not sensitive. Splenomegaly is usually caused by systemic disease rather than by primary splenic disease. Because of exposure below the protective rib cage, splenomegaly results in increased risk of splenic injury or rupture.

DIAGNOSTIC WORKUP & INITIAL MANAGEMENT

History and physical examination
- Note fever, left upper quadrant pain, dyspnea, fatigue, diarrhea, pruritis, and signs of malignancy
- Assess medical history, recent abdominal trauma, recent illness, ingestion of hepatotoxic substances, surgical history, family history, and sexual history
- Complete physical exam, including abdominal, chest and cardiac, skin, head and neck, and rectal exams

Initial diagnostic workup
- Initial laboratory testing begins with a CBC with differential cell counts
  - Decreases in ≥1 cell lineages may indicate hypersplenism
  - Neutrophilia suggests infection
  - Atypical lymphocytes suggest mononucleosis
  - Spherocytes suggest hereditary spherocytosis
  - Teardrop-shaped red blood cells suggest bone marrow invasion
- Further studies may include electrolytes, BUN and creatinine, urinalysis, ESR, liver function tests, coagulation profile, chest radiography, ANA, RF, HIV testing, and sickle cell prep
- Abdominal CT or ultrasound better delineate splenomegaly and may reveal associated abdominal pathology
- Bone marrow biopsy may be indicated to evaluate for leukemia, myelofibrosis, and/or infection

Initial patient management
- Therapy is directed at the underlying etiology:
  - Infectious etiologies require appropriate antibiotic regimens
  - Leukemia and lymphoma are treated with combination chemotherapy
  - SLE and rheumatoid arthritis are treated with steroids and/or cytotoxic agents
  - Hemolytic anemia is treated with steroids
- Benefits of splenectomy must be balanced against the risk of postsplenectomy sepsis (especially from encapsulated bacteria, such as *Streptococcus pneumoniae*, *H. influenzae*, and *N. meningitidis*)
  - Splenectomy may be required for patients who have traumatic spleen injury with persistent bleeding and other hematologic disorders (e.g., immune thrombocytopenic purpura, hereditary spherocytosis)
  - Patients without a spleen are at increased risk of sepsis and should receive regular pneumococcal, meningococcal, and *H. influenzae* vaccinations

DIFFERENTIAL DIAGNOSIS

Infection or inflammation
- Acute hepatitis A, B, or C
- Mononucleosis
- Viral infection (e.g., EBV, cytomegalovirus, HIV)
- Bacterial infection (e.g., cat scratch disease, tuberculosis, histoplasmosis, toxoplasmosis, *Salmonella*, *Mycobacterium avium* complex, Rocky Mountain spotted fever)
- Endocarditis
- SLE
- Rheumatoid arthritis
- Inflammatory bowel disease (IBD)
- Celiac disease
- Acidosis
- Chronic granulomatous disease
- Serum sickness
- Protozoal infection (e.g., malaria, schistosomiasis)
- Kala-azar (visceral leishmaniasis)

Hemolytic anemia
- Hereditary spherocytosis
- Hemoglobinopathies
- Thalassemia major
- Nonspherocytic hemolytic anemias (pyruvate kinase deficiency)

Malignancy
- Leukemia
- Lymphoma
- Metastatic disease
- Lymphoproliferative or myeloproliferative disorder

Extramedullary hematopoiesis
- Thalassemia major
- Osteopetrosis
- Myelofibrosis

Storage/infiltrative diseases
- Histiocytosis
- Amyloidosis
- Lipidoses (e.g., Niemann-Pick, Gaucher's)
- Mucopolysaccharidoses

Congestive
- Chronic congestive heart failure
- Portal hypertension
- Portal or splenic venous thrombosis
- Hepatic fibrosis
- Cirrhosis

Structural
- Trauma
- Hematoma
- Hemangioma or hamartoma
- Cyst or pseudocyst

Other
- Normal variant
- Wandering spleen
- Sickle cell disease
- Polycythemia vera
- Felty's syndrome (rheumatoid arthritis, splenomegaly, granulocytopenia)

Stomatitis

INTRODUCTION

Stomatitis refers to inflammation of the oral mucous membranes and may involve the cheeks, gums, lips, tongue, or roof or floor of the mouth. It may be caused by numerous underlying disorders, many of which are infectious. A careful history and physical examination are often sufficient to narrow the differential diagnosis. In uncertain cases, biopsy the lesions and/or refer to an otolaryngologist, dermatologist, or oral surgeon.

DIAGNOSTIC WORKUP & INITIAL MANAGEMENT

History and physical examination

- The diagnosis is usually evident based on history and clinical observation
- History should focus on the onset, duration, presence and type of pain, and associated symptoms (e.g., hand or foot lesions, dermatologic complaints, fever, past medical history, exposure, and sexual history)
- Physical exam should focus on the eyes, ears, nose, throat, neck, and skin, with a cursory systemic evaluation

Initial diagnostic workup

- For infectious causes, specific microbe identification by culture, antigen detection assays, and histologic studies is necessary, especially in immunocompromised patients
- Laboratory evaluation may include CBC, syphilis testing (RPR), viral titers, ESR, and HIV test
- A biopsy may be necessary for definitive diagnosis
  - If an infectious etiology is being considered, send one piece of the specimen for biopsy in formalin and a second piece in nonbacteriostatic saline for cultures
- Consider referral to a dermatologist, otolaryngologist, or oral surgeon in uncertain cases

Initial patient management

- Aphthous stomatitis generally requires symptomatic treatment only; lesions will spontaneously resolve within 2 weeks
  - Strict oral hygiene (e.g., antiseptic mouthwash)
  - Topical anesthetics may relieve pain
  - Judicious use of topical and oral steroids in severe disease
  - Oral thalidomide is reportedly helpful in severe disease (e.g., AIDS patients)
- Infectious stomatitis should be treated with appropriate antimicrobial treatment and topical antiseptics or anesthetic
  - Coating agents (e.g., milk of magnesia, aluminum hydroxide) may be helpful
- Gangrenous stomatitis is treated with high-dose IV penicillin and correction of underlying malnutrition or debility; surgery may be necessary
- Chronic granulomatous disease is managed by early recognition and aggressive treatment of infections

DIFFERENTIAL DIAGNOSIS

Aphthous stomatitis
- Most common cause of recurrent oral lesions
- Etiology is unknown; it presents as a gray-yellow, tender ulcer in the anterior part of the mouth; similar ulcers may appear in the genital area
- Herpetiform ulcers present as multiple vesicles on the tip or sides of the tongue
- May be associated with Behcet's syndrome and inflammatory bowel disease

Infectious stomatitis
- HSV may present as a primary infection (herpetic gingivostomatitis), with ulcers or vesicles in the oropharynx, or as a secondary infection, with "fever blisters" on the lips
- Herpangina primarily occurs in children and is caused by coxsackievirus; results in 1- to 2-mm vesicles on the soft palate that rupture to become white ulcers; may be associated with palmar and plantar lesions in cases of hand-foot-and-mouth disease
- Syphilis results in painless oral chancres (condyloma latum) on the lips, mucosa, and gingiva
- Varicella (chickenpox)
- Condyloma acuminatum (warts) and molluscum contagiosum lesions resemble their characteristic genital lesions
- Primary HIV infection
- Candidiasis

Stevens-Johnson syndrome
- A serious, potentially fatal skin disorder; a severe form of erythema multiforme
- Although many cases are idiopathic, most cases result from drug reactions (e.g., penicillins, sulfa antibiotics, anticonvulsants, valdecoxib); other etiologies include infections (e.g., HIV, HSV, coxsackievirus, influenza, hepatitis, group A streptococci, diphtheria, mycobacteria, coccidioidomycosis, histoplasmosis, malaria, trichomoniasis), and malignancies
- Following a 1- to 3-day, flu-like prodrome, an erythematous, confluent, morbilliform eruption occurs that rapidly evolves into exfoliation of the skin at the dermal–epidermal junction, resulting in large sheets of necrotic epidermis and shiny, denuded dermal surface

Gangrenous stomatitis (necrotizing ulcerative gingivitis, "trench mouth")
- Primarily affects children with severe malnourishment or debilitation
- The causative agent is most commonly a spirochete (e.g., *Borrelia vincentii*)
- Presents as a painful, red, gingival vesicle and progresses to a necrotic ulcer and cellulitis

Chronic granulomatous disease
- A disorder of phagocytic cells; results in severe, recurrent bacterial and fungal infections
- Granulomas occur in the skin, GI tract, and genitourinary tract
- Associated presentations include skin infections, pneumonia, lymphadenitis, diarrhea, numerous abscesses (e.g., lung, hepatic, splenic, perianal), osteomyelitis, and/or sepsis
- Diagnosed by NBT slide test, in which a drop of blood is added to an activating agent; neutrophils from patients with chronic granulomatous disease do not stain with NBT dye

Behcet's syndrome (recurrent oral and genital ulcers)
- A systemic vasculitis characterized by oral and genital ulcers, uveitis, blindness, arthritis, aneurysms, thrombosis, and/or CNS involvement (e.g., meningitis, neurologic deficits)
- Oral ulceration is the hallmark of the disease and usually the initial clinical symptom; ulcers are painful, nonscarring, and appear in crops

Stomatitis
- Common in immunocompromised patients
- Breakdown of the epithelium results in superinfection by *Candida*, HSV, varicella zoster virus, or cytomegalovirus
- May occur secondary to chemotherapy

Other causes
- Poor oral hygiene, poorly fitted dentures, burns from hot food or drinks, vitamin C deficiency, lichen planus, and various cancers (e.g., mouth cancer, leukemia)

Stridor and Wheezing

INTRODUCTION

Stridor is a harsh, high-pitched, musical sound produced by turbulent airflow through a partially obstructed airway. It typically originates from large airways. It should be distinguished from wheezing, which is a high-pitched, whistling sound produced by turbulent airflow through constricted small airways. The age of the patient is important in determining the specific etiology: Younger patients are more likely to have symptoms of asthma or a foreign body; older patients are more likely to suffer from pulmonary edema, COPD, or cancers.

DIAGNOSTIC WORKUP & INITIAL MANAGEMENT

- Assess vital signs, especially respiratory rate and pulse oximetry
- Administer supplemental oxygen via nasal cannula; be sure to have a nonrebreather mask and Ambu-bag ready as backup
  - Have a low threshold for intubation if the patient is in respiratory distress
- Stridor can progress rapidly; a patient who is developing cyanosis, hypoxemia, or mental status changes has just seconds to minutes before respiratory and cardiac arrest ensue— do not hesitate to call for help, which may include anesthesiologist or ENT specialist

History and physical examination

- Assess for nature of the symptom, and distinguish stridor from wheezing
  - Supraglottic lesions or edema will most commonly cause inspiratory stridor
  - Glottic and subglottic lesions cause biphasic stridor
  - Tracheal and bronchial lesions cause expiratory stridor
- Determine how long the patient has had difficulty breathing or abnormal breath sounds
- Evaluate for trauma, such as recent intubations, inhalation injury, or crush injury to the neck (e.g., while the patient was being restrained)
- Assess mental status
- Evaluate for accessory muscle breathing, and auscultate the neck and chest to determine the type and location of the stridor
- Check the oral cavity, and palpate the neck for signs of infection or asymmetry

Initial workup and management

- Initial laboratory testing may include pulse oximetry, ABG, electrolytes, BUN and creatinine, calcium, and glucose
- If suspect allergic reaction, consider steroids, diphenhydramine, and H_2-blockers (e.g., ranitidine)
- If concern for infection (e.g., Ludwig's angina, parapharyngeal or retropharyngeal abscess), a CBC and blood cultures are indicated
- Chest radiography helps to differentiate respiratory infection from pulmonary edema; shows radiopaque foreign bodies and also a "steeple sign" in patients with croup
- Lateral neck radiography may reveal swelling of the epiglottis in cases of epiglottitis or abscess
- Chest CT with contrast provides excellent views of the lung parenchyma and helps to identify tumors and bronchiectasis
- Bronchoscopy may be diagnostic and therapeutic in cases of obstruction by a foreign body
- Lung biopsy or bronchoalveolar lavage can be performed if suspect malignancy
- Echocardiography may be indicated to evaluate for structural heart disease, valve disease, and left ventricular function

DIFFERENTIAL DIAGNOSIS

Stridor

- Anaphylaxis (may be the most likely cause of emergent stridor in hospitalized patients)
- Congenital etiologies
  - Supraglottic: Laryngomalacia, laryngocele, hemangioma, lymphangioma
  - Glottic: Webs and atresia, hemangioma, vocal cord paralysis
  - Subglottic: Stenosis, cysts, hemangioma
  - Vascular anomalies: Hemangioma, arteriovenous malformation
- Infectious etiologies
  - Parapharyngeal and retropharyngeal abscesses usually occur secondary to dental or tonsillar infections; patients usually appear toxic, with high fever, odynophagia, neck pain, and drooling
  - Croup (laryngotracheobronchitis) is a viral infection resulting in tracheal narrowing caused by airway edema and presents with a "bark-like" cough and hoarseness; the most common cause of acute stridor in children
  - Epiglottitis is an airway emergency most commonly caused by *Haemophilus influenzae* or group A streptococci infection; presents with abrupt onset of high fever, sore throat, hoarseness, dysphagia, and respiratory distress
- Toxins
  - Inhalation of toxic substances (e.g., carbon monoxide) can cause laryngeal edema and stridor; usually easy to obtain this history from the patient, if not obtunded
  - Occasionally, patients can be exposed to an allergenic substance (e.g., penicillin, ACE inhibitors), resulting in laryngeal edema because of anaphylaxis
- Trauma
  - Neck trauma may result in stridor because of laryngeal fractures or laryngeal mucosal injuries
  - Iatrogenic causes must also be considered: Thyroid surgery can injure the recurrent laryngeal nerve; endotracheal intubation or decannulation of tracheostomy tubes can result in subglottic and tracheal stenosis
- Endocrine etiologies
  - Thyroid gland enlargement because of goiter or neoplasm may cause stridor and respiratory difficulty and require thyroidectomy
  - Hypothyroidism and myxedema can cause hoarseness but rarely present with stridor
- Neoplastic etiologies
  - Laryngeal cancer must be considered in heavy smokers and drinkers
- Many systemic diseases can present with stridor secondary to laryngeal lesions: Wegener's granulomatosis, sarcoidosis, amyloidosis
- Foreign body lodged in the upper airway
- Psychogenic (e.g., paroxysmal vocal cord dyskinesia)
- COPD (patients produce expiratory vocalization to prolong time to airway closure and avoid air trapping)
- Heart failure (patients produce expiratory vocalization to prolong increased intrathoracic pressure and unload the left ventricle)

Wheezing

- Asthma: Presents as triad of chronic cough, dyspnea, and wheezing; however, wheezing may be absent in cases of severe obstruction because of insufficient air movement
- Pulmonary edema: Leakage of fluid into the interstitium and alveoli because of elevated capillary pressure (cardiogenic) or abnormal capillary permeability (noncardiogenic)
- COPD
- GERD
- Respiratory infection (upper respiratory infection, bronchiolitis, "atypical" pneumonia)
- Aspirated foreign body: Presents with abrupt onset of unilateral wheezing or stridor (if lodged in the upper airway), cough, and decreased breath sounds
- Allergic reaction or anaphylaxis

Syncope

INTRODUCTION

Syncope is transient loss of consciousness and postural tone with subsequent spontaneous recovery. It is often precipitated by decreased blood flow to the brain. Syncope usually lasts for brief periods of a few minutes. Longer periods are of more concern because of possible major cardiac or neurologic disorders. It accounts for 3% of emergency department visits and 6% of hospital admissions, and nearly $750 million is spent each year in the U.S. to diagnose and treat syncope. Overall mortality is low, but it may be as high as 35% with a cardiac etiology. Of patients with syncope, 30%–45% will not have a definitive diagnosis; of those with undiagnosed causes, almost 50% will eventually be diagnosed with a neurally mediated cause.

DIAGNOSTIC WORKUP & INITIAL MANAGEMENT

History and physical examination

- The patient's and other observers' descriptions of symptoms immediately before and after the episode are key to determining etiology of the syncopal episode
- Evaluate vital signs, including fingerstick blood glucose and pulse oximetry
- Note events surrounding the event: Syncope while moving from supine to standing suggests orthostatic syncope; syncope during exertion is ominous and suggests a cardiac outflow obstruction (e.g., aortic stenosis, hypertrophic obstructive cardiomyopathy, atrial myxoma); syncope during sudden head turning, shaving, or while wearing a tight neck collar suggests carotid sinus hypersensitivity
- Note symptoms immediately before loss of consciousness: Headache may suggest subarachnoid hemorrhage; chest pain, palpitations, and dyspnea suggest acute coronary syndrome, pulmonary embolism, dissection, or cardiac tamponade; abdominal or low back pain suggests AAA or ectopic pregnancy
- Note current medications, including prescription medications and drugs of abuse
- With family history of sudden death, consider inherited etiologies (e.g., hypertrophic obstructive cardiomyopathy, Jervell-Lang-Nielsen syndrome, Romano-Ward syndrome, Brugada syndrome)
- Note previous episodes and earlier medical evaluations to guide the workup
- Any history of cardiovascular disease raises the probability of cardiac etiology
- Rectal exam is necessary in all patients to evaluate for GI bleeding

Initial diagnostic workup

- Primary objective is to identify patients with syncope from a cardiac cause, which carries the highest 1-year mortality (>30%)
- CBC to check for anemia/blood loss
- 12-lead ECG is indicated in all patients; tachyarrhythmias, bradyarrhythmias, or AV blocks raise the likelihood of a cardiac etiology
- In appropriate patients, the following testing may be valuable:
  - Pregnancy testing is indicated in all females of reproductive age
  - Chemistries should be measured in patients on diuretics or who have vomiting or diarrhea
  - Elevated BNP may be a clue to cardiac syncope
  - Chest x-ray in patients with chest pain, dyspnea, or abnormal cardiac exam
  - Head CT in patients who complain of headache immediately before syncope or have focal neurologic findings on exam
  - Echocardiography in patients with exertional syncope; also usually obtained before stress testing to rule out valve lesions (e.g., aortic stenosis, hypertrophic subaortic stenosis)
  - Cardiac monitoring may be necessary if suspect arrhythmia, but diagnostic yield of 24-hour monitoring is low; consider an implantable loop recorder in recurrent cases
  - Tilt-table testing may evaluate for neurally mediated syncope
  - Consider MRI, EEG, or carotid Doppler if suspect TIA, stroke, or seizure disorder

DIFFERENTIAL DIAGNOSIS

Cardiac etiologies

Structural heart disease
- Valvular disease, especially aortic stenosis
- Outlet obstruction (e.g., hypertrophic obstructive cardiomyopathy, hypertrophic subaortic stenosis, atrial myxoma)

Arrhythmias
- Very slow (<30 bpm) or fast (>180 bpm) heart rates may result in decreased cardiac output and diminished blood flow to the brain

Ischemia

Noncardiac etiologies

Neurally mediated disease
- Vasovagal episode is the most common cause of syncope and results from decreased cerebral blood flow; may be triggered by heat, fatigue, stress, hunger, alcohol, or severe pain
- Situational syncope occurs when increased intrathoracic pressure (e.g., cough, micturition, defecation) leads to decreased venous return and diminished blood flow to the brain
- Carotid sinus hypersensitivity may result in syncope during sudden head turning, shaving, or while wearing a tight neck collar

Orthostatic hypotension
- Results from a fall in blood pressure on standing secondary to failure of vasoconstrictor reflexes
- Volume depletion (e.g., dehydration, hypovolemia, hemorrhage)
- Autonomic disorders (e.g., Shy-Drager syndrome)
- Often associated with antihypertensive medications (e.g., diuretics, vasodilators, α- or β-blockers)

Others
- Hypoglycemia
- Anemia
- Pulmonary embolus
- Aortic dissection
- Ectopic pregnancy
- Medications
- Cerebrovascular insufficiency (e.g., TIA, stroke), usually caused by carotid or vertebrobasilar artery disease (including subclavian steal syndrome)
- Subarachnoid or intracerebral hemorrhage
- Psychiatric etiologies

Nonsyncopal diagnoses

Seizures
- In contrast to syncope, patients with seizures may report a premonitory aura and frequently present with postictal confusion
- Labs may reveal lactic acidosis

Drop attack
- Occurs in older patients with neurologic disease (e.g., Alzheimer's dementia)
- In contrast to syncope, patients have abrupt loss of postural tone but no loss of consciousness

Vertigo and dizziness
- In contrast to syncope, patients have no loss of consciousness

Altered mental status
- In contrast to syncope, patients do not spontaneously regain consciousness

Anxiety attack

Migraine

Tachypnea

INTRODUCTION

Tachypnea is defined as an increase in the normal respiratory rate. Normal respiratory rate varies with age (24–38 respirations per minute for children >1 year, and 12–19 respirations per minute for older children and adults). Tachypnea is typically associated with dyspnea (the feeling of inadequate respiration).

DIAGNOSTIC WORKUP & INITIAL MANAGEMENT

- Immediate assessment of airway, breathing, and circulation, including vital signs and pulse oximetry
- Administer supplemental oxygen as needed
- Treat pain, if appropriate
- Evaluate for toxic ingestions and treat immediately as per toxicology protocols

History and physical examination

- History should focus on precipitants, time course, associated symptoms, medical history, and medications
- Perform a focused physical exam

Initial diagnostic workup

- Initial laboratory studies may include CBC, electrolytes, renal function, glucose, urinalysis, blood culture, urine culture, pulmonary function tests, serum aspirin level, and urine toxicology screen
- ECG and cardiac enzymes to rule out myocardial ischemia and infarction
- Chest radiography
- ABG will determine whether the cause is primary respiratory alkalosis or secondary to primary metabolic acidosis
  - Increased A-a gradient suggests pulmonary disease or pulmonary embolism
- V/Q scan may be used to assess for pulmonary embolism and infarction
- Chest CT may be used to better visualize the lung parenchyma and can also be used to evaluate for pulmonary embolism
- Echocardiography is useful if suspect congenital heart disease and pericardial effusion and can also be used to evaluate left ventricular function in patients with congestive heart failure or MI

DIFFERENTIAL DIAGNOSIS

Cardiovascular etiologies
- Pulmonary embolism
- Congestive heart failure
- Acute coronary syndrome or angina
- Hypotension
- Pericardial effusion

Pulmonary etiologies
- COPD
- Asthma
- Pneumonia
- Pneumothorax
- Restrictive lung diseases
  - Interstitial lung disease
  - Thoracic abnormalities (e.g., kyphosis, pneumonectomy)
  - Neuromuscular diseases (e.g., amyotrophic lateral sclerosis, Guillain-Barré syndrome, diaphragmatic paralysis)
- Tuberculosis

Metabolic and toxicologic etiologies
- Diabetic ketoacidosis
  - Associated with dehydration, Kussmaul's respirations (deep breathing with normal or reduced frequency), and acetone breath
- Severe dehydration
  - Vomiting
  - Diarrhea
  - Burns
  - Inadequate fluid intake (e.g., elderly, immobility)
- Salicylate toxicity
  - May be associated with nausea, vomiting, tinnitus, altered mental status, and convulsions
- Metabolic acidosis

Neurologic etiologies
- Stroke
- Head trauma

Medications/drugs
- Sympathomimetics (e.g., cocaine)
- Aspirin
- β-Agonists
- Methylxanthines

Anxiety/hyperventilation
- A common cause of tachypnea affecting up to 10% of the population
- Strong female predominance

Other
- Sepsis
- Hyperthyroidism
- Pheochromocytoma
- Malignancy

Tactile Fremitus

INTRODUCTION

Tactile fremitus is performed by placing your hands firmly on the patient's chest and having the patient repeat a phrase several times so you can feel the vibration of conducted sound through the lungs. Then, examine the rest of the chest in the same fashion. The most commonly used phrase is "99"; "blue moon" is also useful. An increase in fremitus indicates a direct solid communication from the bronchus to the chest wall or a consolidation. A decrease in fremitus indicates the presence of air, fluid, or solid material in the pleural space or obstruction of the bronchi.

DIAGNOSTIC WORKUP & INITIAL MANAGEMENT

History and physical examination
- Assess associated symptoms, medical history, family history, and medications
- Note egophony ("E" to "A" changes)
- Note symmetry of chest movement
- Auscultate and percuss the entire lung area

Initial workup and management
- Attention to airway, breathing, and circulation
- Administer supplemental oxygen as needed
- Initial laboratory testing may include CBC, pulse oximetry, electrolytes, BUN and creatinine, calcium, and glucose
- Consider blood and/or sputum cultures if suspect an infectious etiology
- Chest radiography may reveal pneumothorax, pneumonia, effusion, atelectasis, or other diagnoses
- Consider chest CT if unexplained abnormal chest radiograph or to better delineate fibrosis or causes of effusions
- ABG may be indicated
- Pulmonary function tests may be indicated to identify restrictive or obstructive disease and barriers to diffusion
- Chest tube insertion may be indicated for pneumothorax, hemothorax, or chylothorax

DIFFERENTIAL DIAGNOSIS

Increased fremitus (increased transmission of sound through the chest)

- Consolidative pneumonia (e.g., *Streptococcus pneumoniae*, lobar pneumonias)
- Diffuse alveolitis
- Diffuse fibrosis (e.g., cystic fibrosis)

Decreased fremitus (decreased transmission of sound through the chest)

- Pleural effusion
  - May result from congestive heart failure, pneumonia, cancer, pulmonary embolus, connective tissue disease (e.g., SLE, rheumatoid arthritis), pancreatitis, and renal and liver disease
- Hemothorax
  - May result from chest trauma or instrumentation
- Chylothorax
  - May result from traumatic disruption of the thoracic duct or malignancy
- Pneumothorax
  - May occur spontaneously or following trauma or instrumentation
- Asthma
- Bronchitis
- Emphysema
- Atelectasis
  - May be acute (e.g., postoperative) or chronic (airlessness, infection, bronchiectasis, destruction, fibrosis)
- Foreign body aspiration
- Pleural thickening
- Rhonchal fremitus
  - Results from airway secretions
- Friction fremitus
  - Results from pleural friction rub

Testicular Pain

INTRODUCTION

Acute or chronic scrotal or testicular pain may occur at any age and may or may not be associated with a scrotal or testicular mass. Orchalgia is chronic pain of the testicles or scrotum that typically lasts beyond 3 months. Testicular pain often is accompanied by significant concern on the part of the patient, who worries that this might be cancer. Although most etiologies are neither serious nor emergent, testicular pain must be considered an emergency because of the possibility of testicular torsion or Fournier's gangrene.

DIAGNOSTIC WORKUP & INITIAL MANAGEMENT

History and physical examination

- Note character of onset (sudden or subacute), duration (minutes, hours, or days), location (generalized or localized), quality (sharp or dull, moderate or severe, constant or intermittent), and previous episodes
- Palpate the testicle and spermatic cord to assess for tenderness, effusion, subcutaneous emphysema, size and orientation of testicle, and hernias
- Transilluminate for presence of fluid
- If suspect testicular torsion, emergent detorsion is necessary
  - "Blue dot sign": Bluish discoloration along the upper pole because of infarction and necrosis is seen in 20% of cases of torsion of the testicular appendix
  - "Prehn's sign": Relief of pain on elevation of the testis in cases of epididymitis
- A painless scrotal mass should be considered testicular cancer until proven otherwise
- Masses that are easily separable from the testicle are much more likely to be benign
- Include abdominal, back, genital, and digital rectal exams

Initial diagnostic workup

- Scrotal ultrasound with color Doppler is usually indicated to measure blood flow and evaluate for masses
  - Radionucleotide scintigraphy may also be used to assess blood flow
- Initial testing includes CBC, urinalysis, urethral Gram's stain and culture
  - Presence of urine WBCs or RBCs suggests infection (e.g., epididymitis)
  - Culture for *Neisseria gonorrhoeae* and *Chlamydia trachomatis* in sexually active males before urinalysis
- CT and/or MRI may be warranted

Initial patient management

- Testicular torsion is a surgical emergency
  - If surgery is not available, manual detorsion may be attempted
  - Detorsion maneuver: Infiltrate the spermatic cord with 10–20 ml of 1% lidocaine, then twist the testicle toward the outside of the body on the affected side; successful detorsion is indicated by immediate relief of pain
- Incarcerated inguinal hernias and testicular rupture require immediate surgical repair
- Epididymitis and orchitis are treated with antibiotics
  - Patients <35 years (presumed to be sexually acquired): Treat with ceftriaxone or a fluoroquinolone, plus doxycycline, azithromycin, or tetracycline
  - Patients >35 years: Trimethoprim-sulfamethoxazole or a fluoroquinolone, unless history reveals that infection is sexually acquired
  - Analgesics and scrotal support may be used
- Testicular cancer found on exam or ultrasound should prompt immediate urologic and oncologic consultation for orchiectomy

DIFFERENTIAL DIAGNOSIS

Epididymitis
- A bacterial (chlamydia, enterobacter) or viral infection (mumps, mononucleosis, adenovirus) of adolescent boys and young adults

Testicular torsion
- Twisting of the spermatic cord that results in testicular ischemia and infarction
- Presents with acute onset of severe pain and diffuse tenderness
- Testicle on the affected side is tender, shortened, and lays transversely
- Duration of ischemia (time until detorsion is completed) determines the viability of the affected testicle

Hydrocele
- A collection of fluid (usually nontender) between the parietal and visceral layers of the tunica vaginalis around the testicle

Varicocele
- A mass of dilated veins that may be palpated as a "bag of worms" above the testes
- Presents as a dull ache exacerbated by strenuous exercise
- It is the most common correctable cause of male infertility

Epididymal or testicular appendage torsion
- Subacute onset of pain localized to the upper pole of the testicle
- Primarily seen in prepubertal boys

Referred pain
- Incarcerated inguinal hernia
- Constipation
- Urolithiasis

Scrotal trauma
- Results from a direct blow or saddle injury
- May result in traumatic epididymitis, hematocele, or laceration of the tunica albuginea (testicular rupture)

Fournier's gangrene (necrotizing fasciitis of the perineum)
- Primarily occurs in older men

Vasculitis
- Polyarteritis nodosa
- Henoch-Schönlein purpura
  - A systemic vasculitis resulting in scrotal pain, abdominal pain, arthralgias, nonthrombocytopenic purpura, and renal disease
  - Primarily occurs in prepubertal boys but also seen in adults

Tumor
- A painless scrotal mass is considered a testicular neoplasm until proven otherwise

Other
- Peritonitis
- Postvasectomy syndrome
- Chord lipoma or adenoma

Tinnitus

INTRODUCTION

Tinnitus is a perception of noise (usually ringing, buzzing, or hissing) in the ears, which may be constant or intermittent, temporary or permanent. The pitch and other characteristics of tinnitus should be identified, if possible, to more effectively narrow the differential diagnosis. Additionally, the presence or absence of associated symptoms, including hearing deficits, further narrows the differential diagnosis, and a hearing test is indicated in most cases of tinnitus when the diagnosis is unclear. The degree of distress caused by tinnitus varies widely.

DIAGNOSTIC WORKUP & INITIAL MANAGEMENT

History and physical examination
- Assess onset, duration, and severity; distinguish whether one or both ears are affected
- Assess pitch of the tinnitus, duration, and recent noise exposure
- Include a detailed medication history
- Complete head and neck exam, including neurologic and/or systemic exam if indicated by history
- Evaluate the temporomandibular joint (TMJ) for clicking, popping, and dislocation

Initial diagnostic workup
- Consider CBC to assess for anemia and infection
- Consider thyroid function tests to rule out occult thyroid disease
- Consider glucose tolerance test to rule out occult diabetes mellitus
- Tympanometry is usually indicated to diagnose otitis media and eustachian tube dysfunction
- A full audiology evaluation is warranted if suspect sensorineural etiology
- Head CT is indicated if suspect glomus tumor (delineates base of skull involvement)
- MRI (with enhancement) if suspect Arnold-Chiari malformation, multiple sclerosis, pseudotumor cerebri, or acoustic neuroma
- Consider angiography or MRA if CT and MRI are negative but suspect vascular etiology
- Consider screening for secondary depression or insomnia, because these are common in patients with tinnitus

Initial patient management
- Treat the underlying cause, if possible
- Treat underlying depression and insomnia, if present
- Discontinue ototoxic medications
- Consider referral to otolaryngologist or neurologist
- Consider a hearing aid in cases of presbycusis; cochlear implants may be indicated for severe hearing loss in patients that do not benefit from hearing aids
- Tinnitus retraining therapy may reduce tinnitus by habituation training
- Many medications treat tinnitus, but in randomized trials none has proven particularly effective without significant side effects
- Masking devices may be used to create a low-level sound to decrease or eliminate perceived tinnitus
- Biofeedback or stress reduction may be useful as tolerance to tinnitus decreases with stress and fatigue
- Surgery may be necessary to correct conductive defects with outer or middle ear disease or to remove tumors

DIFFERENTIAL DIAGNOSIS

- Acute or chronic otitis media
- Impacted cerumen
- Eustachian tube dysfunction
  - Patients may complain of an "ocean roar" that waxes and wanes with respirations
- Dysfunctional hearing aid
- Presbycusis (high pitch)
- Idiopathic (low pitch)
- Noise-induced hearing loss (high pitch)
- Ménière's disease
  - Triad of tinnitus, hearing loss, and vertigo
- Ototoxicity secondary to drugs (high pitch)
  - May persist after medication (e.g., aminoglycosides) is discontinued
  - May be dose-related (e.g., aspirin)
- Trauma
  - Commonly associated with airbag impact, whiplash, or barotrauma
  - May be associated with a ruptured tympanic membrane
- Temporomandibular joint (TMJ) syndrome
  - Nonpulsatile tinnitus (Costen's syndrome)
  - Associated jaw symptoms (e.g., pain, clicking)
- Migraine headache
- Vascular disease (e.g., atherosclerosis, diabetic vasculopathy, arteriovenous malformation, small vessel disease, hypertension)
- Stroke
- Otosclerosis
  - Associated with chronic otitis media or tympanic membrane trauma
- Pseudotumor cerebri
- Tumors
  - Glomus tympanicum or jugulare: Pulsatile tinnitus with hearing loss
  - Acoustic neuroma: Unilateral hearing loss and tinnitus, headache
- Infections (e.g., meningitis, Lyme disease, rubella)
- Arteriovenous malformation
- Thyroid disease
- Autoimmune inner ear disease

Less common etiologies
- Paget's disease
- Myoclonus of the palatal muscles
- Fetal insults (infections, toxins)
- Sickle cell disease
- Osteogenesis imperfecta
- Neurosyphilis
- Symptomatic Arnold-Chiari malformation
- Late-onset congenital hearing loss
- Dissecting aneurysm
- Carotid cancer
- Multiple sclerosis

Toothache

INTRODUCTION

Toothache, or tooth pain, is caused when the nerve root of a tooth becomes irritated. Tooth infection, decay, injury, or loss of a tooth are common causes. Pain may also occur after an extraction (removal of a tooth). Pain sometimes originates from other areas and radiates to the jaw (most commonly from the temporomandibular joint (TMJ), ear, or occasionally, cardiac disease), thus being perceived as tooth pain.

DIAGNOSTIC WORKUP & INITIAL MANAGEMENT

History and physical examination

- Include complete ear, nose, throat, mouth, neck, and cardiac exams
- Intraoral exam should include mobility tests, percussion, electric pulp test, and thermal tests (e.g., ice)
  - Tooth mobility is tested by using the back ends of two mouth mirrors on both sides of the tooth
  - Reversible pulpitis pain is sharp, intermittent pain of short duration that is provoked by hot, cold, sweets, or biting; the pain does not linger more than a few seconds when the stimulus is removed
  - Irreversible pulpitis pain lasts for >30 seconds on withdrawal of the stimulus and may occur spontaneously (e.g., when sleeping)
  - If an abscess is present, the tooth may be slightly elevated in its socket and mobile
  - A periapical abscess may have systemic findings (e.g., lymphadenopathy, fever)
  - Toothache or TMJ pain in the morning may result from bruxing (grinding of teeth) at night

Initial diagnostic workup

- Transillumination may show fracture lines in teeth
- Pulp necrosis will not have any response to stimulation or via electrical pulp tester
- Dental radiography may be necessary
- Consider sinus radiography or CT if suspect sinusitis
- Consider referral to a dentist or otolaryngologist

Initial patient management

- Reversible pulpitis from tooth decay can be treated with a restoration (e.g., filling or crown)
- Irreversible pulpitis requires root canal or tooth extraction if the tooth is not salvageable
- Incision and drainage of an abscess will often result in instant relief of pain
- Penicillin is generally sufficient for oral infections (clindamycin if severe)
- Appropriate oral antibiotics (e.g., amoxicillin, trimethoprim-sulfamethoxazole) for bacterial sinusitis or otitis media
- TMJ syndrome may be treated with avoidance of gum chewing and bruxing, a bite block, NSAIDs, or topical ice massage
- Treat headache syndromes and migraine as appropriate (refer also to the *Headache* entry)

DIFFERENTIAL DIAGNOSIS

Dental etiologies
- Pulp pain (pulpalgia) secondary to dental caries
- Traumatic tooth injury (e.g., tooth fracture, restoration fracture, avulsion)
- Traumatic occlusion
  - Secondary to a new tooth restoration or bruxing
  - May be caused by galvanic "shock" due to contact by two dissimilar metals (e.g., a gold crown with an amalgam filling)
- Oral infection
- Periradicular or periapical pain due to infection of the tooth root or abscess formation
- Referred pain from a tooth in the opposing arch
- Dry socket (osteitis)

Non-dental head and neck etiologies
- Sinusitis
  - Maxillary sinusitis is the most common extraoral source of tooth pain
  - All or most teeth in the upper arch may become sensitive secondary to sinusitis
- Headache
- Trigeminal neuralgia
- Salivary gland disorders (e.g., Sjögren's syndrome, systemic lupus erythematosus)

Referred pain
- Angina pectoris or acute coronary syndrome
- Temporomandibular joint syndrome
- Ear disease
- Otitis media
- Mastoiditis

Other
- Barodontalgia due to high altitudes
- "Dental migraine" (may be associated with depression)

Tremor

INTRODUCTION

Tremor, an involuntary, rhythmic oscillation of the hands, palate, or head, is the most common movement disorder. It may be classified as resting tremor or intention tremor. Resting tremor occurs at rest or in a static position (postural tremor). Intention tremor occurs or increases with purposeful activity (e.g., reaching for an object). Tremor can be associated with a cerebellar deficit or be benign familial essential tremors. It may be worsened by caffeine or anxiety and relieved by alcohol ingestion. Tremor is usually not disabling but may be socially embarrassing; severe tremors can interfere with daily activities, especially fine motor skills (e.g., writing) and speech, which may lead to social withdrawal and isolation.

DIAGNOSTIC WORKUP & INITIAL MANAGEMENT

History and physical examination

- Assess onset, exacerbating and relieving factors, medications, family history, and associated symptoms
- Physical exam should give attention to the body parts involved and to the frequency and amplitude of the tremor; test the involved body parts at rest, with changes in posture, and during intended movement

Initial diagnostic workup

- Diagnostic testing should be ordered based on the suspected etiology
- Essential or familial tremor is typically action-induced and may affect the head or voice
- Blood chemistry, hematology, thyroid function tests, and liver function tests may be ordered routinely; toxicology screen may be indicated to rule out drug ingestion
- In patients with suspected Wilson's disease, 24-hour urine copper and serum ceruloplasmin determinations are helpful
- CSF exam for oligoclonal IgG bands is appropriate in patients suspected of having multiple sclerosis
- MRI may be useful if suspect cerebellar tremor, strokes, or multiple sclerosis
- PET or SPECT may be useful in evaluating for parkinsonism
- Other evaluation tools used in research settings include surface EMG, accelerometers, potentiometers, handwriting tremor analysis, and long-term tremor records

Initial patient management

- Mild cases do not require treatment, and most forms of tremor do not have effective medical treatments
- Eliminate predisposing factors as necessary
- Medical therapy can be used as needed (e.g., during social events)
  - Primidone and propranolol are the most commonly used agents to decrease the essential or action tremor
  - Other agents may include topiramate, mirtazapine, and methazolamine
  - Alcohol use may also be effective, but abuse potential may limit clinical utility
- No established treatment for cerebellar tremor; some patients may respond to isoniazid plus pyridoxine
- Parkinsonian tremor (postural or rest tremor) may be treated with anticholinergic medications (e.g., benztropine, trihexyphenidyl) and/or dopamine-replacement therapy (e.g., levodopa plus carbidopa)
- Surgical therapy (e.g., stereotactic thalamotomy, thalamic deep brain stimulation) may be considered in severe cases but is rarely necessary

DIFFERENTIAL DIAGNOSIS

Resting tremors

Parkinson's disease
- Classically referred to as "pill rolling" postural tremor of the hands, but may affect the head, trunk, jaw, or lips
- Occurs at 4–8 cycles per second, usually at rest
- May be the first sign of disease
- Most patients have tremor that is maximal at rest or with distraction

Benign familial (essential) tremor
- Initially presents as a postural distal arm tremor, usually bilateral, and may slowly progress to a resting tremor
- May also involve the head, voice, tongue, and legs
- Positive family history
- No other neurologic findings

Drug- or toxin-induced tremors
- MPTP
- Alcohol

Medications
- β-Agonists
- Lithium
- Amiodarone
- Valproic acid
- Metoclopramide
- Theophylline
- Methylphenidate

Postural tremors
- Elicited when a limb is held up against gravity
- Caused by metabolic conditions (e.g., thyrotoxicosis)

Other
- Voluntary movement (hyperkinetic) tremor
- Wilson's disease
- Stroke
- Cerebellar disease
- Psychogenic tremor (may decrease or disappear when not watched)

Movement tremors

Intention tremor
- Occurs with movement toward a target with terminal accentuation (worse at the end of movement)
- Associated with a cerebellar deficit that would otherwise inhibit the tremor (e.g., multiple sclerosis, midbrain injury or stroke)
- Occurs primarily at the limbs, trunk, and head
- Tremor is absent at rest

Movement that may be confused with a tremor
- Tics (usually unifocal and slower than tremor)
- Chorea (jerky, irregular movements)
- Myoclonus (rapid and irregular)
- Athetosis and dystonia (slow movements)
- Asterixis (caused by inhibition of muscle contractions in patients with hepatic encephalopathy)

Unequal Pulses

INTRODUCTION

A thorough vascular examination is an integral part of every cardiac examination. Unequal pulses or a difference in blood pressure measurements between limbs can signify severe underlying vascular and nonvascular disease and also aid in prompt recognition and management.

DIAGNOSTIC WORKUP & INITIAL MANAGEMENT

History and physical examination

- Elicit risk factors and identify predisposing conditions
- Atrophic changes and dependent rubor in a patient with claudication suggest peripheral artery disease
- Pulsatile abdominal mass and abdominal bruit suggest aortic aneurysm
- New-onset aortic insufficiency with unexplained pericardial effusion and left pleural effusion suggest aortic dissection with possible rupture
- Asymmetric upper extremity blood pressures (difference of >15 mm Hg) suggest aortic dissection, subclavian stenosis, or Takayasu's arteritis; diminished lower extremity blood pressures suggest aortic coarctation, aortic dissection, severe aortoiliac or femoral artery disease, or aortic occlusion
- Compartment syndromes following traumatic injury can cause vascular compromise because of pressure elevation in the surrounding soft tissues

Initial diagnostic workup

- Ankle-brachial index (ABI) of systolic blood pressure of <0.9 is abnormal; values of <0.5 suggest severe peripheral artery disease
  - Patients with renal disease or heavily calcified vessels may have a falsely "normal" ABI
- Chest radiography may reveal widened mediastinum, pleural effusion, and tracheal deviation in cases of aortic aneurysm or dissection; "rib notching" caused by intercostal artery collateral channels may occur in cases of coarctation of the aorta
- CT or MRA may be helpful to diagnose Takayasu's arteritis, aortic aneurysm or dissection, subclavian stenosis, and coarctation of the aorta
- Transesophageal echocardiography may be helpful in the diagnosis of aortic dissection
- Duplex ultrasound may be helpful in assessing subclavian stenosis

Initial patient management

- Atherosclerosis is a systemic disease; many patients with peripheral artery disease have concomitant coronary and carotid artery disease
  - Lifestyle interventions include exercise, smoking cessation, and lipid and glucose control
  - Medical therapy includes aspirin, pentoxifylline, cilostazol, and statins
  - Surgical or endovascular revascularization procedures may be necessary
- Aortic dissection requires prompt, aggressive therapy to lower blood pressure; it should be treated preferentially with β-blockers
- Treat aortic aneurysm with blood pressure reduction; surgical correction may be necessary if symptomatic, large, or rapidly expanding
- Treat Takayasu's arteritis with corticosteroids, methotrexate, and possible revascularization
- Subclavian stenosis may require surgical bypass or endovascular stenting
- Coarctation of aorta is treated with angioplasty or surgical correction
- Compartment syndrome requires immediate decompression by fasciotomy

DIFFERENTIAL DIAGNOSIS

Atherosclerosis/peripheral artery disease
- Most common cause of unequal pulses
- Manifestations may include claudication, rest pain, ischemic ulcers, and gangrene

Aortic dissection
- Sharp, "tearing" chest or back pain
- Etiologies include hypertension, Marfan's syndrome, bicuspid aortic valve, cocaine, and trauma

Aortic aneurysm
- Focal or diffuse dilation 50% larger than normal vessel diameter
- Etiologies include atherosclerosis (most common for abdominal and descending thoracic aneurysms), cystic medial necrosis (most common for ascending aneurysms), connective tissue disorders (Marfan's syndrome, Ehlers-Danlos syndrome), congenital abnormalities (bicuspid aortic valve), syphilitic aortitis, spondyloarthropathies, and vasculitis

Takayasu's disease ("pulseless disease")
- Idiopathic inflammatory disorder of the aorta that results in narrowing of the aortic branches, ultimately causing vascular insufficiency
- Often presents with systemic complaints (e.g., fever, malaise, weight loss, fatigue)

Coarctation of aorta
- Accounts for 6%–8% of congenital heart diseases
- May rarely result in diminished left brachial pulse when the origin of the left subclavian artery is distal to the coarctation
- Narrowing of the aortic arch that results in decreased blood pressure in the lower extremities may present as hypertension in the upper extremities
- May be associated with a bicuspid aortic valve, ventricular septal defect, patent ductus arteriosus, or left ventricular outflow obstruction

Subclavian steal syndrome
- Syncope or dizziness occurs following exercise of the arms

Compartment syndrome
- Increased pressure in a closed compartment may decrease blood pressure to the downstream tissues
- Look for the "five P's": Pain, pallor, pulselessness, paresthesia, and paralysis

Urinary Incontinence

INTRODUCTION

Incontinence, defined as the involuntary loss of urine, is 1 of the 10 most common medical problems in the U.S., with prevalence estimated at 13–60 million Americans, particularly elderly women (it affects up to 30% of women >65 years). Most patients, however, do not seek treatment despite the significant effects on self-esteem and social interactions. Associated health care costs approach $16 billion per year. With newer and more effective anticholinergic medicines coming to the market and the development of less invasive surgical procedures to correct incontinence, patients suffering with this problem have many options from which to choose. In a vast majority of these patients, a durable solution can be found.

DIAGNOSTIC WORKUP & INITIAL MANAGEMENT

History and physical examination

- Note problems holding urine vs. emptying the bladder; leakage of urine with cough, exercise, sneezing, laughing, or lifting; frequency of voiding; number of nocturnal voids; excessively strong urge to void; loss of urine before reaching the toilet; hesitancy, dribbling, slow stream, incomplete voiding, or dysuria; associated bowel habits (e.g., constipation or fecal/flatal incontinence); medications; fluid intake; and medical and surgical history
- Physical exam should include full neurologic and mental status exams, assessment of physical frailness (e.g., use of walking aids, dysfunction secondary to stroke), abdominal exam (e.g., lower quadrant distension, pregnancy, fecal impaction), and genital and rectal exams (in women, evaluate for cystocele, vaginal atrophy, strength of pelvic muscles; in men, assess rectal tone and abnormalities of glans penis and prostate)
- A "cough stress test" may be attempted: Immediate leakage indicates stress incontinence; delayed leakage indicates urge incontinence
- Voiding diaries may be used to track urinary habits; these should document total fluid intake and number and amount of voids over a 24-hour period

Initial diagnostic workup

- Initial testing may include electrolytes, calcium, glucose, urinalysis, and urine culture
- Consider urine cytology in appropriate patients
- Measure postvoiding residual volume by catheterization and/or pelvic ultrasound; volume >100 mL of residual urine is abnormal
- Specialized urodynamic tests (e.g., cystometrography, cystourethrography) are reserved for ambiguous results or treatment failure
- Cystoscopy may be indicated to evaluate for bladder and prostate pathology

Initial patient management

- Goals of treatment are to preserve renal function, optimize quality of life, and treat and/or prevent infections (e.g., UTI) and other reversible causes (e.g., medications)
- Stress incontinence may respond to pelvic exercises (Kegel exercises), electrical stimulation, medications (e.g., α-adrenergics, tricyclic antidepressants, estrogens, duloxetine) to increase urethral tone, local estrogen replacement therapy, or pessaries to prevent urine loss during stress maneuvers; surgical intervention may be indicated for some
- Urge incontinence may respond to behavioral therapy (timed voiding, pelvic floor physical therapy, biofeedback) or medications (estrogens, anticholinergics such as oxybutynin, magnesium, tricyclic antidepressants); surgical intervention may include botox injection, hydrodistension, nerve stimulation, or cystoplasty
- Overflow incontinence is treated by decreasing outlet resistance to improve urine outflow, including drugs to open bladder neck and decrease prostate size; (e.g., α-blockers, 5α-reductase inhibitors); intermittent catheterizations for neuropathic conditions; surgical therapy may include prostatectomy, bladder neck incision, urethral dilation, or urethroplasty

DIFFERENTIAL DIAGNOSIS

Acute, transient incontinence (DIAPERS mnemonic)
- **D**elirium
- **I**nfections of urinary tract
- **A**trophic urethritis or vaginitis
- **P**harmaceuticals (e.g., diuretics, sedatives, anxiolytics, alcohol, β-blockers, ACE inhibitors, antidepressants, antipsychotics) or **P**sychiatric conditions (e.g., depression)
- **E**ndocrine disorders (e.g., hypercalcemia, hyperglycemia)
- **R**estricted mobility or (urinary) **R**etention
- **S**tool (i.e., fecal impaction)

Chronic, persistent incontinence
Stress incontinence
- Leakage of urine on abdominal straining and increases in intra-abdominal pressure (e.g., coughing, sneezing, laughing, exercising, going from sitting to standing position)
- Results from pelvic floor weakness caused by urethral hypermobility or sphincter dysfunction
- Risk factors include vaginal childbirth, episiotomy, urethral trauma (e.g., prostate surgery), hypoestrogenism, genitourinary surgery/radiation, chronic cough, and deconditioning
- More common in women who have had vaginal deliveries

Urge incontinence ("overactive bladder")
- Results from spontaneous bladder contractions, caused by central neurologic disorders (e.g., detrusor hyperreflexia), local bladder disorders (e.g., cystitis, bladder cancer), or idiopathic
  - Detrusor hyperreflexia is a disorder of involuntary bladder contractions caused by a neurologic lesion above the sacral spinal cord (e.g., multiple sclerosis, Parkinson's, stroke, spinal cord injury, hydrocephalus)
- Presentation may include leakage of urine associated with a strong urge to void, having to run to the restroom, urinary frequency and urgency, nocturia, or suprapubic discomfort
- Commonly associated with reversible causes (e.g., UTI, increased fluid intake), neurologic etiologies (e.g., neuropathy, hyperreflexia), poor bladder contractility, and increased sphincter relaxation

Overflow incontinence
- Overdistension of the bladder caused by outlet obstruction (e.g., prostate hyperplasia, prostate cancer, prolapse, stricture) or contractility dysfunction/atonic bladder (e.g., neurologic disorders such as diabetic/alcoholic neuropathy, spinal stenosis, anticholinergics)
- Associated with leakage of urine on abdominal straining, weak stream, urinary hesitancy or intermittency, nocturia, urinary dribbling, palpable bladder, no sensation of bladder filling (neurogenic), or suprapubic discomfort from a full bladder (obstruction)
- Most cases are age-related and idiopathic
- May result from loss of cortical inhibition of the micturition reflex (e.g., stroke, Parkinson's)
- Local bladder etiologies include bladder tumors, stones, and infections

Functional incontinence
- A normal urinary system affected by external factors (e.g., poor mental status or mobility)

Physiologic changes of aging
- These predispose, but do not cause, incontinence: Decreased bladder capacity and shortened urethra, increased involuntary bladder muscle contractions, decreased detrusor contractility, decreased mobility and functional capacity

Mixed incontinence
- Combined elements of stress and urge incontinence are common in older females
- Combined elements of overflow and urge incontinence are most common in men and frail nursing-home patients

Other
- Continuous leakage may indicate fistula (e.g., vesicovaginal fistula) or ectopic ureter
- Postvoid dribbling in women may indicate urethral diverticulum or vaginal pooling of urine

Urinary Stream, Decreased

INTRODUCTION

A perceived or observed decrease in the strength of flow of the urinary stream is a common complaint. This is often concerning to a patient because of the uncomfortable slowing of urination, associated dribbling or incomplete emptying, and fears of a serious underlying medical disorder. Benign prostatic hyperplasia is by far the most common etiology in men and is often accompanied by nocturia, urgency, frequency, dribbling, and incomplete emptying.

DIAGNOSTIC WORKUP & INITIAL MANAGEMENT

History and physical examination

- Note difficulty initiating urinary stream (hesitancy) versus fully emptying the bladder (dribbling, slow stream, incomplete voiding); incontinence; frequency of urination; nocturia; excessively strong urge to urinate; dysuria; associated bowel habits (e.g., constipation); medications; fluid intake; and medical and surgical history
- Include abdominal, back, genital (palpate the penis for areas of tenderness or induration), neurologic, and digital rectal exams
- Note previous urinary tract instrumentation and STDs

Initial diagnostic workup

- Consider placing a urinary catheter to assess for obstruction and postvoid residual volume (normal, <100 mL); acute urinary retention must be treated immediately to prevent additional injury and to relieve pain
- Initial laboratory testing includes urinalysis and culture, CBC (may reveal leukocytosis in cases of infection), BUN and creatinine (elevated in acute renal failure, such as with obstruction), and electrolytes
- Consider PSA screening, which is elevated in prostate cancer and prostatitis; may be mildly elevated in benign prostatic hyperplasia
- Consider urine cytology and alkaline phosphatase (elevated in metastatic prostate cancer)
- Uroflowmetry: Calculate urine flow rate during timed void (normal, 20–25 mL/second; <10 mL/s indicates obstruction)
- Consider renal ultrasound to rule out hydronephrosis
- Consider abdominal and pelvic CT to evaluate for urolithiasis and cancer
- Consider cystoscopy (to rule out cancer and anatomic problems), retrograde urethrography (to assess for strictures), voiding cystourethrography (pressure/volume curves), and transrectal ultrasound with needle biopsy (prostate cancer)

Initial patient management

- If necessary, interventions that decrease outlet resistance to improve urine flow include:
  - Medications to open the bladder neck and decrease prostate size (e.g., α-adrenergic blockers, 5α-reductase inhibitors)
  - Intermittent bladder catheterizations or indwelling Foley catheter may be necessary for neuropathic conditions
  - Surgical therapy may include prostatectomy, bladder neck incision, urethral dilation, or urethroplasty
- Eliminate causal medications (e.g., anticholinergics), if possible

DIFFERENTIAL DIAGNOSIS

Physical outlet obstruction
- Benign prostatic hyperplasia is the most common cause of decreased urinary stream in men >40 years
- Urolithiasis
- Urethral stricture
- Chronic urethritis
- Pelvic malignancy
  - Prostate cancer
  - Bladder neck cancer
  - Urethral cancer
- Bladder neck contracture
  - Congenital
  - Acquired (e.g., postprostatectomy)
- Urethral or bladder foreign body
- Medications (e.g., α-agonists)
- Phimosis or meatal stenosis
- Urethral polyp
- Posterior urethral valves
- Post-pelvic surgery
- Pregnancy
- Trauma
- Blood clots

Neurogenic causes
- Anesthetics
- Medications (e.g., α-agonists, β-agonists, antihistamines, dicyclomine, diazepam, tricyclics, anticholinergics)
- Spinal cord trauma
- Herniated disk
- Multiple sclerosis
- Spina bifida
- Stroke
- Brain tumor
- Parkinson's disease
- Myasthenia gravis
- Diabetes mellitus
- Nerve injury secondary to pelvic surgery (e.g., prostatectomy)

Other
- Intravascular volume depletion
- Acute renal failure
- Aortic aneurysm
- Uterine leiomyoma
- Ruptured bladder or urethra

Urine Output, Decreased

INTRODUCTION

Decreased urine output (oliguria) is defined as <0.5 mL/kg per hour per day, or <400 mL/day. The absence of urine output (anuria) is defined as <100 mL/day. The presence of oliguria may indicate clinically significant acute renal failure, whereas anuria always signals severe renal injury or complete urinary obstruction. It is important to quickly determine whether a patient is simply dehydrated or suffering from a more severe disorder.

DIAGNOSTIC WORKUP & INITIAL MANAGEMENT

History and physical examination

- Evaluate vital signs to assess for hypo- or hypertension, hypo- or hyperthermia, tachycardia, or respiratory distress that could explain decreased output
  - Note that hospitalized patients may have increased metabolic and fluid requirements as a result of their illness (e.g., burns, surgery, sepsis)
- In hospitalized patients, review the flow sheets for urine output measurements
- Evaluate inputs (solids, liquids, IV medications and fluids); urine output may be decreased by inappropriate intake (failing to provide IV fluids to patients not taking oral fluids)
- Obtain a urinary history: Assess for hesitancy, urge, incomplete or frequent voiding, dysuria, hematuria, any previous history of difficulty voiding, or history of prostate disease
  - Men with urinary retention warrant rectal exam to evaluate for prostate hyperplasia
- Assess for diseases that can affect renal function (e.g., hypertension, diabetes, CHF, SLE)
- Note recent administration of nephrotoxic drugs (NSAIDs, ACE inhibitors, aminoglycosides)
- Note recent surgical instrumentation in the pelvic area
- If a Foley catheter is in place, note amount of urine, color of the urine, presence or absence of blood and sediment, and if catheter has been flushed recently
- Review baseline creatinine to estimate baseline GFR, and compare with recent measurements for evidence of deteriorating renal function

Initial patient management

- Address any hemodynamic instability
- If the patient does not have a Foley catheter, place one, and record the urine output
  - If a catheter cannot be inserted, a mechanical obstruction is likely (usually a large prostate)
  - If initial urine output is >200 mL, acute urinary retention is likely, and the patient will need the Foley catheter for at least 24 hours while an etiology is determined
  - If the initial urine output is <200 mL, acute urinary retention is not likely, and a workup should be initiated to determine the nature of the decreased urine output
- If the patient appears euvolemic or hypovolemic, consider a fluid bolus; exercise caution, however, in patients with impaired cardiac function
- Order a basic metabolic panel, urinalysis, and urine culture if suspect UTI
  - If the patient has a history of colicky abdominal pain and has blood on urinalysis, consider abdominal and pelvic CT to evaluate for urolithiasis
  - If the patient has an acute increase in creatinine, treat for acute renal failure
- If anuria, attempt to flush the catheter with 100–200 mL of sterile saline; if the catheter does not flush easily or flushes without return, the catheter is either clogged or misplaced; in such cases, deflate the balloon, and insert a new Foley catheter
  - If a blood clot has obstructed the catheter, consider placing a dual-lumen catheter, and begin continuous bladder irrigation to prevent further clotting
  - Consider renal ultrasound to evaluate for bilateral hydronephrosis

DIFFERENTIAL DIAGNOSIS

Prerenal failure
- Responsible for 30% of all cases of acute renal failure
- Consider causes of volume depletion (e.g., hemorrhage, decreased oral intake, GI losses, dehydration, fever), decreased effective circulating volume (e.g., cirrhosis, CHF, septic shock), or renal vasoconstriction (e.g., contrast dye, cyclosporine)

Intrinsic renal failure
- Most common form of acute renal failure (50% of cases); results from glomerular and/or tubular injury
- Often iatrogenic as a result of medications administered in hospital; common drugs include NSAIDs, ACE inhibitors, and aminoglycosides
- Major etiologies to consider: Acute tubular necrosis (secondary to poor renal perfusion, drugs, or contrast agents), glomerulonephritis, TTP, vasculitis, interstitial nephritis (e.g., drugs, infection, idiopathic), rhabdomyolysis, multiple myeloma, or atheromatous emboli
- Contrast nephropathy remains a significant concern for those undergoing cardiac catheterization or radiographic studies utilizing iodinated IV dye (high-risk comorbidities include diabetes, chronic kidney disease, dehydration, multiple myeloma); hydration before, during, and after procedures and use of *N*-acetylcysteine may prevent renal injury

Postrenal obstruction
- Results from processes that increase renal tubular pressures by blocking urine outflow (e.g., enlarged prostate, urethral stricture, pelvic mass, urolithiasis, surgical complications)
- Inpatients can develop renal stones during hospitalization
- Consider benign prostatic hyperplasia in older men and medications that interfere with urinary outflow (e.g., anticholinergics, narcotics)

Obstruction or malfunction of the Foley catheter
- Foley catheter allows easy determination of urine output but significantly increases the risk for UTIs
- Catheters can be misplaced, or the orifice can become clogged with debris or clots

Neurogenic bladder
- Inability of the bladder to contract properly, causing acute or chronic urinary retention
- Acute urinary retention most often results from a medication effect; review chart for anesthetics (postoperative patients), β-agonists, α-agonists, antihistamines, benzodiazepines, tricyclic antidepressants, anticholinergics, and narcotics
- Consider neurologic emergencies (e.g., cord compression, stroke)
- Various comorbid conditions can cause urinary retention (e.g., diabetes, multiple sclerosis, Parkinson's disease, myasthenia gravis)

Paraphimosis or phimosis
- A relatively uncommon diagnosis, but should be considered in older patients
- Phimosis is the inability to retract the foreskin proximally over the glans, most often because of poor hygiene or balanitis; paraphimosis is a urologic emergency characterized by an inability to reduce the retracted foreskin, which can compromise the blood supply to the glans penis

Pregnancy
- Consider bilateral ureteral obstruction by enlarging uterus
- Bladder injury during cesarean section may present with decreased urine output and intra-abdominal urine leakage
- Bladder and urethral ruptures have been reported after normal vaginal delivery
- Consider obstetrical emergencies (e.g., preeclampsia, abruptio placentae, amniotic fluid embolism)

Urticaria (Hives)

INTRODUCTION

Urticaria (hives) is a common clinical presentation characterized by transient (typically disappearing within a few hours), itchy, erythematous dermal wheals. They are polymorphic, round, or irregularly shaped with central clearing and are well-circumscribed, raised, and range in size from a few millimeters to several centimeters in diameter. Urticarial lesions affect the superficial dermis. In contrast, angioedema is a swelling of the deeper dermis and subcutaneous tissues and often mucosa (e.g., lips). It is episodic and recurrent, and it may occur alone or in association with urticaria.

DIAGNOSTIC WORKUP & INITIAL MANAGEMENT

History and physical examination

- Family history of angioedema, anaphylaxis, etc.
- Seasonal or activity-related (work/home) symptoms
- Note whether urticaria occurs after ingestion of certain foods or with physical stimuli (e.g., exercise, pressure)
- Pay specific attention to potential triggers (e.g., foods, medications, environmental exposures)
- Physical exam should evaluate for underlying occult infections (e.g., UTI, vaginal yeast infection, tinea)
- Firmly trace the blunt tip of a cotton applicator across the patient's back; those with dermatographism will develop a pruritic urticarial wheal within 5 minutes
- Determine if the patient has isolated urticaria, urticaria with angioedema, or isolated angioedema

Initial diagnostic workup

- In patients with acute urticaria, no lab workup is necessary; however, a symptom diary may be useful
- In patients with chronic urticaria, concerning features of the history and physical exam should prompt diagnostic evaluation; CBC with differential, thyroid function tests, and ESR comprise a cost-effective screen
  - Additional testing for patients with elevated ESR may include liver function tests, serum protein electrophoresis, hepatitis serologies, complement levels, ANA, IgE antibodies, or serum studies for celiac disease
- Consider punch biopsy if vasculitis is possible (e.g., painful urticaria lasting >12–24 hours)
- If clinical suspicion exists, consider age-appropriate malignancy screening
- If a cause cannot be found, consider referral to a dermatologist to rule out an occult etiology, although many cases will ultimately be deemed idiopathic

Initial patient management

- Identify and remove the offending trigger, if possible; consider an elimination diet to pinpoint suspicious foods
- H_1-receptor blockers (e.g., hydroxyzine, diphenhydramine, loratadine, fexofenadine) have the quickest onset and are often the initial choice for symptomatic relief; refractory cases may respond to addition of H_2-receptor blockers (e.g., ranitidine, cimetidine)
  - Cyproheptadine has been shown to be helpful for cold-induced urticaria
  - Doxepin exerts both H_1- and H_2-receptor blockade and may be particularly effective
- Leukotriene inhibitors may be beneficial as add-on therapy with antihistamines
- Corticosteroids and epinephrine may be necessary for severe attacks with associated angioedema; prescribe an epinephrine pen (Epi-Pen) for patients with angioedema

DIFFERENTIAL DIAGNOSIS

Idiopathic urticaria without angioedema

- Most common diagnosis in patients with hives
- Most cases are immunologically-mediated:
  - Type I reaction (IgE hypersensitivity): Reaction to foods, drugs, latex, venom, and other allergens results in histamine release from mast cells, local vasodilation and edema, and inflammatory response with wheals and erythema
  - Type II reaction (cytotoxic antibody): Transfusion reaction
  - Type III reaction (antigen–antibody complex): Reaction to serum sickness
  - Type IV reaction (delayed-type sensitivity): Reaction to drugs, foods, or animal exposures
  - Other cases involve autoimmune diseases (e.g., vasculitis, thyroiditis, SLE), infections (e.g., *H. pylori*, viruses), and malignancies (e.g., lymphoma)
- Nonimmune cases may be caused by physical entities (e.g., dermatographism, cold, sun exposure), direct mast cell degranulation caused by certain drugs (e.g., opiates, NSAIDs, vancomycin, radiocontrast media), and foods with high histamine content (e.g., shellfish)

Chronic urticaria

- Episodes occur at least twice weekly for >6 weeks
- 25% of patients with one episode of urticaria will progress to chronic urticaria
- Idiopathic in 50% of cases; resolves spontaneously within 2 years in 80% of patients

Occult infection

- Sinusitis
- Oral infection
- Cholecystitis
- Vaginitis
- Prostatitis
- Hepatitis
- HIV
- Tinea manum or pedis

Drugs

- Common drugs include radiocontrast media, penicillin, salicylates, benzoates, and azo dyes
- May result in life-threatening urticaria and acute angioedema that can lead to anaphylaxis

Urticaria secondary to physical stimuli

- Dermatographism (physical urticaria arising in the distribution of a scratch or rubbed skin)
- Cold exposure
- Exercise (cholinergic)
- Vibratory pressure
- Sun exposure (solar urticaria)

Hereditary or acquired deficiency of complement factor C1

- Generally appears as episodic angioedema in the absence of urticaria (consider hereditary or acquired complement deficiency only in the absence of urticaria)

Urticarial vasculitis

- Presents as urticaria lasting >12–24 hours
- Associated with autoimmune disease (e.g., SLE)

Other

- Malignancy
- Contact dermatitis or atopic dermatitis
- Mastocytosis
- Vasculitis
- Bullous pemphigoid
- Muckle-Wells syndrome
- Familial cold autoinflammatory syndrome
- Angioedema-urticaria-eosinophilia syndrome
- Thyroid disease
- Insect bite
- Hepatitis B
- Erythema multiforme
- Dermatitis herpetiforme
- Cellulitis
- Schnitzler's syndrome

Vaginal Bleeding (Abnormal)

INTRODUCTION

Normal menses is defined as bleeding of <80 mL over 2–7 days at 21- to 35-day intervals. Variation of normal menses often occurs during perimenarche, perimenopause, and in situations such as initiation of oral contraceptive pills. Abnormal variations include oligomenorrhea (menses >35 days apart), polymenorrhea (menses <21 days apart), menorrhagia (menses of a duration >7 days or with blood loss >80 mL), metrorrhagia (irregular menses), and menometrorrhagia (increased flow at irregular intervals). Postmenopausal bleeding is never normal, although the cause is often benign. Remember that not all vaginal bleeding is from the genital tract or uterus; consider also bladder (e.g., bladder cancer) and GI sources (e.g., hemorrhoids).

DIAGNOSTIC WORKUP & INITIAL MANAGEMENT

- Acute, life threatening bleeding must be treated emergently with IV estrogen or other medications, fluids and/or blood replacement, curettage, and possible ligation of the uterine artery or hysterectomy

History and physical examination

- Note the number of pads used (>1 per hour is worrisome) and passage of clots
- History should include menarchal, menstrual, and sexual history; history of pregnancies, births, abortions, STDs, and contraceptive use; also inquire about recent fever, uterine pain, systemic disorders, gynecologic surgeries, medication use, trauma, and abuse
- Physical exam should include vital signs, evaluation of skin for signs of abuse and coagulopathy, palpation of the thyroid, signs of androgen excess (e.g., hirsutism, deep voice, acanthosis nigricans), and examination of the heart, lungs, and abdomen
- Gynecologic exam must be performed in all patients (avoid bimanual exam in gravid females during the 2nd and 3rd trimesters until placenta previa is ruled out): Evaluate the vaginal walls and cervix for lacerations, polyps, friability, and motion tenderness; evaluate the uterus for size (fibroids, pregnancy); evaluate the ovaries for size and tenderness; consider rectal exam if there is no blood in the vaginal canal or coming from the cervical os
- Presentation of vaginal bleeding may relate to the vaginal bleeding itself or subsequent anemia; anemia may present with tachycardia, orthostasis, dizziness, light-headedness, or syncope; chest pain and shortness of breath may occur in severely anemic patients
- May present as heavy menses with clot passage, midcycle spotting, or dyspareunia
- Take cervical cultures or DNA probe for gonorrhea and chlamydia; cervical cytology and colposcopy may be indicated in outpatients to follow up for any visualized cervical lesions

Initial workup and management

- Consider a wet prep (for trichomoniasis), CBC, coagulation studies, and TSH; consider testosterone, DHEA-S, prolactin level, and fasting insulin level if suspect polycystic ovarian syndrome, ovarian disease, or adrenal disease; consider iron studies
- Pregnancy testing is indicated in all women unless documented to be postmenopausal
- Consider coagulation studies, peripheral smear, clotting factor assays, liver function tests, serum progesterone, and BUN and creatinine to evaluate for coagulopathy, hepatic, or renal disease
- Gynecology may recommend further imaging or evaluation, which may include endometrial biopsy, ultrasound, sonohysterography, hysteroscopy, and laparoscopy
- Diagnostic dilatation and curettage may be indicated in some patients
- Treat the underlying etiology as appropriate
- Nonacute bleeding is often treated with oral contraceptives to regulate bleeding (consider dosage change if already on oral contraceptives); other treatments include cyclic progesterone (will not prevent pregnancy), NSAIDs, GnRH agonists, intrauterine progesterone, anti-fibrinolytic agents, or endometrial ablation

DIFFERENTIAL DIAGNOSIS

Uterine lesions
- Fibroid tumor is the most common cause of menorrhagia
- Leiomyosarcoma
- Endometrial hyperplasia and dysfunctional uterine bleeding
- Endometrial, vaginal, and vulvar atrophy are the most common causes if postmenopausal
- Endometrial cancer accounts for as much as 5% of cases of postmenopausal bleeding
- Adenomyosis uteri (endometrium infiltrates myometrium)
- Endometriosis
- Uterine arteriovenous malformation

Anatomic lesions
- Vaginal or genital tract laceration or trauma
- Postcoital trauma
- Foreign body (often an intrauterine device)

Vaginal and cervical lesions
- Cervical polyps or cancer
- Vaginal or vulvar cancers

Gastrointestinal and bladder etiologies
- Hemorrhoids
- Colon or rectal cancer
- Bladder cancer
- Bladder or GI tract fistula (e.g., as occurs in Crohn's disease, diverticulitis)

Infectious etiologies
- STDs (e.g., trichomoniasis, HIV, pelvic inflammatory disease)
- Pelvic infection (e.g., cervicitis, UTI, endometritis)

Pregnancy-related etiologies
- Normal spotting
- Threatened or inevitable abortion
- Ectopic pregnancy
- Placenta previa
- Placental abruption
- Gestational trophoblastic disease
- Hydatiform mole
- Bloody show
- Infection
- Postpartum etiologies (e.g., uterine atony, lacerations, endomyometritis)

Systemic etiologies
- Coagulopathies: Platelet dysfunction (e.g., thrombocytopenia, leukemia, aspirin, NSAIDs), clotting factor abnormality (e.g., hemophilia, von Willebrand's disease, hepatic or renal disease, anticoagulant use)
- Leukemia

Endocrine etiologies
- Hypo- or hyperthyroidism
- Anovulatory cycles (e.g., perimenarchal or perimenopausal)
- Polycystic ovarian syndrome
- Adrenal or ovarian dysfunction
- Hyperprolactinemia

Iatrogenic etiologies
- Medications (e.g., anticoagulant therapy, hormone replacement therapy, opiates, tricyclic antidepressants, metoclopramide, phenothiazines, reserpine, ginseng) and radiation therapy

Vaginal Discharge

INTRODUCTION

Vaginal discharge is one of the most common primary care complaints, accounting for ~10 million office visits yearly. It is often accompanied by concerns about the presence of an STD. The most common causes of vaginal discharge are candidiasis ("yeast" infection), bacterial vaginosis, and trichomoniasis. In women with vaginal symptoms, 25%–50% have bacterial vaginosis, 20%–40% have vaginal candidiasis, 5%–35% have trichomoniasis, and many cases remain undiagnosed. Whenever one STD is identified, a search for all other STDs is indicated in an effort to treat the individual patient as well as to prevent spread to others. If an STD is identified, the patient should be encouraged to inform all sexual partners of the diagnosis.

DIAGNOSTIC WORKUP & INITIAL MANAGEMENT

History and physical examination

- A focused history and physical exam are crucial, including a complete sexual and exposure history and a full abdominal and pelvic exam
- Associated symptoms include odor, irritation, dyspareunia, bleeding, or pruritus
- Discharges are characterized by color (clear, white, green, gray, or yellow), consistency (thin, thick, or curd-like), and amount (more or less than usual)
- Signs include erythema, excoriation, or discharge on the perineum or introitus

Initial diagnostic workup

- Evaluate the appearance, pH, odor, and microscopic exam of the discharge (see chart)
  - Wet mount and KOH test of the discharge are imperative
  - pH of the discharge may aid in diagnosis
  - Discharge should be sampled from the vaginal side wall, midway to the vagina
  - Whiff test is done by smelling the discharge after KOH is added; a positive test reveals a fishy odor characteristic of bacterial vaginosis

	pH	Discharge	Odor	Microscopy
Trichomonas	>4.5	yellow-green, copious	present	motile, flagellated
Bacterial vaginosis	>4.5	white-grey	fishy	clue cells
Candida	<4.5	white, curd-like	none	pseudohyphae
Gonorrhea/chlamydia	>4.5	mucopurulent	varies	PMNs
Atrophic vaginitis	>5.0	thin, gray, watery	none	few epithelial cells

- Initial laboratory testing may include CBC, urinalysis, urine culture, β-hCG, and cultures or DNA probe (Gen-Probe) for *N. gonorrhea* and *Chlamydia*
- Consider Pap smear
- Test and treat for other STDs when one STD is found (HIV, hepatitis B and C, syphilis)
- Resources include the CDC National Prevention Information Network (info@cdcnpin.org or www.cdcnpin.org) and the American Social Health association (www.ashatd.org)

Initial patient management

- Bacterial vaginosis: Oral metronidazole for 7 days, metronidazole vaginal gel for 5 days, clindamycin for 7 days, or 2% clindamycin vaginal cream for 7 days
- Avoid alcohol during (and for 24 hours after) treatment with metronidazole to avoid possible disulfuram-like reactions
- Trichomoniasis: Oral metronidazole (single dose or 7 days) or tinidazole (single dose)
- Treat sexual partners in patients with trichomoniasis
- Candidiasis: Fluconazole, itraconazole, or intravaginal azoles
- Treat recurrent candidiasis with 6-month suppression therapy with oral or topical agents

DIFFERENTIAL DIAGNOSIS

Physiologic

- Many women have a consistent, slightly clear, non–odor producing discharge either midcycle or premenstrually, particularly if on oral contraceptives
- Normal pH of the vagina is <4.5; normal vaginal flora is heterogeneous and predominated by lactobacilli
- A change in odor, consistency, or color of discharge may signify infection or other pathology
- Increased discharged is associated with pregnancy

Sexually transmitted disease (STD)

- Gonorrhea and chlamydia
  - May be associated with pelvic pain, dysmenorrhea, and dyspareunia
- Trichomoniasis
  - Caused by *Trichomonas vaginalis* (a motile, single-celled parasite)
  - May be associated with a "strawberry cervix" with punctate erythema
  - May see flagellated oval organisms on wet mount
  - Risk factors include multiple sexual partners, history of previous STDs, or coinfection with other sexually transmitted infections
- Herpes simplex

Bacterial vaginosis

- Overgrowth of the normal vaginal flora, including *Gardnerella vaginalis*, *Bacteroides*, *Mobiluncus*, *Mycoplasma hominis*, and other anaerobes
- Not considered an STD
- Has a characteristic fishy odor
- May increase the risk of preterm delivery, preterm rupture of membranes, and endometritis in pregnant women

Atrophic vaginitis

- Common in postmenopausal women, especially those not on hormone replacement therapy
- Associated with poor coital lubrication and dyspareunia
- Dysuria may result from atrophic urethral tissue

Alteration of normal vaginal flora and/or inflammatory response

- Candidiasis
  - Caused by overgrowth of *Candida albicans*, *Candida glabrata*, or *Candida tropicalis*
  - May be associated with recent antibiotic use, poorly controlled diabetes, pregnancy, and immunocompromised states
  - Presents with an intensely pruritic, inflamed, and erythematous introitus
- Doderlein's cytolysis
  - Caused by an overgrowth of lactobacilli

Foreign body vaginitis

- Retained tampon is a common cause

Noninfectious irritant or allergic contact vaginitis

- Offending substances include soaps, chemical irritants, latex, semen, feminine pads, and perfumes

Cervicitis

- Usually caused by *N. gonorrhea* or *Chlamydia*

Other

- Cervical dysplasia, cancer, or polyps
- Vaginal or vulvar cancer
- Vaginal or vulvar trauma

Vision Loss

INTRODUCTION

Visual loss is a common presenting complaint with a protean differential diagnosis; it may occur as a result of lesions throughout the visual pathway, including the retina, orbit, optic nerve or chiasm, optic radiations, occipital cortex, or visual association cortex. It may be unilateral or bilateral, transient or persistent, of sudden or gradual onset, and painless or painful. Vision loss in one eye may be followed quickly by ensuing vision loss of the other eye, rendering the patient completely blind (e.g., untreated temporal arteritis). In some situations, vision loss may be reversible with timely intervention. Vision loss may be a harbinger of more serious, even life-threatening, conditions (e.g., brain tumor, meningitis, giant cell arteritis, cavernous sinus thrombosis, mucormycosis).

DIAGNOSTIC WORKUP & INITIAL MANAGEMENT

History and physical examination

- Focus on neurologic complaints and the acuity of onset
- Determine if visual loss is central or peripheral, unilateral or bilateral, constant or intermittent, progressive or stable
- Evaluate for age, tempo and duration of visual disturbance, whether unilateral or bilateral, history of trauma, photophobia, headache, pain (especially temporal pain), previous episodes, alcohol/drug and tobacco use, and medications; assess medical history for diabetes, hypertension, carotid or cardiac disease, arrhythmia (particularly atrial fibrillation), cancer, hyperlipidemia, stroke, vertigo, migraine, collagen vascular disease or other systemic inflammatory disease (e.g., SLE), syphilis, and ocular disease
- Obtain vital signs with particular attention to blood pressure
- Exam includes thorough eye exam, evaluation of cranial nerves, visual acuity, funduscopic exam, intraocular pressure, ocular media opacity (corneal edema, dystrophy, anterior chamber or vitreous cells, cataracts), and head and neck exam to assess for trauma or other readily identifiable cause for the visual change (e.g., temporal artery pain)
- Using a penlight, examine conjunctiva and iris, assess for corneal opacity (whitening), and stain with fluorescein to evaluate for a corneal abrasion
- Using an ophthalmoscope, assess the red reflex, optic disc, retinal vessels, and macula

Initial workup and management

- Emergent ophthalmology consultation may be indicated for patients with acute visual changes, including the following possible diagnoses:
  - Temporal arteritis: Immediate administration of steroids (oral prednisone) is indicated; ESR will be elevated; biopsy is necessary for definitive diagnosis
  - Acute angle-closure glaucoma: An ophthalmologic emergency; iridotomy required
  - Corneal abrasion or ulcer: Abrasions require topical antibiotic ointments; steroids should be strictly avoided because they increase the risk of secondary bacterial infection
  - HSV or cytomegalovirus retinal infections: Treat with acyclovir; avoid steroids because they increase the risk of systemic spread
- Fluorescein exam can be a high-yield test in the diagnosis of corneal abrasion
- Consider CT of the head to evaluate for stroke (infarction of the occipital lobe or any area along the optic tract can cause visual loss or visual changes)
- Consider CT or MRI of the brain and orbits, with and without contrast
- Carotid Doppler ultrasound and cardiac echocardiography if suspect ischemia
- ERG and visual-evoked potentials (retinal dystrophies, optic neuropathies)
- Lab testing may include glucose, Hb_{A1c}, PPD, RPR, ACE level, vitamin B_{12} and folate, and screening for vascular risk factors (e.g., lipids, coagulation screen, vasculitis screen, ESR)
- Consider carotid endarterectomy for transient monocular blindness if carotid stenosis is >70% in the carotid artery unilateral to the visual loss

DIFFERENTIAL DIAGNOSIS

Lesions (may occur anywhere along the visual pathway)
- Retina: Detached retina, retinitis pigmentosa, macular degeneration
- Orbital: Mass lesions, vitreous hemorrhage, corneal opacities
- Optic nerve: Mass lesion, autoimmune (e.g., optic neuritis), toxins, ischemia (e.g., embolism, temporal arteritis), carotid stenosis, giant cell arteritis, hyperviscosity, optic atrophy, hypotension, severe disc edema, tobacco/alcohol amblyopia, ischemic optic neuropathy
- Optic chiasm: Usually from compressive mass lesions (e.g., pituitary adenoma, aneurysm, meningioma, craniopharyngioma)
- Optic radiation: Mass lesion, ischemia, intracerebral hemorrhage
- Visual cortex: Unilateral visual loss may result from mass lesions, vascular disease (e.g., stroke, hemorrhage, venous thrombosis); bilateral transient visual loss may result from migraine, vertebrobasilar insufficiency, prolonged hypertension or hypotension, drug-induced (e.g., cyclosporine toxicity), seizure, or postictal phenomenon

Transient vision loss (<24 hours)
- Papilledema can result in visual changes caused by compression of the optic nerve
- Retinal migraine (migraine variant that affects the retinal artery and ciliary circulation)
- Hypotension or othostatic hypotension (vertebrobasilar artery insufficiency)
- Amaurosis fugax: Unilateral visual change lasting minutes
- Vertebrobasilar artery insufficiency (lasts minutes, bilateral)
- Impending central retinal vein occlusion
- Ocular ischemic syndrome (carotid occlusive disease)
- Transient acute increase in intraocular pressure (e.g., acute angle-closure glaucoma, retrobulbar or peribulbar hemorrhage)

Sudden, painless vision loss lasting >24 hours
- Ischemic optic neuropathy
- Temporal arteritis (visual loss is generally sudden and occurs on the same side as the headache; may progress to opposite eye if not treated)
- Retinal detachment (e.g., trauma, aging)
- Retinal artery or vein occlusion
- Vitreous or aqueous hemorrhage (hyphema): Usually occurs following trauma; may result from coagulopathy (hemophilia, anticoagulation)
- Other retinal or CNS disease (e.g., cortical blindness caused by occipital lobe stroke)
- Prolonged exposure to intense UV light (e.g., skiers, boaters, welders)

Gradual, painless vision loss lasting >24 hours
- Cataract
- Refractive error
- Open-angle glaucoma
- Chronic retinopathy (e.g., age-related macular degeneration, diabetic retinopathy)
- Chronic corneal disease (e.g., corneal dystrophy)
- Optic neuropathy or atrophy (e.g., compressive lesion, toxic-metabolic, radiation)
- Retinitis pigmentosa
- Pseudotumor cerebri

Painful vision loss lasting >24 hours
- Acute angle-closure glaucoma (intense pain with red eye, nausea, vomiting, diaphoresis)
- Optic neuritis (unilateral pain with extraocular motion)
- Orbital apex/superior orbital fissure/cavernous sinus syndrome
- Uveitis
- Corneal hydrops (keratoconus)
- Corneal abrasion or ulcer
- Herpes simplex or zoster infection
- Consider onchocerciasis ("river blindness") caused by *Onchocerca volvulus*

Hysteria/conversion disorder

Vomiting

INTRODUCTION

Vomiting is a complex, coordinated reflex orchestrated by neural mechanisms that originate in the chemoreceptor trigger zone and the vomiting center of the medulla. The chemoreceptor trigger zone, contained in the area postrema on the floor of the 4th ventricle, is particularly sensitive to chemical stimuli. It also is readily accessible to emetic substances, because the blood-brain barrier is poorly developed in this area. The vomiting center, located in the dorsolateral border of the reticular formation, coordinates the emetic response during the act of vomiting; it receives and integrates excitatory inputs from vagal sensory fibers in the GI tract, labyrinths, higher centers in the cortex, chemoreceptor trigger zone, and intracranial pressure receptors.

DIAGNOSTIC WORKUP & INITIAL MANAGEMENT

- Severe vomiting requires immediate intervention
- Evaluate airway, breathing, and circulation
  - If airway compromise is possible, ensure a secure airway; note risk of aspiration
  - Ensure adequate IV access with ≥18-gauge IV line, and begin IV fluids
- Patients should avoid oral intake until stabilized, especially if likely to require surgery or endoscopy
- Consider a nasogastric tube for decompression

History and physical examination

- Note whether vomiting is acute or chronic
- Evaluate medical history (e.g., cancer, renal failure, immunodeficiency, coronary artery disease, CHF), new medications (including oral electrolytes), abdominal surgeries, and substance abuse; assess recently administered medications and timing of meals, and compare to the chronology of the vomiting
- Note any temporal relationship with eating
- Note irritative foods or medications taken on an empty stomach
- Assess contents and nature of the emesis (e.g., bloody, bilious, projectile, digested vs. undigested food, fecal odor, acidic odor)
- Note associated nausea; vomiting tends to relieve nausea if the cause is irritative substances in the stomach but does not usually alleviate that caused by a central effect (e.g., gastritis, gastroenteritis, uremia, certain drugs)
- Note associated symptoms (e.g., fever, diarrhea, abdominal pain, headache)

Initial workup and management

- Laboratory testing may include electrolytes, glucose, liver function tests, hematocrit, amylase and lipase, urinalysis, pregnancy testing in females, and toxicology screen
- ECG, cardiac enzymes, and telemetry if a cardiac etiology is considered
- Consider abdominal radiographic series (e.g., flat and upright) to evaluate for obstruction or perforation
- CT of the abdomen and pelvis is an appropriate test if suspect pancreatitis or anatomic obstruction
- Cine-esophagram or barium swallow may be indicated if dysphagia and vomiting
- Emergent head CT is indicated if suspect increased intracranial pressure
- Consider benzodiazepine administration, folic acid, and fluids for alcohol withdrawal
- If suspect adrenal failure, give IV hydrocortisone (100 mg) until a diagnosis is confirmed
- IV proton pump inhibitors may be indicated to reduce stomach acidity in gastric bleeding
- Consider IV or rectal antiemetics (e.g., promethazine); monitor for extrapyramidal effects and mental status change, especially in the elderly and patients with liver failure
- Consider serotonin antagonists (e.g., ondansetron) for refractory cases or vomiting caused by chemotherapy
- Hematemesis requires emergent gastroenterology consultation and ICU admission

DIFFERENTIAL DIAGNOSIS

Gastrointestinal disease
- Hepatobiliary disease
- Pancreatic disease (e.g., pancreatitis)
- Gastritis and peptic ulcers (especially in ICU or trauma patients)
- Peritonitis (e.g., ruptured appendix, ascites caused by liver disease, peritoneal dialysis)
- Gastroenteritis (most common cause of vomiting at any age)
- GI obstruction
  - Adhesions
  - Malignancy
  - Volvulus
  - Pyloric stenosis
  - Intussusception
- GI motility disorders
  - Diabetes
  - Achalasia
  - Peritonitis
  - Scleroderma
  - Amyloidosis

Iatrogenic
- Systemic drug effects are very common in hospitalized patients; nearly any medication can be implicated, including digitalis, opiates, theophylline, salicylates, nicotine patch, quinidine, potassium preparations, chemotherapy, antibiotics, and antihypertensives
- Severe constipation caused by medications (e.g., narcotics, iron) can also lead to vomiting
- Postoperative vomiting

Central etiologies of nausea and vomiting
- Uremia
  - Nausea and vomiting may be worse in the morning
  - In chronic dialysis patients, evaluate for rising creatinine or missed dialysis sessions
- Pregnancy (hyperemesis gravidarum)
- Hypercalcemia
- Drugs (e.g., chemotherapeutics)

Endocrine disorder or electrolyte disturbance
- Etiologies include hypothyroidism, parathyroid disease, hypokalemia, hypercalcemia, metabolic alkalosis, diabetic ketoacidosis, and adrenal failure

Toxic ingestions
- Syrup of ipecac, alcohol, salicylates, iron, arsenic

Head and neck etiologies
- Migraine
- Middle ear disturbance (e.g., Ménière's disease, labyrinthitis, benign positional vertigo)
- Acute angle-closure glaucoma

Other
- Motion sickness
- Acute myocardial ischemia or infarction
- Alcohol or opiate withdrawal
- Increased intracranial pressure (e.g., head trauma, brain tumor or abscess, hydrocephalus)
- Pyelonephritis
- Testicular or ovarian torsion
- Carbon monoxide poisoning
- Psychogenic or self-induced vomiting
- Malingering

Weight Gain

INTRODUCTION

Weight gain is a common complaint. The key to diagnosis is often a thorough history and physical examination. It is important to quantify the degree and rapidity of weight gain by comparing old weights in the chart and questioning the patient. Physical examination will help to differentiate fluid retention from increase in adipose tissue.

DIAGNOSTIC WORKUP & INITIAL MANAGEMENT

History and physical examination

- Assess baseline weight and rapidity of weight gain
- Assess dietary history, but be aware that patient estimates of food intake are often inaccurate; a food diary may be helpful
- Assess medications, tobacco and alcohol history, menstrual history, and review of systems
- Screen for depression
- Note body habitus (e.g., Cushing's syndrome often presents with moon facies, buffalo hump, and thin extremities; "apple" vs. "pear" shape)
- Note body hair distribution (scarce in hypothyroidism; hirsutism in polycystic ovarian syndrome and Cushing's syndrome)
- Note skin appearance (abdominal striae and easy bruising in Cushing's syndrome; acanthosis nigricans in diabetes)
- Assess for peripheral edema and ascites (as may occur in CHF, nephrotic syndrome, liver disease, or preeclampsia)

Initial diagnostic workup

- Initial laboratory testing may include:
  - CBC (leukocytosis in Cushing's syndrome; thrombocytopenia in preeclampsia)
  - Fasting glucose (elevated in diabetes and Cushing's syndrome)
  - BUN and creatinine (rule out renal failure)
  - Urinalysis (excessive proteinuria and lipiduria in nephrotic syndrome; proteinuria in preeclampsia and diabetes)
  - TSH (hypothyroidism)
  - Lipid profile (hypercholesterolemia in nephrotic syndrome, Cushing's syndrome, diabetes)
  - Albumin (decreased in nephrotic syndrome and liver disease)
  - Urine pregnancy test in females
- Further studies may include 24-hour urine (if urinalysis reveals proteinuria), liver function tests (elevated in liver disease and preeclampsia), dexamethasone suppression test (rule out Cushing's syndrome), chest radiography and/or echocardiography (rule out CHF if suspect pulmonary edema from exam), abdominal ultrasound and/or CT (rule out liver or renal disease), and/or pelvic ultrasound (rule out polycystic ovaries)

Initial patient management

- Treat underlying medical disorders as necessary
- Discontinue or change offending medications, if possible
- Weight from fluid overload can be treated with diuretics or other medications
- Weight from an increase in adipose tissue can be lost by a low-calorie diet and exercise

DIFFERENTIAL DIAGNOSIS

Physiologic weight gain
- Pregnancy

Medication side effect
- Oral contraceptives
- Corticosteroids and androgenic steroids
- Antidepressants
- Benzodiazepines
- Hypoglycemic agents
- Anticonvulsants

Imbalance in caloric intake vs. expenditure
- Primary obesity caused by overeating and sedentary lifestyle
- Overeating secondary to nicotine withdrawal, depression, or binge phase of bulimia nervosa
- Hypothyroidism (decreased metabolic rate)
- Hyperthyroidism (increased appetite)
- Diabetes mellitus (type 2)
- Polycystic ovarian syndrome
- Cushing's syndrome

Fluid-related weight gain
- Premenstrual syndrome
- Nephrotic syndrome
- Acute or chronic liver disease
- Congestive heart failure
- Preeclampsia/eclampsia

Less common etiologies
- Hypothalamic lesions
  - Tumor (e.g., craniopharyngioma)
  - Infection
  - Head trauma
  - Infiltrative or inflammatory lesions
  - Postneurosurgery or postirradiation
- Acromegaly (growth hormone excess, usually from a pituitary tumor)
- Growth hormone deficiency
- Insulinoma
- Genetic syndromes resulting in obesity in children
  - Prader-Willi syndrome
  - Laurence-Moon-Bardet-Biedl syndrome
  - Alstrom's syndrome
  - Cohen's syndrome
  - Down's syndrome
  - Carpenter's syndrome
  - Grebe syndrome
  - Beckwith-Wiedemann syndrome
- Adiposogenital dystrophy syndrome
- Congenital leptin deficiency
- Leptin resistance

Weight Loss

INTRODUCTION

Unexplained, involuntary weight loss (defined as loss of 5% of baseline body weight over 6–12 months) is a concerning clinical presentation, because it is nearly always a sign of a serious medical or psychiatric illness. Numerous studies independently associate unintentional weight loss with various adverse health outcomes, including decreased functional status and increased mortality. Weight maintenance requires a balance between calories ingested/absorbed and calories expended/lost. Determining if the imbalance has to do with intake, absorption, or expenditure is the initial step in determining the source of an imbalance.

DIAGNOSTIC WORKUP & INITIAL MANAGEMENT

History and physical examination

- History should confirm whether the weight loss is voluntary or involuntary; assess body image and concerns about body fat; determine if appetite is increased or decreased; inquire about changes in lifestyle, physical activity, and bowel patterns (e.g., floating, smelly stools are a clue to fat malabsorption); and assess medications, herbal remedies, illegal drug use, travel history, social issues, stressors, and family history of malignancies
- Assess diet and caloric intake (in patients with adequate caloric intake, endocrine and malabsorption disorders are more likely)
- Note general appearance, including temporal wasting; record weight, and measure heart rate and blood pressure
- Pay particular attention to thyroid, lymph node, and abdominal exams; as always, a thorough exam of all organ systems is warranted

Initial diagnostic workup

- Initial laboratory tests may include CBC, serum chemistries, glucose (to rule out diabetes), thyroid function tests, ESR, and albumin and/or prealbumin
- Consider a toxicology screen
- HIV testing may be indicated if risk factors are present
- Chest radiography in smokers and others at risk for pulmonary disease
- Age-appropriate cancer screening may include mammography, fecal occult blood testing, flexible sigmoidoscopy, or colonoscopy
- Morning (AM) cortisol and ACTH stimulation test if suspect adrenal insufficiency
- Consider upper GI endoscopy, colonoscopy, and GI consultation

Initial patient management

- Identify and address the underlying cause
- Appetite disturbance of depression may be reversed by antidepressant medications
- Pancreatic enzymes for pancreatic malabsorption
- Referral to nutritionist if necessary
- Referral to social services if necessary
- Anorexia of malignancy and AIDS can be treated with megestrol acetate or dronabinol
- Aggressive treatment of anorexia nervosa, including evaluation for electrolyte and cardiac disorders and consultation with a psychiatrist or psychologist

DIFFERENTIAL DIAGNOSIS

Malignancy
- Weight loss is mediated by enhanced production of cytokines (e.g., TNF-α, interleukin-6)

Gastrointestinal and malabsorption disorders
- Celiac disease
- Crohn's disease
- Cystic fibrosis
- Peptic ulcer disease

Depression
- Most common cause of weight loss in outpatient populations; weight loss is one of the criteria for a diagnosis of depression

HIV infection
- Weight loss may be associated with secondary infections or GI disease

Hypercalcemia
- Usually occurs in patients with cancer

Advanced cardiac and pulmonary disease
- CHF ("cardiac cachexia")
- COPD

Chronic drug use
- Alcohol
- Nicotine
- Opiates
- CNS stimulants (including cocaine)
- Lead exposure

Hyperthyroidism
- Weight loss results from increased appetite and increased energy expenditure

Uncontrolled diabetes mellitus
- Cells are unable to use glucose; glucose "spills" into the urine

Hyperemesis gravidarum
- Pathologic exaggeration of early pregnancy nausea
- Presents with elevated β-hCG and estrogen levels

Adrenal insufficiency
- Anorexia, nausea, and fatigue are common

Anorexia nervosa
- May present with low potassium (caused by vomiting), low albumin, parotid enlargement, lesions on knuckles and diminished tooth enamel from induced vomiting, and menstrual irregularities
- Patients often deny food restriction and/or purging

Failure to thrive (infants)
- Parental neglect/emotional deprivation
- Improper mixing of formula
- Significant heart (shunts) or lung disease
- Inborn errors of metabolism
- Intestinal parasites

Failure to thrive (adults)
- Inability to obtain or limited access to food
- Often occurs in socially isolated elderly persons

Wide Pulse Pressure

INTRODUCTION

Pulse pressure is the difference between systolic and diastolic blood pressures. Wide pulse pressure is defined as a difference >60–70 mm Hg. It often results from conditions that produce an increase in stroke volume or in diastolic runoff. It can be an innocent finding or a harbinger of serious, life-threatening disease, so prompt recognition and appropriate management are important.

DIAGNOSTIC WORKUP & INITIAL MANAGEMENT

History and physical examination
- Assess present illness (if any), medical and cardiovascular history, associated symptoms, and medications
- Perform a complete cardiovascular exam, with an additional, focused exam as indicated
- Evaluate for cardiac causes, especially if murmurs or abnormal pulses are present

Initial diagnostic workup
- Initial laboratory testing may include CBC, electrolytes, TSH, and lipid panel
- Obtain blood cultures if suspect endocarditis
- ECG may reveal left ventricular hypertrophy, complete heart block, atrial fibrillation, and evidence of coronary artery disease (e.g., Q wave, ST elevations)
- Echocardiography (transesophageal or transthoracic) may reveal left ventricular hypertrophy, aortic regurgitation, aortic dissection, valve vegetation, or pericardial effusion
  - Transesophageal echocardiography is very sensitive and specific for diagnosing aortic dissection, because it can evaluate both anatomically (dissection flap) and physiologically (flow difference between true and false lumen)
- Chest radiography will show widening of the mediastinum and enlargement of the aortic knob in cases of aortic dissection
- CT or MRI may be indicated to evaluate for aortic dissection and other pathologies
- Aortography may be indicated in cases of aortic regurgitation or aortic dissection
- If suspect atherosclerosis, evaluate risk factors and consider stress testing and cardiac catheterization

Initial patient management
- Assess hemodynamic stability
- Treat emergent causes as necessary
  - Immediate medical or surgical management of aortic dissection
  - Use β-blockers with caution in severe aortic regurgitation to avoid prolonging ventricular diastolic filling time and precipitating CHF
  - Immediate blood cultures and IV antibiotic therapy for endocarditis
- Evaluate and treat underlying causes of anemia, fever, hyperthyroidism, increased intracranial pressure, and chronic disease
- Chronic atrial regurgitation may require aortic valve replacement if there is associated aortic root dilation, concurrent endocarditis, failure of medical therapy, or left ventricular dysfunction

DIFFERENTIAL DIAGNOSIS

Atherosclerosis
- Large arteries stiffen with age, resulting in increased systolic blood pressure and widened pulse pressure

Chronic aortic regurgitation
- Causes include rheumatic heart disease, idiopathic aortic root dilatation, Marfan's syndrome, and endocarditis
- Exam may reveal an early diastolic "blowing" murmur
- Corrigan's (water-hammer) pulse: Rapid rise and rapid fall
- Hill's sign: Systolic blood pressure of the lower extremities is $\geq$20 mm Hg more than systolic blood pressure in the arms
- de Musset's sign: Head bobs with each heartbeat
- Acute aortic regurgitation does not result in widened pulse pressure

Thyrotoxicosis
- Associated with nervousness, sweating, heat intolerance, tachycardia, weight loss
- Thyroid nodules may be present

Increased cardiac output states
- Fever, anemia, anxiety, pregnancy

Patent ductus arteriosus
- Presents with "bounding" pulses and continuous, "machine-like" murmur throughout diastole and systole

Complete heart block
- Often secondary to MI or coronary artery disease

Sinus bradycardia
- Identified by the heart rate in sinus rhythm with a rate <60 bpm
- P waves have normal contour and occur before each QRS complex; PR interval is constant
- May be caused by intrinsic cardiac dysfunction (e.g., sinus node dysfunction) or secondary to the influence of extrinsic, noncardiac factors (e.g., medications)

Systemic arteriovenous fistula
- Tachycardia may be the only clue

Aortic dissection
- A tear in the aortic wall that originates from the intima
- Hypertension, Marfan's syndrome, and pregnancy are common predisposing factors
- A common site is the ascending aorta (50%) and is often fatal
- Type A involves the ascending aorta; more prevalent in patients with hypertension, carries a worse prognosis, and mandates immediate surgery
- Type B involves the aorta distal to the origin of the left subclavian artery; more prevalent in patients with atherosclerosis, carries a slightly better prognosis, and can be managed medically, endovascularly, or surgically, depending on severity and extent

Endocarditis
- All patients require serial exams to assess for changes in murmurs or new heart failure and serial ECGs to assess for new heart block, all of which suggest a complication
- Begin organism-specific IV antibiotics as soon as cultures and sensitivities are available
- Penicillins, often in combination with gentamicin, remain cornerstones for therapy for susceptible streptococci; penicillin or ampicillin for enterococci; nafcillin or cefazolin for staphylococci

Increased intracranial pressure
- Bradycardia is often associated with a rise in systolic blood pressure (Cushing's response)
- Prompt CT as well as involvement of neurology and neurosurgery may be necessary

Index

Androgenetic alopecia, 19
Aneurysm
    aortic, in unequal pulse differential
        diagnosis, 334–335
    left ventricular, 83
    ruptured abdominal aortic, 7, 15
    thoracic aortic, 83
Angiodysplasia, 119
Angioedema, 342
Anisocoria, 273, 275
Ankle, swelling and pain of, 196–197
Anorexia nervosa, 355
Anosmia, 24–25
Anticoagulant drugs, 39
Antiplatelet drugs, 39
Antipsychotic drugs, 72
Anuria, 340
Anxiety
    in dyspnea differential diagnosis, 97
    in tachypnea differential diagnosis,
        323
Anxiety disorders, 26–27
Aortic aneurysm
    ruptured abdominal
        in abdominal guarding differential
            diagnosis, 7
        in abdominal pain differential
            diagnosis, 15
    thoracic, 83
    in unequal pulse differential
        diagnosis, 334–335
Aortic dissection
    in unequal pulse differential
        diagnosis, 334–335
    in wide pulse pressure differential
        diagnosis, 357
Aortic insufficiency, 131
Aortic regurgitation
    in orthopnea differential diagnosis,
        233
    in paroxysmal nocturnal dyspnea
        differential diagnosis, 247
    in wide pulse pressure differential
        diagnosis, 357
Aortic sclerosis, 131
Aortic stenosis, 131
    in orthopnea differential diagnosis,
        233
    in paroxysmal nocturnal dyspnea
        differential diagnosis, 247

Aortoenteric fistula, 119
Aphasia, 28–29
    Broca's, 29
    defined, 74
    Wernicke's, 29
Aphthous stomatitis, 316–317
Appendicitis
    in abdominal guarding differential
        diagnosis, 7
    in abdominal pain differential
        diagnosis, 15
Apraxia, defined, 74
Argyll Robertson pupils, 273
Arrhythmias
    in palpitation differential diagnosis,
        239
    in syncope differential diagnosis, 321
    in tachycardia differential diagnosis,
        135
Arteriovenous malformations, in
    hematemesis differential diagnosis, 117
Arteritis
    giant cell, 194–195
    Takayasu's, 53, 334–335
    temporal, 127
Arthritis
    in elbow pain differential diagnosis,
        199
    in foot/toe pain differential diagnosis,
        204–205
    in knee pain differential diagnosis,
        201
    in low back pain differential
        diagnosis, 211
    in neck stiffness differential diagnosis,
        224–225
    rheumatoid
        in toe/foot pain differential
            diagnosis, 204
        in wrist/hand pain differential
            diagnosis, 206–207
    septic, in foot/toe pain differential
        diagnosis, 204–205
    in shoulder pain differential
        diagnosis, 203
    in wrist/hand pain differential
        diagnosis, 206–207
Ascites
    in abdominal distension differential
        diagnosis, 5

Breathing disorders (*continued*)
orthopnea, 232–233
paroxysmal nocturnal dyspnea,
246–247
tachypnea, 322–323
Broca's aphasia, 28–29
Bronchiectasis, in rales differential
diagnosis, 278
Bronchiolitis, in rales differential
diagnosis, 278
Bronchitis
in nonproductive cough differential
diagnosis, 62–63
in productive cough differential
diagnosis, 65
Bronchospasm, in rales differential
diagnosis, 279
Brown-Sequard syndrome, 143
Brudzinski's sign, 224
Bruit
abdominal, 2–3
carotid, 52–53
Bullous diseases, 231
Bullous skin lesions, 310–311
Bursitis
in elbow pain differential diagnosis, 199
in knee pain differential diagnosis, 201
in shoulder pain differential
diagnosis, 203

C

Cafe-au-lait macule, 309
Calcific tendonitis, 203
Calcium
hypercalcemia, 154–155
hypocalcemia, 156–157
Cancer
in abnormal vaginal bleeding
differential diagnosis, 345
breast, 47
colon, 119
in hepatomegaly differential
diagnosis, 149
in hypercalcemia differential
diagnosis, 155
in lymphadenopathy differential
diagnosis, 213
in neck mass differential diagnosis,
222–223

in night sweats differential diagnosis,
227
pain syndrome in, 59
in pelvic mass differential diagnosis,
248–249
in pigmented skin lesion differential
diagnosis, 308–309
in pruritus differential diagnosis, 269
in purpura differential diagnosis,
277
in rectal mass differential diagnosis,
280–281
in scrotal mass differential diagnosis,
294–295
in sore throat differential diagnosis,
313
in splenomegaly differential diagnosis,
315
in stridor differential diagnosis, 319
in weight loss differential diagnosis,
355
Candida intertrigo, 299
Candidiasis, vaginal, 346–347
Cardiac asthma, 247
Cardiac pump failure, in hypotension
differential diagnosis, 183
Cardiac tamponade, in displaced PMI
differential diagnosis, 83
Cardiomegaly, 50–51
Cardiomyopathy
hypertrophic, 131
in orthopnea differential diagnosis,
233
Cardiovascular disease, heartburn due
to, 138–139
Carey-Coombs murmur, 131
Carotid artery stenosis, 52–53
Carotid bruits, 52–53
Carpal tunnel syndrome, 204–205
Catecholamine excess, in palpitation
differential diagnosis, 239
Cauda equina syndrome, in paraplegia
differential diagnosis, 243
Cavernous sinus thrombosis, 265
Cellulitis
dissecting, of scalp, 290–291
orbital, 265
in peripheral edema differential
diagnosis, 104–105
Central diabetes insipidus, 261

Hemothorax, in tactile fremitus
    differential diagnosis, 325
Henoch-Schönlein purpura, 327
Hepatic venous hum, 3, 131
Hepatomegaly, 148–149
    in abdominal distension differential
        diagnosis, 5
    defined, 148
Herpes simplex virus, 310–311
    in genital lesion differential diagnosis,
        298–299
    in oral ulcer differential diagnosis,
        231
Herpes zoster, 37
Hidradenitis suppurativa, 17
Hippus, 273, 275
Hirsutism, 150–151
Histoplasmosis, 231
Hives, 267, 342–343
Hoarseness, 152–153
Homan's sign, 105
Horner's syndrome
    in miosis differential diagnosis,
        272–273
    in ptosis differential diagnosis,
        270–271
Human immunodeficiency virus (HIV)
    in pruritus differential diagnosis, 269
    in weight loss differential diagnosis,
        355
Huntington's disease, in chorea
    differential diagnosis, 57
Hydrocele, 295, 327
Hydrocephalus, 240–241
Hypercalcemia, 154–155
    in weight loss differential diagnosis,
        355
Hyperemesis gravidarum, 355
Hyperglycemia, 168–159
    in blurred vision differential diagnosis,
        41
Hyperkalemia, 162–163
Hypernatremia, 166–167
Hyperosmolar hyperglycemic coma, 159
Hyperosmotic hyponatremia, 168–169
Hyperparathyroidism, 154–155
Hyperpigmentation, skin, 170–171
Hyperprolactinemia, 21
Hyperreflexia, 174–175
Hypersensitivity reaction

    in hives differential diagnosis,
        342–343
    in lymphadenopathy differential
        diagnosis, 213
    types of, 343
Hypersomnia, 178–179
Hypertension, 180–181
    drug-induced, 181
    intracranial, 241
    portal, 117
    primary, 181
    secondary, 181
Hypertensive emergency, defined, 180
Hypertensive urgency, defined, 180
Hyperthermia, 110
Hypertrichosis, 150–151
Hypertrophic cardiomyopathy, 131
Hyperventilation
    in dizziness differential diagnosis, 85
    in tachypnea differential diagnosis,
        323
Hypervolemia, 168–169
Hypesthesia, 184–185
Hypoalbuminemia, 157
Hypocalcemia, 156–157
Hypoglycemia, 160–161
    in dizziness differential diagnosis, 85
Hypogonadism, in gynecomastia
    differential diagnosis, 121
Hyponatremia, 168–169
Hypoparathyroidism, 157
Hypopigmentation, skin, 172–173
Hyporeflexia, 176–177
Hyposmotic hyponatremia, 168–169
Hypotension, 182–183
    orthostatic, 321
    postural, 84–85
Hypothermia, 186–187
Hypothyroidism, in hypothermia
    differential diagnosis, 187
Hypovolemia, 168–169, 183

I

Ichtyosis vulgaris, 87
IGF-2–secreting tumors, 161
Ileus, 42–43
Iliotibial band syndrome, 201
Illusions, defined, 124
Impetigo, bullous, 311